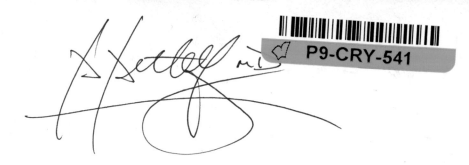

SPECIALTY BOARD REVIEW
Anesthesiology

Third Edition

SPECIALTY BOARD REVIEW
Anesthesiology
Third Edition

THOMAS P. BEACH, MD
Chief, Department of Anesthesiology
Children's Hospital
Columbus, Ohio

Clinical Associate Professor
Department of Anesthesiology
Ohio State University
Columbus, Ohio

APPLETON & LANGE
Norwalk, Connecticut/San Mateo, California

Copyright © 1990 by Appleton & Lange
A Publishing Division of Prentice Hall;
Copyright © 1978 by Arco Publishing Co., Inc.;
Copyright © 1984 by Appleton-Century-Crofts

91 92 93 94 / 10 9 8 7 6 5 4 3 2

Prentice Hall International (UK) Limited, *London*
Prentice Hall of Australia Pty. Limited, *Sydney*
Prentice Hall Canada, Inc., *Toronto*
Prentice Hall Hispanoamericana, S.A., *Mexico*
Prentice Hall of India Private Limited, *New Delhi*
Prentice Hall of Japan, Inc., *Tokyo*
Simon & Schuster Asia Pte. Ltd., *Singapore*
Editora Prentice Hall do Brasil Ltda., *Rio de Janeiro*
Prentice Hall, *Englewood Cliffs, New Jersey*

ISBN 0-8385-8620-1

Acquisitions Editor: R. Craig Percy
Production Editor: Charles F. Evans

PRINTED IN THE UNITED STATES OF AMERICA

To

Joan

Contents

Introduction

If you are planning to prepare for the American Board of Anesthesiology (ABA) written or oral examination, then *Specialty Board Review: Anesthesiology, 3rd edition* is designed for you. Here, in one package, is a comprehensive review resource with 1800 Board-type multiple-choice questions with referenced, paragraph-length discussions of each answer. In addition, the last 350 questions have been set aside as a Practice Test for self-assessment purposes.

All of the questions, answers, explanations, and references have been extensively revised and updated for this edition of this review book. In addition, there are approximately 250 new questions, reflecting the change in the ABA examination and recent updates in the specialty.

ORGANIZATION OF THIS BOOK

Specialty Board Review: Anesthesiology, 3rd edition is divided into 14 chapters, all of which are designed to contribute to your review. The first five chapters (Part I) are devoted to the basic science component of the ABA examination. The next nine chapters (Part II) review the clinical science component. The final section (Part III) is a two-part Practice Test, which simulates an exam situation. Each of the chapters in Parts I and II consists of questions, then answers and explanations. These components are discussed below in terms of what they contain and how you can use them in the most effective manner.

Questions

Each chapter in this book contains two different types of multiple-choice questions (or "items," in testing parlance). In general, about 50 percent of these are "one best answer–single item" questions and 50 percent are "multiple true-false items." In some cases, a group of two or three questions may be related to a situational theme. In addition, some questions have illustrative material (graphs, x-rays, tables) that require understanding and interpretation on your part. Moreover, questions may be of three levels of difficulty: (1) rote memory question, (2) memory question that requires more understanding of the problem, and (3) a question that requires understanding *and* judgment. It is the judgment question that we have tried to emphasize throughout this text. Finally, some of the items are stated in the negative. In such instances, we have printed the negative word in capital letters (eg, "All of the following are correct EXCEPT;" "Which of the following choices is NOT correct;" and "Which of the following is LEAST correct").

One best answer–single item question. This type of question presents a problem or asks a question and is followed by five choices, only **one** of which is entirely correct. The directions preceding this type of question will generally appear as below:

DIRECTIONS (Question 1): Each of the numbered items or incomplete statements in this section is followed by answers or by completions of the statement. Select the <u>ONE</u> lettered answer or completion that is <u>BEST</u> in each case.

An example for this item type follows:

1. An obese 21-year-old woman complains of increased growth of coarse hair on her lip, chin, chest, and abdomen. She also notes menstrual irregularity with periods of amenorrhea. The most likely cause is

    (A) polycystic ovary disease
    (B) an ovarian tumor
    (C) an adrenal tumor
    (D) Cushing's disease
    (E) familial hirsutism

In this type of question, choices other than the correct answer may be partially correct, but there can only be one *best* answer. In the question above (taken from *Appleton & Lange's Review for National Boards Part II*), the key word is "most." Although ovarian tumors, adrenal tumors, and Cushing's disease are causes of hirsutism (described in the stem of the question), polycystic ovary disease is a much more common cause. Familial hirsutism is not associated with the menstrual irregularities mentioned. Thus, the *most* likely cause of the manifestations described can only be "(A) polycystic ovary disease."

TABLE 1. STRATEGIES FOR ANSWERING ONE BEST ANSWER–SINGLE ITEM QUESTIONS*

1. Remember that only one choice can be the correct answer.
2. Read the question carefully to be sure that you understand what is being asked.
3. Quickly read each choice for familiarity. (This important step is often not done by test takers.)
4. Go back and consider each choice individually.
5. If a choice is partially correct, tentatively consider it to be incorrect. (This step will help you lessen your choices and increase your odds of choosing the correct choice/answer.)
6. Consider the remaining choices and select the one you think is the answer. At this point, you may want to quickly scan the stem to be sure you understand the question and your answer.
7. Fill in the appropriate circle on the answer sheet. (Even if you do not know the answer, you should at least guess—you are scored on the number of correct answers, so **do not leave any blanks**.)

*Note that steps 2 through 7 should take an average of 70 seconds total. The actual examination is timed for an average of 70 seconds per question.

Multiple true–false items. These questions are considered more difficult (or tricky), and you should be certain that you understand and follow the code that always accompanies these questions:

DIRECTIONS (Question 7): For each of the items in this section, ONE or MORE of the numbered options is correct. Choose the answer

> A if only 1, 2 and 3 are correct,
> B if only 1 and 3 are correct,
> C if only 2 and 4 are correct,
> D if only 4 is correct,
> E if all are correct.

This code is always the same (i.e., "D" would never say "if 3 is correct"), and it is repeated throughout this book at the top of any page on which multiple true–false item questions appear.

SUMMARY OF DIRECTIONS				
A	B	C	D	E
1, 2, 3 only	1, 3 only	2, 4 only	4 only	All are correct

A sample question follows:

7. A 12-year-old boy complains of severe pruritus, especially at night, and is found to have scabies. Effective management includes
   (1) treating household pets
   (2) treating normal-appearing skin
   (3) using griseofulvin
   (4) treating asymptomatic family members

You first need to determine which choices are right

and wrong, and then which code corresponds to the correct numbers. In the example above, 2 and 4 are both effective management procedures, and therefore (C) is the correct answer to this question.

TABLE 2. STRATEGIES FOR ANSWERING MULTIPLE TRUE–FALSE ITEM QUESTIONS

1. Carefully read and become familiar with the accompanying directions to this tricky question type.
2. Carefully read the stem to be certain that you know what is being asked.
3. Carefully read each of the numbered choices. If you can determine whether any of the choices are true or false, you may find it helpful to place a "+" (true) or a "–" (false) next to the number.
4. Focus on the numbered choices and your true/false notations, and use the following sequence to logically determine the correct answer:
   a. Note that in the answer code choices 1 *and* 3 are *always* both either true or false together. If you are sure that either one is incorrect, your answer must be C or D.
   b. If you are sure that choice 2 and *either* choice 1 *or* 3 are incorrect, your answer must be D.
   c. If you are sure that choices 2 and 4 are incorrect, your answer must be B.*

*Remember, you only have an average of 70 seconds per question. Note that the following two combinations cannot occur: choices 1 and 4 both incorrect; choices 3 and 4 both incorrect.

Answers, Explanations, and References

In each of the sections of this book, the question sections are followed by a section containing the answers, explanations, and references to the questions. This section (1) tells you the answer to each question; (2) gives you an explanation/review of why the answer is correct, background information on the subject matter, and why the other answers are incorrect; and (3) tells you where you can find more in-depth information on the subject matter in other books and/or journals. We encourage you to use this section as a basis for further study and understanding.

If you choose the correct answer to a question, you can then read the explanation (1) for reinforcement and (2) to add to your knowledge about the subject matter (remember that the explanations usually tell not only why the answer is correct, but also why the other choices are incorrect). **If you choose the wrong answer** to a question, you can read the explanation for a learning/reviewing discussion of the material in the question. Furthermore, you can note the reference cited (eg, *2:345*), look up the full source in the References on page xv (eg, Wylie WD, Churchill–Davidson HC. *A Practice of Anaesthesiology*, 5th ed. Chicago: Year Book Medical Publishers, Inc.; 1984), and refer to the page cited (p 345) for a more in-depth discussion.

Practice Test

In the 350-question Practice Test at the end of the book the questions are grouped according to question type (one best answer–single item, then multiple true–false items), with the subject areas integrated. This format mimics the actual exam and enables you to test your skill at answering questions in all of the areas under simulated examination conditions.

HOW TO USE THIS BOOK

There are two logical ways to get the most value from this book. We will call them Plan A and Plan B.

In Plan A, you go straight to the Practice Test and complete it according to the instructions. Analyze your areas of strength and weakness. This will be a good indicator of your initial knowledge of the subject and will help to identify specific areas for preparation and review. You can now use the first 14 chapters of the book to help you improve your relative weak points.

In Plan B, you go through chapters 1 through 14 checking off your answers, and then comparing your choices with the answers and discussions in the book. Once you have completed this process, you can take the Practice Test to see how well prepared you are. If you still have a major weakness, it should be apparent in time for you to take remedial action.

In Plan A, by taking the Practice Test first, you get quick feedback regarding your initial areas of strength and weakness. You may find that you have a good command of the material indicating that perhaps only a cursory review of the first 14 chapters is necessary. This, of course, would be good to know early in your exam preparation. On the other hand, you may find that you have many areas of weakness. In this case, you could then focus on these areas in your review—not just with this book, but also with the cited references and with your current textbooks and journals.

It is, however, unlikely that you will not do some studying prior to taking the ABA exam (especially since you have this book). Therefore, it may be more realistic to take the Practice Test after you have reviewed the first 14 chapters (as in Plan B). This will probably give you a more realistic type of testing situation since very few of us just sit down to a test without studying. In this case, you will have done some reviewing (from superficial to in-depth), and your Practice Test will reflect this studying time. If, after reviewing the first 14 chapters and taking the Practice Test, you still have some weaknesses, you can then go back to the first 14 chapters and supplement your review with your texts.

THE AMERICAN BOARD OF ANESTHESIOLOGY

History
Anesthesiology is a relatively new specialty, and therefore the American Board of Anesthesiology is also relatively young.

The American Society of Anesthesiologists had its beginnings in 1911 in the New York area when two groups merged to form the New York Society of Anesthetists. The group grew and by 1935 was national in scope. In 1936 the name was changed to the American Society of Anesthetists, and the society was incorporated.

The American Society of Anesthesiology, Inc. grew out of a committee representing the American Society of Anesthetists, Inc., the American Society of Regional Anesthesia, Inc., and the Section on Surgery of the American Medical Association. In 1937, the American Board of Anesthesiology, Inc., was formed as an affiliate of the American Board of Surgery, Inc. In 1941, the board was approved as a separate entity.

The purposes of the board are as follows*:

1. To maintain the highest standards of practice of anesthesiology by fostering educational facilities and training in anesthesiology. For present purposes anesthesiology is defined as a practice of medicine dealing with but not limited to:

   A. The assessment of, consultation for and preparation of patients for anesthesia.
   B. The provision of insensibility to pain during surgical, obstetric, therapeutic, and diagnostic procedures and the management of patients so affected.
   C. The monitoring and restoration of homeostasis during the perioperative period, as well as homeostasis in the critically ill, injured, or otherwise seriously ill patient.
   D. The diagnosis and treatment of painful syndromes.
   E. The clinical management and teaching of cardiac and pulmonary resuscitation.
   F. The evaluation of respiratory function and application of respiratory therapy in all its forms.
   G. The supervision, teaching, and evaluation of performance of both medical and paramedical personnel involved in anesthesia, respiratory and critical care.
   H. The conduct of research at the clinical and basic science levels to explain and improve the care of patients insofar as physiologic function and the response to drugs are concerned.
   I. The administrative involvement in hospitals, medical schools, and outpatient facilities necessary to implement these responsibilities.

2. To establish and maintain criteria for the designation of a specialist in anesthesiology.
3. To advise the Accreditation Council for Graduate Medical Education (ACGME) concerning the

*The American Board of Anesthesiology, Inc. *Booklet of Information*, 1989.

training required of individuals seeking certification as such requirements relate to residency training programs in anesthesiology.

4. To establish and conduct those processes by which the Board may judge whether physicians who voluntarily apply should be issued certificates indicating that they have met the required standards for certification as a consultant in anesthesiology. A consultant anesthesiologist possesses adequate measures of knowledge, judgement, clinical and character skills, and personality suitable for assuming independent responsibility for patient care and for serving as an expert with the ability to deliberate with others providing advice and opinions in areas related to the practice of anesthesia including all subspecialties and for functioning as the leader of the anesthesia care team.

5. To establish and conduct those processes by which the Board may judge whether physicians who voluntarily apply should be issued certificates indicating that they have met the required standards for certification of special qualifications in critical care medicine.

6. To serve the public, medical profession, hospitals and medical schools by preparing lists for publication of physicians certified by the Board.

Certification

To be certified as a Diplomate of the American Board of Anesthesiology, each applicant must:

1. Hold a permanent and unrestricted license to practice medicine or osteopathy in one state of the United States or in Canada whose registration is unexpired.

2. Fulfill all the requirements of the four-year Continuum of Education in Anesthesiology.

3. Have on file with the American Board of Anesthesiology a satisfactory Certificate of Clinical Competence covering the final six-month period of Clinical Anesthesia training.

4. Satisfy all examination requirements of the Board.

Information concerning the board and its requirements may be obtained from:

The American Board of Anesthesiology, Inc.
100 Constitution Plaza
Hartford, Connecticut 06103-1721
Telephone: (203) 522-9857

Examination Preparation

Ideally, preparation for the examination should begin during training. During this period, time spent in a *systematic* approach to the body of knowledge will be well rewarded.

A *Content Outline of the In-Training Examination,* by the American Board of Anesthesiology and the American Society of Anesthesiologists is available to cover the knowledge that should be gained during the training period. It serves as a grid for the questions to be covered in the examination and also serves as an outline for study.

Textbooks provide a good background of information. Popular texts include a basic text by Dripps et al, and comprehensive texts edited by Miller and a newer one by Barash et al. Many monographs are available on subspecialties, eg, pain control, obstetric, and pediatric anesthesia. These are invaluable for "fleshing out the skeleton."

The best source of current information are journals and meetings. The newest data and latest techniques are reported in these two sources, and one must be familiar with them. Tape recordings of presentations at many major meetings are available.

An invaluable source of information is the Annual Refresher Course given each year in conjunction with the ASA meeting in October. A series of one-hour lectures is given for two days. A syllabus is available covering all the lectures. This book is available each year—it is of good quality, up-to-date, and inexpensive. *It is a must for board preparation*. If you cannot attend the lectures the book may be purchased from the ASA.

Format of Examination

Written Examination. The written examination of the American Board of Anesthesiology is of the objective, multiple-choice form. It is a comprehensive test that covers the wide field related to anesthesiology.

The questions are designed to test the information gained while in training and knowledge expected of physicians in general. "Trick" or ambiguous questions are avoided.

The test consists of a total of 350 questions to be answered in seven hours. The test is split into two sessions of three and one-half hours each to complete 175 questions. You should plan your time accordingly. There are two types of questions used: one best answer–single item type and multiple true–false type. These are discussed earlier in this introduction.

In this book only these two types of questions are used.

Oral Examination. While the written examination is designed to measure knowledge, the oral examination is meant to measure the ability to use that knowledge in the clinical setting. This requires the ability to assimilate data and put it to use. One must be able to assess the information presented, sort out the priorities, and arrive at an anesthetic plan. This may also involve the ability to discuss the problems intelligently and convincingly. The ability to adapt to changing developments is also assessed.

The oral examination consists of two 30-minute examination periods with a break between periods. Two examiners interview each candidate during each period.

Only one examines at a time, and the time is evenly divided between the examiners.

Each session starts with the presentation of a case report for discussion. All candidates receive the same report for discussion at that period. The approach of the candidate will determine, in part, further questions that may be asked.

A typical case report:
A 26-year-old woman enters the obstetric suite with a diagnosis of abruptio placenta. She last ate 1 hour before her arrival at the hospital. She is actively bleeding. She states that she is a Jehovah's Witness and does not want any blood or blood products under any circumstances.

The discussion can take many routes: preparation, anesthetic of choice, complications, etc.

Subsequent questions may result from the candidate's response.

It is important to think before you answer. Do not try to read the examiner's mind: do not try to figure out *why* he or she is asking that question. Answer the question as you understand it, and if you do *not* understand it, ask for clarification.

If you do not know much about regional anesthesia, do not take that path. You are bound to get further questions!

If you do not know the answer, simply say "I do not know." You are better off moving to an area in which you have some knowledge than digging yourself deeper into a hole.

References

Below is a numbered list of reference sources pertaining to the material in this book.

On the last line of each explanation there appears a number combination that identifies the reference source and the page or pages where the information relating to the question and the correct answer may be found. The first number, in **bold,** refers to the textbook or journal in the list below, and the second number refers to the page of that textbook or journal.

For example: (**2**:*345*) is a reference to the second book in the list, page 345 of Wylie's *A Practice of Anaesthesia.*

1. Miller RD (ed). *Anesthesia,* 2nd ed. New York: Churchill Livingston; 1986
2. Wylie WD, Churchill–Davidson HC. *A Practice of Anaesthesia,* 5th ed. Chicago: Year Book Medical Publishers, Inc.; 1984
3. Bendixen HH, et al. *Respiratory Care.* St. Louis: C. V. Mosby Company; 1965
4. Burrows, B, et al. *Respiratory Insufficiency.* Chicago: Year Book Medical Publishers, Inc.; 1983
5. Wilson RS. Use and abuse of double lumen endotracheal tubes. *ASA Annual Refresher Course Lectures,* Lecture 173, 1986
6. Nichols D. Respiratory control in the newborn and young children. *ASA Annual Refresher Course Lectures,* Lecture 162, 1986
7. Wilson R. Technique of mechanical ventilation based on patient need. *ASA Annual Refresher Course Lectures,* Lecture 172, 1985
8. Goudsouzian NG, Karamanian A. *Physiology for the Anesthesiologist,* 2nd ed. New York: Appleton-Century-Crofts; 1984
9. Benumof JL. *Anesthesia for Thoracic Surgery.* Philadelphia: W.B. Saunders Company; 1987
10. Tremper K. The measurement and maintenance of oxygen transport. *ASA Annual Refresher Course Lectures,* Lecture 222A, 1987
11. Nunn JF. Effects of anesthesia on the respiratory system. *ASA Annual Refresher Course Lectures,* Lecture 254, 1987
12. Marshall BE. Etiology and management of perioperative pulmonary edema. *ASA Annual Refresher Course Lectures,* Lecture 146, 1986
13. Brown M. Assessment and treatment of the patient with hypoxemia. *ASA Annual Refresher Course Lectures,* Lecture 132, 1986
14. Shapiro BA. PEEP therapy in acute lung injury. *ASA Annual Refresher Course Lectures,* Lecture 173, 1985
15. Stoelting RK. *Pharmacology and Physiology in Anesthesia Practice.* Philadelphia: J.B. Lippincott Company; 1987
16. Martin JT. *Positioning in Anesthesia and Surgery,* 2nd ed. Philadelphia: W.B. Saunders Company; 1987
17. Klein EF. Management of the patient with traumatic chest injuries. *ASA Annual Refresher Course Lectures,* Lecture 176, 1985
18. Reves JG, Hart A. Anesthesia and myocardial ischemia. *IARS Review Course Lectures,* 1988:66
19. Thomas, SJ. *Manual of Cardiac Anesthesia.* New York: Churchill Livingston; 1984
20. Gravenstein JS, Paulus DA. *Monitoring Practice in Clinical Anesthesia.* Philadelphia: J.B. Lippincott Company; 1982
21. Tarhan S. *Cardiovascular Anesthesia and Postoperative Care.* Chicago: Year Book Medical Publishers, Inc.; 1982
22. Shoemaker WC, et al. *Textbook of Critical Care.* Philadelphia: W.B. Saunders Company; 1984
23. Curling PE. Cardiac transplantation: Perianesthetic management. *ASA Annual Refresher Course Lectures,* Lecture 144, 1987
24. Campbell FW. Anesthetic management of the patient with congestive heart failure. *ASA Annual Refresher Course Lectures,* Lecture 432, 1987
25. Merin RG. Effects of inhalation anesthetic on the cardiovascular system. *ASA Annual Refresher Course Lectures,* Lecture 136, 1987
26. Ryan JF, et al. Myoglobin after a single dose of succinylcholine. *N. Engl J Med.* 285:824, 1971

27. Kalow W, Genest K. A method for the detection of atypical forms of human serum cholinesterase: Determination of dibucaine numbers. *Can Anaesth Soc J.* 35:339, 1967

28. Thomson IA. Cardiopulmonary bypass. *ASA Annual Refresher Course Lectures,* Lecture 136, 1988

29. Nathan HJ. Nitrous oxide worsens myocardial ischemia in isoflurane-anesthetized dogs. *Anesthesiology.* 68:407, 1988

30. Davis RF. Acute post-operative hypertension. *ASA Annual Refresher Course Lectures,* Lecture 245, 1988

31. Pulmonary terms and symbols (A Report of the ACCP-ATS Joint Commission on Pulmonary Nomenclature). *Chest.* 67:583, 1975

32. Shapiro BA, et al. *Clinical Application of Respiratory Care,* 3rd ed. Chicago: Year Book Medical Publishers, Inc.; 1985

33. Mangano DT. Evaluation of cardiac risk. *ASA Annual Refresher Course Lectures,* Lecture 131, 1988

34. Comroe JA. *Physiology of Respiration.* Chicago: Year Book Medical Publishers, Inc.; 1974

35. McLeskey CH. Physiologic changes in the aging patient. *ASA Annual Refresher Course Lectures,* Lecture 275, 1988

36. Hines R. Right ventricular function and failure. *ASA Annual Refresher Course Lectures,* Lecture 521, 1988

37. Rees DI, Wansborough SR. One-lung anesthesia: Percent shunt and arterial oxygen tension during continuous insufflation of oxygen to the nonventilated lung. *Anesth Analg* (Cleveland). 61:507, 1982

38. Wade JG, et al. Effect of carotid endarterectomy on carotid receptor and baroreceptor function in man. *N Engl J Med.* 282:823, 1970

39. Miller ED. Systemic and pulmonary hypertension: Anesthetic considerations. *ASA Annual Refresher Course Lectures,* Lecture 225, 1985

40. Fairley HB. Management of respiratory failure. *ASA Annual Refresher Course Lectures,* Lecture 141, 1973

41. Churchill-Davidson HC. A philosophy of relaxation. *Anesth Analg* (Cleveland). 52:495, 1973

42. Schmid ER, Rehder K. General anesthesia and the chest wall. *Anesthesiology.* 55:668, 1981

43. Orkin FK, Cooperman LH (eds). *Complications in Anesthesiology.* Philadelphia: J.B. Lippincott Company; 1983

44. West JB. Causes of carbon dioxide retention in lung disease. *N Engl J Med.* 284:1232, 1971

45. Salvatore AJ, et al. Postoperative hypoventilation and hypoxemia in man following hyperventilation. *N Engl J Med.* 280:467, 1970

46. Bonchek LI. Salivary enlargement during induction of anesthesia. *JAMA.* 209:1716, 1969

47. Clark WG, et al. *Goth's Medical Pharmacology.* 12th ed. St. Louis: The C.V. Mosby Company; 1988

48. Price HL, Price ML. Has halothane a predominant circulatory function? *Anesthesiology.* 27:764, 1966

49. Bahlman SH, et al. The cardiovascular effects of nitrous oxide—Halothane anesthesia in man. *Anesthesiology.* 35:274, 1971

50. Smith TW. Digitalis glycosides. *N Engl J Med.* 288:719, 1973

51. MacIntosh R, et al. *Physics and the Anaesthetist,* 3rd ed. Philadelphia: F.A. Davis Company; 1963

52. Cottrell JE, Turndorf H. *Anesthesia and Neurosurgery,* 2nd ed. St. Louis: The C.V. Mosby Company; 1986

53. West JB. *Respiratory Physiology.* Baltimore: Williams & Wilkins Company; 1985

54. Brobeck JR (ed). *Best and Taylor's Physiological Basis of Medical Practice,* 10th ed. Baltimore: The Williams & Wilkins Company; 1979

55. West JB. *Pulmonary Pathophysiology.* Baltimore: The Williams & Wilkins Company; 1977

56. Guyton AC. *Textbook of Medical Physiology,* 7th ed. Philadelphia: W.B. Saunders Company; 1986

57. Barash PG. Cardiovascular monitoring—Myth and reality. *IARS Review Course Lectures,* 1989

58. Cullen B. Anesthesia for the patient with a major burn. *ASA Annual Refresher Course Lectures,* Lecture 266, 1985

59. Moncrief JA. Burns. *N Engl J Med.* 288:444, 1973

60. Kaplan JA. How to monitor the cardiac patient for noncardiac surgery. *ASA Annual Refresher Course Lectures,* Lecture 432, 1986

61. Eger EI, Saidman LJ. Hazards of nitrous oxide anesthesia in bowel obstruction and pneumothorax. *Anesthesiology.* 26:61, 1965

62. American College of Surgeons. *Manual of Preoperative and Postoperative Care,* 2nd ed. Philadelphia: W.B. Saunders Company; 1971

63. Donegan JH. CPR updates for adults. *ASA Annual Refresher Course Lectures,* Lecture 431, 1988

64. Jenkins JG, et al. Evaluation of pulmonary function in muscular dystrophy patient requiring spinal surgery. *Crit Care Med.* 10:645, 1982

65. Mihm FG. Analysis of information derived from pulmonary artery catheter monitoring. *ASA Annual Refresher Course Lectures.* Lecture 156, 1987

66. Marshall BE, Wyche MQ. Hypoxemia during and after anesthesia. *Anesthesiology.* 37:178, 1972

67. Kasnitz P, et al. Mixed venous oxygen tension and hyperlactatemia. *JAMA.* 236:570, 1976

68. Gravenstein N. Monitoring fluid and cardiovascular status during anesthesia. *ASA Annual Refresher Course Lectures.* Lecture 164, 1987

69. Bedford RF. Complications of invasive monitoring. *ASA Annual Refresher Course Lectures*, Lecture 212, 1987

70. Parks LK, Bergman NA. Hypoxia as a manifestation of neurogenic pulmonary dysfunction. *Anesthesiology*. 45:93, 1976

71. Thomas SJ. Anesthetic management of the patient with non-coronary heart disease. *ASA Annual Refresher Course Lectures*, Lecture 133, 1988

72. Wilson RS. Monitoring the lung. *Anesthesiology*. 45:135, 1976

73. Edwards H, King TC. Cardiac tamponade from central venous catheters. *Arch Surg*. 117:965, 1982

74. Braunwald E. *Heart Disease*, 3rd ed. Philadelphia: W.B. Saunders Company; 1988

75. Barash PG, et al. (eds). *Clinical Anesthesia*. Philadelphia: J.B. Lippincott Company; 1989

76. Mason JW. Amiodarone. *N Engl J Med*. 316:455, 1987

77. Vitez TS, et al. Chronic hypokalemia and intraoperative dysrhythmias. *Anesthesiology*. 63:130, 1985

78. Rotheram EB, et al. CNS disorder during mechanical in chronic pulmonary disease. *JAMA*. 189:993, 1964

79. Hodgkin JE, et al. Chronic obstructive airway disease. *JAMA*. 232:1243, 1975

80. Belinkoff S. The recovery room and respiratory care. *Int Anesthesiol Clin*. 9:21, 1971

81. Jacobs HB, et al. Transtracheal catheter ventilation. *Chest*. 65:36, 1974

82. Lochning RW, et al. Circulatory collapse from anesthesia for diaphragmatic hernia. *Arch Surg*. 90:109, 1965

83. Cronnelly R. Why, when and how to reverse muscle relaxants. *ASA Annual Refresher Course Lectures*, Lecture 143, 1986

84. Savarese JJ. The newer muscle relaxants. *ASA Annual Refresher Course Lectures*, Lecture 142, 1986

85. Murat I, et al. Isoflurane attenuates baroreflex control of heart rate in human neonates. *Anesthesiology*. 70:397, 1989

86. Braunwald E. Regulation of the circulation. *N Engl J Med*. 290:1124, 1420, 1974

87. Braunwald E. Determinants and assessment of cardiac function. *N Engl J Med*. 296:86, 1977

88. Azar II. The use of muscle relaxants in patients with neuromuscular disease. *ASA Annual Refresher Course Lectures*, Lecture 144, 1986

89. Hug CC. Pharmacokinetics and dynamics at the extremes of age. *ASA Annual Refresher Course Lectures*, Lecture 161, 1988

90. Stoelting RK. Pre-operative medication. *ASA Annual Refresher Course Lectures*, Lecture 164, 1988

91. White PF. Induction agents: Old and new. *ASA Annual Refresher Course Lectures*, Lecture 532, 1988

92. Cullen BF. Drug interactions. *ASA Annual Refresher Course Lectures*, Lecture 166, 1988

93. Albert SN, et al. Pitfalls in blood volume measurement. *Anesth Analg* (Cleveland). 44:805, 1965

94. Shapiro HM. Cerebral blood flow and anesthetics. *ASA Annual Refresher Course Lectures*, Lecture 154, 1988

95. Skillman JJ. *Intensive Care*. Boston: Little, Brown and Company; 1975

96. Kapur PA. Calcium channel blockers. *ASA Annual Refresher Course Lectures*, Lecture 246, 1988

97. Stanski DR. Pharmacokinetic basis for intravenous infusion anesthesia. *ASA Annual Refresher Course Lectures*, Lecture 162, 1988

98. Lawson NW. Use of inotropes and vasopressors. *ASA Annual Refresher Course Lectures*, Lecture 162, 1988

99. Covino BG. How local anesthetics work and what is their toxicity. *ASA Annual Refresher Course Lectures*, Lecture 116, 1987

100. Warner LO, et al. Negative pressure pulmonary oedema secondary to airway obstruction in an intubated infant. *Can J Anaesth*. 35:507, 1988

101. Robin ED. Pulmonary edema. *N Engl J Med*. 290:499, 1973

102. Basta SJ. Clinical selection of muscle relaxants. *ASA Annual Refresher Course Lectures*, Lecture 121, 1987

103. Ramirez A, Abelmann WH. Cardiac decompensation. *N Engl J Med*. 290:499, 1974

104. Stoelting RK. The use of vasopressors and inotropic drugs in anesthesia. *ASA Annual Refresher Course Lectures*, Lecture 241, 1987

105. Smith TW. Digitalis. *N Engl J Med*. 318:358, 1988

106. Cottrell JE. Induced hypotension. *ASA Annual Refresher Course Lectures*, Lecture 156, 1988

107. Sladen RN. Perioperative management of the patient with renal failure. *ASA Annual Refresher Course Lectures*, Lecture 172, 1988

108. Chernow B. Perioperative management of endocrine problems: thyroid, adrenal cortex, pituitary. *ASA Annual Refresher Course Lectures*, Lecture 216, 1988

109. Merin RG, Buffington CW. Is isoflurane dangerous for the patient with coronary artery disease? *ASA Annual Refresher Course Lectures*, Lecture 236, 1988

110. Hirschman CA. Perioperative management of the patient with asthma. *ASA Annual Refresher Course Lectures*, Lecture 264, 1988

111. Royster RL. Management of cardiac rhythm disturbance. *ASA Annual Refresher Course Lectures*, Lecture 522, 1988

112. Artru AA. New concepts concerning anesthetic effects on intracranial dynamics. *ASA Annual Refresher Course Lectures,* Lecture 133, 1987

113. Burton AC. *A Physiology and Biophysics of the Circulation,* 2nd ed. Chicago: Year Book Medical Publishers, Inc.; 1972

114. Price HL. A dynamic concept of the distribution of thiopental in the human body. *Anesthesiology.* 21:40, 1960

115. Cohn JN. Blood pressure and cardiac performance *Am J Med.* 55:351, 1973

116. Braunwald E, et al. Mechanisms of contraction of the normal and failing heart. *N Engl J Med.* 277:853, 910, 1012, 1967

117. Cohn JN. Indications for digitalis therapy. *JAMA.* 299:1911, 1974

118. Behrman RE, Vaughan VC. *Nelson's Textbook of Pediatrics,* 13th ed. Philadelphia: W.B. Saunders Company; 1987

119. Gorlin R. Practical cardiac hemodynamics. *N Engl J Med.* 296:203, 1977

120. Defalque RJ. The anesthesiologist's role in the management of chronic pain. *Anesthesiology Rev.* 4:19, 1977

121. Khalili AA, Ditzler JW. Neurolytic substances in the relief of pain. *Med Clin North Am.* 52:161, 1968

122. Field J, et al. Limitations in the use of the pulmonary capillary wedge pressure. *Chest.* 70:451, 1976

123. Kerr FW. Pain. *Mayo Clin Proc.* 50:685, 1975

124. Defalque RJ. Treatment of causalgia. *JAMA.* 209:259, 1969

125. Redick LF, Walton KN. Physiologic changes during transurethral resection of the prostate. *Anesth Analg* (Cleveland). 46:618, 1967

126. Stephen CR, Wingard DW. Questions and answers. *Anesth Analg* (Cleveland). 51:656, 1972

127. Azar I. Transurethral prostectomy syndrome. *ASA Annual Refresher Course Lectures,* Lecture 126, 1988

128. Kopell HP, Thompson WA. Peripheral entrapment neuropathies of the lower extremity. *N Engl J Med.* 262:56, 1960

129. Ganong WF. *Review of Medical Physiology,* 14th ed. Los Altos: Lange Medical Publications; 1989

130. Editorial. Enterohepatic circulation. *N Engl J Med.* 284:48, 1971

131. Dripps RD, et al. *Introduction to Anesthesia.* 6th ed. Philadelphia: W.B. Saunders Company; 1982

132. Vanatta JC, Fogelman MJ. *Moyer's Fluid Balance,* 2nd ed. Chicago: Year Book Medical Publishers, Inc.; 1976

133. Jenkins MT, et al. Questions and answers on anesthesia for thyroid surgery. *Clin Anesth.* 3:200, 1963

134. Stehling LC. Anesthetic management of the patient with hyperthyroidism. *Anesthesiology.* 41:585, 1974

135. Ammon JR. Perioperative management of the diabetic patient. *ASA Annual Refresher Course Lectures,* Lecture 215, 1988

136. Simon AB. Perioperative management of the pacemaker patient. *Anesthesiology.* 46:127, 1977

137. Wollman H. The Humpty Dumpty phenomenon. *Anesthesiology.* 33:379, 1970

138. Kanter SF, Samuels SI. Anesthesia for major operations on patients who have had transplanted hearts, a review of 29 cases. *Anesthesiology.* 26:65, 1977

139. Kaplan JA. Recent developments in cardiac anesthesia. *ASA Annual Refresher Course Lectures,* Lecture 135, 1988

140. Dundee JW, et al. The hazard of thiopental anesthesia in porphyria. *Anesth Analg* (Cleveland). 41:567, 1962

141. Reves, JG, et al. Anesthetic considerations for coronary artery surgery. *Anesthesiology Rev.* 4:19, 1977

142. Forestner JE, Raj PP. Inadvertent epidural injection of thiopental: A case report. Anesth Analg (Cleveland). 54:406, 1975

143. Petty C, Bageant T. Lack of thiopental effect on the oxyhemoglobin dissociation curve. *Anesth Analg* (Cleveland). 54:406, 1975

144. Pender JW. Dissociative anesthesia. *JAMA.* 215:1126, 1971

145. Stanley TH, et al. Effects of ventilatory techniques during cardiopulmonary bypass on post-bypass and postoperative pulmonary compliance and shunt. *Anesthesiology.* 46:391, 1977

146. Gardner RC. Blood loss after fractures of the hip. *JAMA.* 208:1005, 1969

147. Sudhir KG, et al. Intraoperative awakening for early recognition of possible neurologic sequelae during Harrington-Rod spinal fusion. *Anesth Analg* (Cleveland). 55:526, 1976

148. Feldman SA. *Muscle Relaxants.* Philadelphia: W.B. Saunders Company; 1979

149. Bennett EJ. Muscle relaxants, myasthenia, and mustards. *Anesthesiology.* 46:220, 1977

150. Bernstein RL. Anesthetic management of patients with scoliosis. *ASA Annual Refresher Course Lectures,* Lecture 276, 1987

151. Amaranath L. Relation of anesthesia to total hip replacement and control of operative blood loss. *Anesth Analg* (Cleveland). 54:651, 1975

152. Gauthier JL, Hamelberg W. Hip fractures. *Anesth Analg* (Cleveland). 42:609, 1963

153. Michenfelder JD, et al. Neuroanesthesia. *Anesthesiology.* 30:65, 1969

154. Newfield P. Anesthetic considerations in patients with increased intracranial pressure. *ASA Annual Refresher Course Lectures,* Lecture 176, 1987

155. Cooperman LH, Price HL. Pulmonary edema in the operative and postoperative period. *Ann Surg.* 172:883, 1970

156. Miller RD. Antagonism of neuromuscular block. *Anesthesiology.* 44:318, 1976

157. Miller RD. Comparative times to peak effect and durations of action of neostigmine and pyridostigmine. *Anesthesiology.* 41:27, 1974

158. Ali HH, Savarese JJ. Monitoring of neuromuscular function. *Anesthesiology.* 45:216, 1976

159. Murphy TM. Management of chronic pain syndromes. *IARS Review Course Lectures,* 1988:11

160. Marsh ML, et al. Neurosurgical intensive care. *Anesthesiology.* 47:149, 1977

161. *Blood Transfusion Therapy.* American Association of Blood Banks, 1983

162. Gieseke AH. Anesthesia in diabetes mellitus. *Anesthesiology Rev.* 2:11, 1975

163. Cook DR. Anesthesia for organ transplantation. *IARS Review Course Lectures,* 1987:23

164. *Transfusion Alert.* National Blood Resource Education Program. May 1989

165. Walts LF, Rusin WD. The influence of succinylcholine on the duration of pancuronium blockade. *Anesth Analg (Cleveland).* 56:22, 1977

166. Stoelting RK, et al. Circulatory responses and halothane concentrations during gallbladder or gastric traction with and without neuromuscular blockade. *Anesth Analg (Cleveland).* 55:388, 1976

167. Jones AE, Pelton DA. An index of syndromes and their anaesthetic implications. *Can Anaesth Soc J.* 23:207, 1976

168. Tsang HS. Less commonly recognized hazards of atropine as preanesthetic medication. *Anesthesiology Rev.* 4:15, 1977

169. Rosenthal M. Perioperative management of the patient with end-stage liver disease. *ASA Annual Refresher Course Lectures,* Lecture 171, 1988

170. Dorsch JA, Dorsch SE. *Understanding Anesthesia Equipment,* 2nd ed. Baltimore: Williams & Wilkins Company; 1984

171. Bukstein EJ. *Electronics for Medical Personnel.* New York: Bobbs-Merrill Co., Inc.; 1972

172. El-Baz N, et al. High frequency positive-pressure ventilation for tracheal reconstruction supported by tracheal T-tube. *Anesth Analg (Cleveland).* 61:796, 1982

173. Carron H, Korbon GA. Common nerve blocks in anesthetic practice. *Semin Anesthesia.* 2:30, 1983

174. Murphy TM. Complications of regional anesthesia. *Semin Anesthesia.* 2:58, 1983

175. Greene NM. *Physiology of Spinal Anesthesia.* 2nd ed. Baltimore: Williams & Wilkins Co.; 1969

176. Katz J, et al. *Anesthesia and Uncommon Diseases,* 2nd ed. Philadelphia: W.B. Saunders Company; 1981

177. Ryan JF. *A Practice of Anesthesia for Infants and Children.* New York: Grune & Stratton; 1986

178. Smith RM. *Anesthesia for Infants and Children,* 4th ed. St. Louis: C.V. Mosby Company; 1980

179. Stehling LC, Zauder HL. *Anesthetic Implications of Congenital Anomalies in Children.* New York: Appleton-Century-Crofts; 1980

180. Berry FA. (ed). *Anesthetic Management of Difficult and Routine Pediatric Patients.* New York: Churchill Livingstone; 1986

181. Powers SR. Inappropriate use of diuretics in surgical patients. *Arch Surg.* 110:1439, 1975

182. Berry FA, Gregory GA. Do premature infants require anesthesia for surgery? *Anesthesiology.* 67:3, 1987

183. Moore RA, et al. Atlantoaxial subluxation with symptomatic spinal cord compression in a child with Down's syndrome. *Anesth Analg (Cleveland).* 66:89, 1987

184. Ramanathan S. *Obstetric Anesthesia.* Philadelphia, Lea & Febiger; 1988

185. Mahler DL. Elementary statistics for the anesthesiologist. *Anesthesiology.* 28:749, 1967

186. Bergen RP. Lost or broken teeth. *JAMA.* 221:119, 1972

187. Aidinis SJ, et al. Anesthesia for brain computed tomography. *Anesthesiology.* 44:420, 1976

188. Bonica JJ. Acupuncture anesthesia in the People's Republic of China. *JAMA.* 229:1317, 1974

189. Bonica JJ (ed). *Obstetric Analgesia and Anesthesia.* New York: Springer-Verlag: 1972

190. Scott DL. Awareness during general anesthesia. *Can Anaesth Soc J.* 19:173, 1972

191. Price HL, Price ML. Has halothane a predominant circulatory action? *Anesthesiology.* 27:764, 1966

192. Ronnov-Jennen V, Tjernlund A. Hepatotoxicity due to treatment with papaverine. *N Engl J Med.* 281:1333, 1969

193. McHardy G, Balart LA. Jaundice and oxyphenisatin. *JAMA.* 211:83, 1970

194. Summary of National Halothane Study. *JAMA.* 197:775, 1966

195. Ng TY, Kirimli BI. Hazards in use of anode endotracheal tube. *Anesth Analg (Cleveland).* 54:710, 1975

196. Snow JC, et al. Corneal injuries during general anesthesia. *Anesth Analg (Cleveland).* 54:465, 1975

197. Cooper JB, et al. Preventable anesthesia mishaps: A study of human factors. *Anesthesiology.* 49:399, 1978

198. Poon YK. A life-threatening complication of cricothyroid membrane puncture. *Anesth Analg (Cleveland).* 55:298, 1976

199. Zsigmond EK, et al. Arterial hypoxemia caused by intravenous ketamine. *Anesth Analg (Cleveland).* 55:311, 1976

200. Kim SS, Hodgkinson R. Acute ethanol intoxication and its prolonged effect on a full-term infant. *Anesth Analg* 55:602, 1976

201. Keenan RL. Anesthetic disasters: causes, incidence, preventability. *ASA Annual Refresher Course Lectures,* Lecture 242, 1988

202. Chantigian RC. Neonatal resuscitation. *ASA Annual Refresher Course Lectures,* Lecture 216, 1987

203. Snow JC, et al. Broken disposable needle during an axillary approach to block the brachial plexus. *Anesth Analg* 53:89, 1974

204. Lee CM. Acute hypotension during laparoscopy. *Anesth Analg* 54:142, 1975

205. Cottrell JE, et al. Hazards of disposable rebreathing circuits. Anesth Analg 55:743, 1976

206. Denlinger JK, Nahrwold ML. Cardiac failure associated with hypocalcemia. *Anesth Analg* 55:34, 1976

207. Bartlett RH, et al. Respiratory maneuvers to prevent postoperative pulmonary complications. *JAMA* 224:1017, 1973

208. Danforth DN, Scott JR (eds). *Obstetrics and Gynecology,* 5th ed. Philadelphia: J.B. Lippincott Company; 1986

SPECIALTY BOARD REVIEW
Anesthesiology
Third Edition

PART I
Basic Science

CHAPTER 1

Respiration
Review

ANATOMY

The respiratory tract begins at the nose and ends at the alveolus. Each of the anatomic divisions in the upper airway (nose, mouth, and pharynx) and the lower airway (larynx to alveolus) may be affected and is important to the conduct of an anesthetic.

The nose acts as a filter and as a warming and humidifying organ for incoming air. The nose may be the site of increased airway resistance if the turbinates swell or if polyps are present. In the newborn, choanal atresia may be life threatening, since the newborn is an obligate nose breather. *up to 3 mons*

The mouth and pharynx may be the site of pathology that impairs ventilation in the awake and, especially, the anesthetized state. The tongue, tonsils, and adenoids may impede good air exchange and make airway maintenance a problem. The upper airway must be kept patent any time a patient is asleep.

Cilia are present throughout the tracheobronchial tree. Their function is to rid the tracheobronchial tree of secretions. This is done by a wavelike motion of the tiny hair cells, which are covered by two layers of mucus. These layers trap foreign substances and propel them to the opening of the glottis to be expelled. Ciliary function may be affected by low humidity, anesthetic gases, and smoke.

The larynx is a cartilaginous structure that is the entry to the lower airway. It is covered by a flaplike structure, the epiglottis. The epiglottis closes over the glottis during swallowing to prevent the entry of foreign substances. The epiglottis may become swollen, causing airway obstruction. The larynx overlies the 6th cervical vertebra.

The vocal cords are two folds of mucous membrane that attach to the thyroid cartilage and the arytenoids. They are innervated by the recurrent laryngeal and superior laryngeal nerves. These nerves are subject to surgical trauma, and this may lead to cord palsies. Total bilateral laryngeal nerve palsy will leave the cords partially abducted. A partial palsy may cause complete adduction and closure of the larynx. In the adult, the vocal cord level is the narrowest site of the tracheobronchial tree. In the

child until about age 10, the narrowest site is at the level of the cricoid cartilage.

The trachea is formed of cartilaginous rings that are shaped like a C, the open part of the C being posterior. The cricoid ring is the only complete ring in the trachea. The trachea is about 10 to 13 cm long in the adult. In the newborn, it is about 4 cm long.

The trachea bifurcates at the carina into the left and right bronchi. The carina is at the level of the 5th thoracic vertebra. Dichotomous branching takes place, producing bronchi, bronchioles, segmental bronchioles, and terminal bronchioles. The cross-sectional area is increased at each bifurcation, giving a large surface area for air conduction and, eventually, air exchange. The bifurcations end at the alveolus, the ultimate site of air exchange. The right lung is divided into an upper, a middle, and a lower lobe. The left lobe has an upper lobe, a lingular portion, and a lower lobe. The bronchus to the left lung is more narrow and comes off the trachea at a more acute angle than the bronchus to the right. This is true in the infant and the adult.

The blood supply to the lung is from the bronchial arteries and the pulmonary artery. The bronchial arteries are typical arteries supplying nutrition to structures, whereas the pulmonary arteries are involved in gas exchange from the lungs. Each alveolus is supplied by a branch of the pulmonary artery that effects gas exchange. The pulmonary arterial circulation is a low pressure system and is subjected to many pressure and humoral influences.

The muscles of ventilation are the diaphragm, the intercostal muscles, and the accessory muscles. The diaphragm is innervated by the phrenic nerve and is the most important muscle of ventilation. The intercostal muscles change the configuration of the rib cage and make ventilation more efficient. One can survive without the function of the intercostal muscles, since the diaphragm is so efficient.

The accessory muscles are the neck muscles that are important at extremes of ventilation, eg, exercise and respiratory distress. The alae nasi, which flare the nostrils, and the abdominal muscles also are included as accessory muscles.

CONTROL OF VENTILATION

Ventilation control involves a complex system of chemical sensors and reflexes. The respiratory center measures these inputs and responds appropriately.

The *central medullary center*, which lies on the ventral aspect of the medulla, responds to increased hydrogen ion in the cerebral extracellular fluid. When CO_2 diffuses into the extracellular fluid, it combines with water to form carbonic acid, which in turn dissociates into hydrogen ion and bicarbonate. The hydrogen ion stimulates the respiratory center, and ventilation increases. This is the main regulator of ventilation and cerebral extracellular fluid pH. Studying a standard CO_2 response curve (Figure 1–1) shows how this applies. The solid line shows the normal response to increasing CO_2. At a P_{CO_2} of 40 torr, the minute ventilation is about 6 L/minute. At a P_{CO_2} of 45 torr, the minute ventilation has increased to about 22 L/minute. The slope of the line as well as the baseline may shift. A shift of the baseline implies a change in the apneic threshold. Under anesthesia, both may shift as shown in Figure 1–1. This places the anesthetized patient at a disadvantage in maintaining P_{CO_2}.

The peripheral chemoreceptors are the carotid and aortic bodies. The carotid bodies lie at the bifurcation of the common carotid artery. At this level, they are exposed to a high flow of blood directly from the heart. The principal response of the carotid bodies is to decreased oxygen tension and is more important at a P_{O_2} below 60 torr. The total effect of the carotid bodies on ventilation amounts to about 15% of the total ventilatory response.

In patients who have had bilateral carotid endarterectomy, there is no response by the carotid bodies and there may be a rise in P_{CO_2} of about 5 to 6 torr. In addition, these patients do not respond to hypoxemia, and care must be taken to ensure adequate oxygenation at times of stress, eg, in the recovery room.

There is little evidence that the aortic bodies are important in humans.

RESPIRATORY MECHANICS

When we breathe, air enters the lungs because of the negative pressure that has been created by the muscles of respiration, principally the diaphragm. Other muscles, eg, the intercostals, the abdominal muscles, and the scalenes, are important also. The accessory muscles play a larger role as ventilation increases. The power of the diaphragm and the accessory muscles is sufficient to develop a negative force of over 80 torr. It is important to keep these muscles in play when possible. There are many influences that will interfere with good air exchange: limited excursion of the diaphragm, poor movement of the rib cage, lung disease, and obstruction to air flow.

Compliance is defined as volume change per unit of pressure change. The unit of measurement is liters per centimeter of water. It is a static measurement. Compliance changes may be due to the lung or the chest wall. The combination is total pulmonary compliance.

Resistance is defined as pressure differential required for a unit of flow change. The unit is centimeters of water per liter per second. It is, therefore, a dynamic measurement. Resistance may be affected by changes in the airways or changes in the pattern of flow, ie, whether the flow is laminar or turbulent.

LUNG VOLUMES AND CAPACITIES

You should be familiar with the various volumes and capacities as they are measured by a spirometer (Figure 1–2). In addition, the concepts of dead space, closing volume, and closing capacity are important. *Dead space* is air that is moved in and out of the lung without participating in ventilation. It may be anatomic dead space, alveolar dead space, or physiologic dead space, which contains components of the two. *Closing volume* is the lung volume at which airways begin to close. The value is high at extremes of age. If the value is excessive, it will encroach on tidal volume, and the alveoli will not open. Shunting then will occur.

VENTILATION–PERFUSION MATCHING

The lung is functionally divided into three zones based on the difference in the relative perfusion and ventilation in the three zones (Figure 1–3). In zone 1, there is ventilation in excess of perfusion. This zone is high in dead space. In zone 2, ventilation and blood flow depend on the state of ventilation—if the alveolar pressure is high, little blood flow occurs; if the pressure is low, blood flow can occur. In zone 3, there is higher blood flow, and the blood flow is due to the arterial–venous difference. Ventilation/perfusion ratios (V/Q) at the apex of the lung (zone 1) are high. The ratios at the base are low. Various respiratory maneuvers can affect the ventilation and perfusion and must be considered in the conduct of an anesthetic.

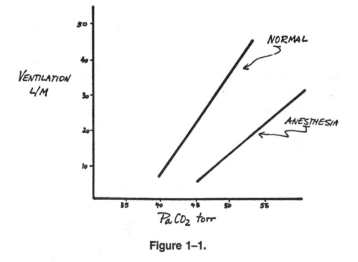

Figure 1–1.

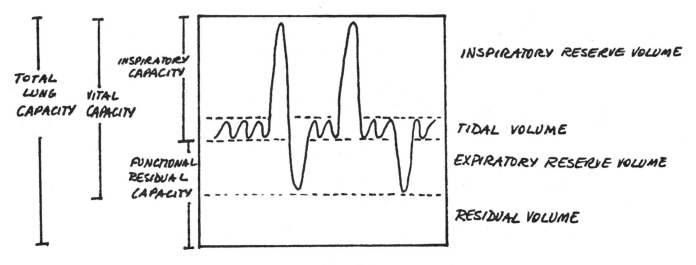

Figure 1–2.

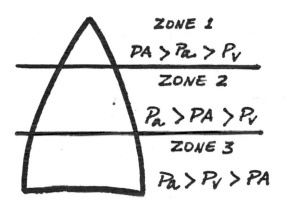

Figure 1–3.

OXYGEN TRANSPORT

Oxygen transport involves the transport to the tissues of oxygen that is combined with hemoglobin, oxygen in solution, and the cardiac output. The bulk of oxygen is combined with hemoglobin, and that amount that can be carried is reflected in the oxyhemoglobin dissociation curve (Figue 1–4).

Saturation of hemoglobin can be affected by many factors, eg, type of hemoglobin, temperature, CO_2 tension, pH, and level of 2, 3-DPG. Again, various maneuvers may have an adverse effect on oxygen-carrying ability. We may take steps to increase oxygen-carrying capacity of the blood and counteract that by doing something to lower cardiac output, resulting in lower oxygen availability to the tissues.

CARBON DIOXIDE TRANSPORT

Carbon dioxide is produced in the tissues and is transported in four forms:

1. In physical solution
2. As carbonic acid; this reaction takes place in the plasma and in the red cell
3. As bicarbonate ion, the major buffer in the body
4. As carbamino groups; these groups are protein molecules carried principally in the red cell

The greatest bulk is in the bicarbonate form.

OTHER ITEMS FOR STUDY

You should be familiar with flow–volume loops and their use in the diagnosis of lung disease.

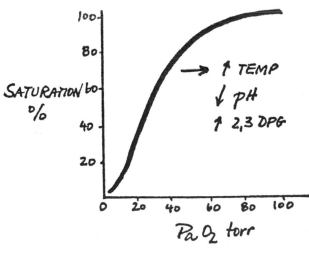

Figure 1–4.

Questions

1. If one measured pleural pressure, one would find that the pressure was

   (A) highest at the apex of the lung
   (B) highest at the base of the lung
   (C) equal at all levels
   (D) unrelated to body position
   (E) completely unpredictable from one level to another

2. The LaPlace law is important in pulmonary physiology because

   (A) it describes the motion of the diaphragm
   (B) it describes the angles of the bronchi
   (C) it describes the bucket handle movement of the ribs during ventilation
   (D) it describes the pressure relationships within the alveoli
   (E) it describes resistance in large airways

3. Surfactant is a substance that

   (A) is produced in the liver of the newborn
   (B) is important in newborns but has little importance in the adult
   (C) is produced by the basement membrane of the lung
   (D) lowers surface tension in the lung
   (E) is a long-chained carbohydrate molecule

4. The functional residual capacity (FRC) is defined as the combination of

   (A) tidal volume and residual volume
   (B) tidal volume and expiratory reserve volume
   (C) inspiratory reserve volume and tidal volume
   (D) residual volume and expiratory reserve volume
   (E) residual volume and inspiratory reserve volume

5. The maximum volume of air inhaled from the end-inspiratory level is referred to as

   (A) tidal volume
   (B) inspiratory capacity
   (C) inspiratory reserve volume
   (D) vital capacity
   (E) functional residual capacity (FRC)

6. Functional residual capacity (FRC) can be measured by

   (A) direct measurement
   (B) use of an esophageal balloon
   (C) body plethysmography
   (D) x-ray examination
   (E) spirometry

7. At functional residual capacity (FRC)

   (A) the pressure difference between the alveoli and atmosphere is zero
   (B) the pressure difference between the alveoli and atmosphere is positive
   (C) the pressure difference between the alveoli and atmosphere is negative
   (D) the total pulmonary vascular resistance is very high
   (E) no further inspiration is possible

8. The cilia of the respiratory tract

   (A) are part of the type II pneumocytes
   (B) are not affected by drugs
   (C) are inhibited by the presence of an uncuffed endotracheal tube
   (D) propel a double layer of mucus toward the larynx
   (E) are not affected by temperature

9. Factors contributing to increased airway pressure under anesthesia include all of the following EXCEPT

   (A) an increase in the caliber of the airways
   (B) a decrease in functional residual capacity

(C) the supine position

(D) the presence of an endotracheal tube

(E) pharyngeal obstruction

10. In the adult, the tracheobronchial tree

(A) divides at an uneven angle, making foreign bodies more apt to go to the left side

(B) divides into right and left bronchi, the left bronchus being narrower and longer

(C) is relatively fixed and immovable with respiration

(D) is lined with squamous epithelium

(E) is protected by circular cartilaginous rings throughout

11. The human larynx

(A) lies at the level of the 2nd through 5th cervical vertebrae

(B) in the adult, is narrowest at the level of the cricoid cartilage

(C) is innervated solely by the recurrent laryngeal nerve

(D) is protected anteriorly by the wide expanse of the cricoid cartilage

(E) lies within the thyroid cartilage

12. Humidification of inhaled air or gases is

(A) more efficient with an endotracheal tube in place

(B) increased with the administration of atropine

(C) more efficient in an open system than a closed system

(D) at its optimum with the patient breathing through the nose

(E) at its optimum with the patient breathing through a tracheostomy

13. The principal muscle(s) of respiration is (are) the

(A) diaphragm

(B) intercostals

(C) abdominals

(D) sternomastoids

(E) scalenes

14. Distribution of ventilation in the lung is such that

(A) the apical portions are better ventilated

(B) the diaphragmatic areas are better ventilated

(C) the central or hilar areas are better ventilated

(D) all areas are ventilated equally

(E) ventilation is not affected by position

15. Inspiratory force is

(A) a measurement of reserve of ventilatory effort

(B) dependent on conscious effort

(C) normal is between 5 and 10 cm of H_2O below atmospheric pressure

(D) difficult to measure

(E) normal if between 5 and 10 cm of H_2O above atmospheric pressure

16. A patient is admitted for an intestinal bypass procedure for treatment of morbid obesity. His height is 65 inches, and his weight is 134 kg. He is diagnosed as having the pickwickian syndrome. You would expect his tests to show

(A) alveolar hyperventilation, anemia, and hypoxemia

(B) alveolar hyperventilation, erythrocytosis, and hypoxemia

(C) decreased expiratory reserve volume and higher intraabdominal pressure when supine

(D) lower work of breathing

(E) unimproved respiratory condition after weight reduction

17. The pickwickian syndrome is one example of primary alveolar hypoventilation. Which of the following is NOT a cause of primary alveolar hypoventilation?

(A) central nervous system infection

(B) hyperthyroidism

(C) schizophrenia

(D) head trauma

(E) syringomyelia of the spinal cord

18. All of the following components contribute to physiologic shunt EXCEPT

(A) bronchial veins

(B) pleural veins

(C) thebesian veins

(D) abnormal arterial–venous communications

(E) nonperfused alveoli

19. During one-lung anesthesia with a double-lumen tube

(A) no shunting occurs in the unventilated lung

(B) no alveoli are in continuity with the proximal airways

(C) CO_2 removal is difficult

(D) insufflation of oxygen leads to decreased shunting

(E) it is not possible to administer oxygen to the collapsed lung

20. After bilateral carotid endarterectomy, a patient will

(A) have no respiratory changes

(B) show no change in arterial carbon dioxide

(C) respond to hypoxia with hyperventilation

(D) be more susceptible to hypoxemia

(E) always develop hypertension

21. Adequacy of alveolar ventilation is determined by measuring

    (A) the oxygen gradient
    (B) oxygen tension
    (C) oxygen saturation
    (D) cardiac output
    (E) carbon dioxide tension ✓

22. Measurement of arterial oxygen tension

    (A) requires use of the Henderson-Hasselbalch equation
    (B) uses the Clark electrode ✓
    (C) uses the Severinghaus electrode
    (D) is not affected by temperature
    (E) is performed on clotted blood

$pH = 24 \times \frac{pco_2}{Hco_3}$

23. Mechanisms that may cause hypoxemia under anesthesia include all of the following EXCEPT

    (A) hypoventilation
    (B) hyperventilation
    (C) increase in functional residual capacity (FRC) ✓
    (D) supine position
    (E) increased airway pressure

24. In a patient with a fixed shunt, a decrease in cardiac output will

    → (A) decrease the arterial oxygenation
    (B) decrease the arterial carbon dioxide tension
    (C) have little effect on oxygenation
    (D) increase dead space ✓
    (E) increase urinary output

25. After a 2-hour anesthetic with hyperventilation, a patient breathing room air will

    (A) return to normal parameters within 30 minutes
    (B) remain hypocarbic for 2 hours
    (C) become hypoxemic if not treated with oxygen ✓
    (D) become hypoxemic and hypercarbic
    (E) be well oxygenated if the air exchange is unimpaired by drugs

26. Carbon dioxide retention in chronic lung disease is

    (A) due primarily to ventilation/perfusion (V/Q) abnormality ✓
    (B) due primarily to shunting
    (C) due primarily to alveolar hypoventilation
    (D) due primarily to increased dead space
    (E) treated best by increasing alveolar ventilation

27. Tracheal mucus flow is

    (A) impeded by deviation from ambient oxygen tension
    (B) decreased in patients with chronic obstructive lung disease
    (C) not important as a cleansing mechanism

    (D) unrelated to ciliary activity
    (E) more active after a patient smokes a cigarette

28. All of the following are true of closing volume EXCEPT that

    (A) it is measured by a single-breath nitrogen technique
    (B) it is useful in determining disease of small airways
    (C) it is decreased at the extremes of age ✓
    (D) closing volume plus residual volume equals closing capacity
    (E) it is measured at phase IV on the nitrogen washout curve

29. Breathing 100 percent oxygen may lead to all of the following EXCEPT

    (A) lung damage
    (B) decreased volume of air-containing space
    (C) retinopathy of prematurity
    (D) hyperventilation in the patient with obstructive lung disease ✓
    (E) atelectasis

30. The central chemoreceptors responsible for respiratory control are

    (A) located in the midbrain
    (B) responsive primarily to change in carbon dioxide
    (C) responsive primarily to change in hydrogen ion concentration ✓
    (D) responsive primarily to hypoxemia
    (E) activated by chronic hypercapnia

31. The peripheral chemoreceptors are

    (A) located in the medulla oblongata
    (B) poorly perfused and, therefore, respond slowly to changes in the oxygen content of the blood
    (C) primarily responsible for the hypoxic drive to respiration ✓
    (D) influenced by oxygen content rather than oxygen tension
    (E) maximally stimulated by arterial oxygen tension over 250 torr

32. Compliance refers to

    (A) a change in volume per unit change in pressure ✓
    (B) a change in pressure per unit change in volume
    (C) the reciprocal of conductance
    (D) a change in volume per unit change in pressure per unit of time
    (E) a measurement of tracheal movement

33. Oxygen toxicity (hyperoxia) exhibits all of the following EXCEPT

    (A) substernal distress
    → (B) increased vital capacity

(C) atelectasis
(D) retinopathy of prematurity
(E) tracheobronchitis

34. In assessing a patient's need for mechanical ventilation, the most important consideration is the

    (A) arterial oxygen tension
    (B) arterial carbon dioxide tension
    (C) pH
    (D) rate of change of the disease process and the consequences of continued hypoventilation
    (E) age of the patient

35. Oxygen toxicity

    (A) develops after breathing 100% oxygen for 12 hours
    (B) is not dose related
    (C) develops after 36 hours of exposure to 25% oxygen
    (D) is due specifically to the oxygen molecule
    (E) is so important that 100% oxygen should never be used

36. General anesthesia alters the mechanical properties of the chest wall, leading to

    (A) increased functional residual capacity (FRC)
    (B) increased lung volume
    (C) decreased elastic recoil of the lung
    (D) decreased compliance
    (E) no change in lung physiology

37. The oxyhemoglobin dissociation curve describes the relationship of oxygen saturation to oxygen tension. All of the following are true EXCEPT that

    (A) at an oxygen tension of 60 torr, the saturation is approximately 90%
    (B) the curve is shifted to the left with a more acid pH
    (C) the curve is shifted to the right with an increase in carbon dioxide tension
    (D) the curve is shifted to the left with a decrease in temperature
    (E) the curve is shifted to the right with increased levels of 2,3-DPG

38. A 35-year-old male enters the hospital with a diagnosis of restrictive pulmonary disease. The pulmonary test result compatible with this diagnosis is

	FORCED VITAL CAPACITY (FVC)	FORCED EXPIRATORY VOLUME IN 1 SECOND (FEV$_1$)	FEV$_1$/FVC%
(A)	normal	decreased	decreased
(B)	decreased	decreased	normal
(C)	decreased	decreased	increased
(D)	increased	increased	normal
(E)	normal	decreased	normal

Questions 39 through 41

An 18-year-old male was involved in an automobile accident that resulted in a cervical cord injury at the C-5 level, with paresthesias and motor weakness, a tender abdomen with an equivocal abdominal tap for blood, and a fracture of the femur. He is being treated with oxygen, 40% by mask, and skeletal traction. He is being evaluated for splenic injury. Initial arterial blood gas results are: pH 7.40, P_{CO_2} 42 torr, and P_{O_2} 96 torr. Over the next 2 hours, his weakness becomes more profound, and repeat arterial blood gas results are: pH 7.35, P_{CO_2} 46 torr, and P_{O_2} 84 torr.

39. At this time, you should

    (A) observe for another hour and reevaluate
    (B) measure his vital capacity—if it is below 8ml/kg, intubate and ventilate
    (C) measure his vital capacity but do not intubate and ventilate, since that may cloud the abdominal findings
    (D) obtain an immediate chest film and evaluate it before making a decision
    (E) increase oxygen delivery by mask

40. His respiratory changes may be caused by all of the following EXCEPT

    (A) hypoventilation due to cord injury
    (B) hypoventilation due to upper abdominal injury
    (C) fat embolus
    (D) respiratory depression secondary to oxygen administration
    (E) pulmonary contusion

41. This patient would be a prime candidate for respiratory failure even in the absence of a leg fracture because

    (A) he has a decreased ability to cough
    (B) his lesion is high enough to predispose to aspiration
    (C) his treatment may lead to pulmonary oxygen toxicity
    (D) he may have blood loss from his other injuries
    (E) he is being kept supine for evaluation

Questions 42 and 43

Pulmonary function test results for a 25-year-old, 70-kg male are:

Vital capacity: 2800 ml
Inspiratory capacity: 3600 ml
Tidal volume: 500 ml
Dead space: 300 ml
O_2 saturation: 93%
O_2 tension: 82 torr [fraction of inspired oxygen (F_{IO_2}) 0.21]
CO_2 tension: 48 torr

42. These values show that the patient has

(A) a normal P_{O_2}
(B) an abnormal inspiratory capacity
(C) a low P_{CO_2}
(D) a decreased vital capacity
(E) an abnormal O_2 saturation ✓

43. Treatment of this patient should be directed toward

(A) decreasing dead space ✓
(B) improving tidal volume
(C) maintaining the status quo
(D) decreasing atelectasis
(E) slowing ventilation

Questions 44 and 45

Please refer to the following figure:

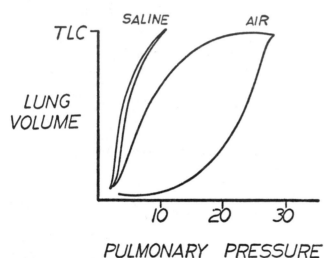

44. In the graph shown, the inflation and deflation curves differ. This is

(A) due to the pull of the thoracic cage
(B) referred to as hysteresis
(C) an abnormal condition in humans
(D) seen only in patients with obstructive lung disease
(E) a measurement of dead space

45. In the graph, there is a marked difference between the curve for air and the curve for saline. This can be attributed to the

(A) effect of pollutants in the air
(B) effect of surface tension on lung elasticity
(C) method of measurement
(D) position of the esophageal balloon used in measurement
(E) presence of diseased lung tissue

46. The definitive test of adequacy of ventilation is

(A) listening to the esophageal stethoscope
(B) watching the rise and fall of the chest
(C) analyzing arterial blood gases ✓
(D) measuring tidal volume with a spirometer
(E) using an apnea monitor

47. Pulmonary vascular resistance $R = \frac{P}{F}$

(A) is entirely dependent on the cardiac output
(B) is entirely dependent on the pressure in the pulmonary artery
(C) is equal to pressure divided by radius of the artery
(D) depends on the state of vasomotion, flow, and pressure
(E) is not affected by cardiac output

48. Hypoxic pulmonary vasoconstriction

(A) is not important in the intact human being
(B) is active only at high altitude
(C) causes more blood flow to the base of the lung
(D) causes higher dead space/tidal volume ratio than in the nonhypoxic lung
(E) diverts blood flow from hypoxic to nonhypoxic ✓ lung areas

49. The work of breathing

(A) is increased in the anesthetized patient breathing spontaneously
(B) involves effort to overcome resistance in the airways only
(C) involves effort to overcome elastic forces only
(D) is at its lowest at a respiratory rate of 25 breaths per minute
(E) is increased in the patient with restrictive disease if the respiratory rate is increased ✓

50. Measurements that can be obtained by spirometry include all of the following EXCEPT

(A) tidal volume
(B) closing volume ✓
(C) expiratory reserve volume
(D) inspiratory reserve volume
(E) vital capacity

51. Anatomic dead space

(A) is independent of lung size
(B) is about 1 ml/kg body weight
(C) is not affected by equipment
(D) combined with alveolar dead space constitutes ✓ physiologic dead space
(E) is of less importance in the newborn than the adult

52. The term P_{50} in reference to the oxyhemoglobin dissociation curve

   (A) refers to the position on the curve at which the Po_2 is 50 torr
   (B) normally has a value of 27 torr ✓
   (C) describes an enzyme system in hemoglobin
   (D) is constant
   (E) is affected only by type of hemoglobin

53. Carbon dioxide transport involves all of the following EXCEPT

   (A) water ✓
   (B) bicarbonate ion
   (C) carbonic anhydrase
   (D) hemoglobin
   (E) carboxyhemoglobin ✓

54. The Bohr effect refers to the

   (A) effect of carbonic anhydrase on the uptake of CO_2
   (B) ability of the blood to pick up more CO_2 when the oxygen tension is low *Haldane effect*
   (C) amount of hydrogen in solution in the blood
   (D) effect of Pco_2 on the saturation of oxygen ✓
   (E) presence of catalytic enzymes in the blood

55. Hypercapnia under anesthesia may be a result of

   (A) hyperventilation
   (B) decreased dead space ventilation *causes ↓ CO_2*
   (C) decreased carbon dioxide production
   (D) use of an Ayre T-piece at less than peak inspiratory flow rate
   (E) increase in pulmonary artery pressure

Questions 56 through 58

Please refer to the following figure:

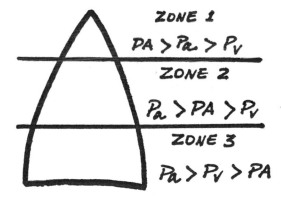

ZONE 1
$PA > Pa > P_V$

ZONE 2
$Pa > PA > P_V$

ZONE 3
$Pa > P_V > PA$

56. In zone 1 of the lung

   (A) no air is moving
   (B) circulation is highest
   (C) venous pressure is high
   (D) dead space is high ✓
   (E) shunting is high

57. In zone 2 of the lung

   (A) there is good blood flow regardless of ventilation
   (B) venous pressure is high
   (C) dead space is high
   (D) the pulmonary vessels are collapsed
   (E) the blood flow is determined primarily by pulmonary artery pressure and alveolar pressure ✓

58. In zone 3 of the lung

   (A) blood flow is governed by the arteriovenous difference ✓
   (B) dead space is high
   (C) there is high alveolar pressure
   (D) venous pressure is very low
   (E) little blood flow occurs

59. Henry's law

   (A) describes the movement of molecules according to their molecular weight
   (B) describes the transfer of oxygen to the hemoglobin molecule
   (C) describes the solubility of a gas ✓
   (D) describes the enzymatic breakdown of a molecule in the lung
   (E) describes the dissolution of a solid in a liquid

60. Boyle's law

   (A) describes the molecular motion of a liquid
   (B) describes the relation of pressure and volume of a gas ✓
   (C) describes the relation of pressure and temperature of a gas
   (D) describes the diffusion of a gas across membranes
   (E) describes the solution of a solid in a liquid

61. The main buffering system of the body is

   (A) hemoglobin
   (B) bicarbonate ✓
   (C) phosphate
   (D) sulfate
   (E) plasma proteins

62. Hemoglobin as a buffer

   (A) is the primary noncarbonic buffer ✓
   (B) is unimportant
   (C) acts only on respiratory pH changes
   (D) acts as the intact hemoglobin molecule, not as a salt
   (E) is a stronger acid than carbonic acid

PV = PV

63. Recognition of hypoxemia in the recovery room

    (A) depends on the detection of cyanosis
    (B) depends on the detection of respiratory responses
    (C) depends on the detection of circulatory responses
    (D) is most dependable with arterial blood gases
    (E) is done better with a transcutaneous oxygen monitor than with a pulse oximeter

64. Hypoxemia in the recovery room may be due to all of the following EXCEPT

    (A) increased functional residual capacity (FRC)
    (B) shivering
    (C) decreased cardiac output
    (D) intrapulmonary shunt
    (E) decreased vital capacity

65. Hypoventilation in the recovery room

    (A) should always be treated with narcotic reversal
    (B) is more common after inhalation anesthesia than intravenous anesthesia
    (C) is uncommon after upper abdominal procedures
    (D) is best detected by arterial blood gases
    (E) is always accompanied by increases in blood pressure

66. A patient who is breathing 100% oxygen

    (A) completely eliminates the nitrogen in the lung in two breaths
    (B) eliminates nitrogen rapidly, dependent on the volume of the breaths
    (C) eliminates nitrogen regardless of presence of disease
    (D) eliminates nitrogen faster if he or she is a smoker
    (E) eliminates nitrogen faster if he or she is older

67. Signs of hypoxemia include all of the following EXCEPT

    (A) decreased ventilatory effort in response to chemoreceptor stimulation
    (B) increased heart rate in response to sympathetic stimulation
    (C) cyanosis
    (D) decreased heart rate due to direct effect of hypoxemia on the heart
    (E) increased blood pressure due to sympathetic stimulation

68. During apneic ventilation

    (A) the time elapsed before desaturation occurs is independent of the patient's oxygen status before the onset of apnea
    (B) all arrhythmias are due to hypoxemia
    (C) the carbon dioxide tension is not important

    (D) the carbon dioxide level rises about 3 torr/minute
    (E) pulse oximetry is not helpful

69. Boyle's law

    (A) states that pressure is directly proportional to volume
    (B) states that pressure is directly proportional to temperature
    (C) states that pressure is inversely proportional to volume
    (D) states that pressure is inversely proportional to temperature
    (E) states that volume is directly proportional to temperature

70. Charles' law

    (A) states that pressure is directly proportional to volume
    (B) states that volume is inversely proportional to temperature
    (C) states that pressure is inversely proportional to volume
    (D) states that pressure is inversely proportional to temperature
    (E) states that volume is directly proportional to temperature

71. Graham's law

    (A) states that diffusion is proportional to temperature
    (B) states that diffusion is proportional to pressure
    (C) states that diffusion is proportional to molecular weight
    (D) states that diffusion is inversely proportional to molecular weight
    (E) states that diffusion is directly proportional to temperature and pressure

72. All of the following are important in oxygen transport EXCEPT

    (A) oxygen content
    (B) oxygen tension
    (C) cardiac output
    (D) hemoglobin level
    (E) carboxyhemoglobin level

73. The Haldane effect refers to

    (A) the effect of the cytochrome system on oxygen uptake
    (B) the shift in the CO_2 dissociation curve caused by altered levels of oxygen
    (C) the shift of the CO_2 curve due to temperature
    (D) the shift of the oxyhemoglobin curve due to blood pressure
    (E) the shift of the CO_2 response curve due to drugs

74. In the normal upright lung

    (A) the blood flow is greatest at the apex
    (B) the ventilation is greatest at the apex
    (C) the ventilation/perfusion (V/Q) ratio is higher at the apex
    (D) the level of lung area is not critical to ventilation
    (E) the P_{O_2} is lower at the apex

75. Intrapulmonary shunting refers to

    (A) anatomic dead space
    (B) alveolar dead space
    (C) ventilation in excess of perfusion
    (D) perfusion in excess of ventilation
    (E) wasted ventilation

76. The cuff of an endotracheal tube should be inflated to what pressure to prevent aspiration while not causing underlying ischemia?

    (A) 20 torr
    (B) 30 torr
    (C) 40 torr
    (D) 50 torr
    (E) 60 torr

77. If a patient is allowed to breathe 100% oxygen under anesthesia

    (A) intrapulmonary shunting may increase
    (B) the oxygen tension will always increase
    (C) the P_{O_2} will rise due to increased dead space
    (D) lung units with high ventilation/perfusion (V/Q) ratios will become shunt units
    (E) the oxygen tension will rise due to an increase in functional residual capacity (FRC)

78. Physiologic dead space calculation

    (A) uses the Bohr equation
    (B) requires the measurement of pulmonary artery oxygen tension
    (C) requires the measurement of mixed venous CO_2
    (D) requires the measurement of inspired CO_2 tension
    (E) requires a body plethysmograph

79. Thiopental, administered in an anesthetic dose, has all of the following respiratory effects EXCEPT

    (A) apnea
    (B) respiratory depression
    (C) impaired response to CO_2 stimulation
    (D) bronchoconstriction
    (E) initial hyperpnea followed by respiration depression

80. As one moves from the apex of the lung to the dependent portions

    (A) the alveoli become larger

    (B) the caliber of the air passages becomes larger
    (C) pleural pressure decreases
    (D) compliance becomes greater
    (E) ventilation of the alveoli becomes less due to decreased compliance

81. All of the following nerves are important in the motor supply of the larynx EXCEPT

    (A) the superior laryngeal nerve
    (B) the inferior laryngeal nerve
    (C) the internal laryngeal branch of the superior laryngeal nerve
    (D) the external laryngeal branch of the superior laryngeal nerve
    (E) the recurrent laryngeal nerve

82. The musculature of the bronchioles

    (A) runs along one side of the bronchus only
    (B) becomes thinner as it proceeds distally
    (C) becomes thinner relative to the thickness of the bronchiole as it proceeds distally
    (D) has little effect on the diameter of the bronchiole
    (E) has no relationship with the elastic fibers

83. The Hering-Breuer reflex

    (A) has little importance in the adult human
    (B) causes a deep inspiration after a total expiration in the laboratory animal
    (C) causes a deep inspiration after a cough
    (D) has a major role in the control of ventilation
    (E) is stimulated by barbiturates

84. The position of the vocal cords after bilateral cutting of the recurrent laryngeal nerve is

    (A) closed in the midline
    (B) in complete abduction
    (C) the same whether the nerve is completely or incompletely severed
    (D) open in midposition
    (E) both aligned to the left, since the left is the dominant branch of the nerve

85. The carbon dioxide response curve describes the pattern of ventilation following challenge by various concentrations of carbon dioxide. Which of the following is true?

    (A) the anesthetized patient under anesthesia will show the same effects regardless of the agent
    (B) the slope of the response may change, but the position of the curve remains the same
    (C) the position and slope are the same in adults and infants
    (D) increased work of breathing leads to a steeper slope
    (E) the slope of the line measures the patient's sensitivity to carbon dioxide

86. All of the following will influence the carbon dioxide response curve EXCEPT

   (A) individual responses
   (B) hypoxemia
   (C) chronic bronchitis
   (D) drugs
   (E) nitrous oxide at 50% concentration

87. All of the following statements about the diaphragm are true EXCEPT that it

   (A) is innervated by the phrenic nerve
   (B) gets it principal innervation from the 3rd, 4th, and 5th cervical nerves
   (C) has an excursion of about 1.5 cm with normal tidal breathing
   (D) has an excursion that changes with changes of posture
   (E) has a peripheral tendon by which it attaches to the rib cage

88. Circulation to the lung

   (A) consists entirely of the pulmonary artery and its branches
   (B) consists of the pulmonary artery and the bronchial arterial system, which are of equal importance
   (C) is under high pressure relative to the left side of the heart
   (D) consists of two systems, but the bronchial system is expendable
   (E) consists of the pulmonary artery, which nourishes the bronchioles, and the bronchial arteries, which progress only to the level of the second branching of the bronchioles

89. Metabolic effects of the lung do NOT include

   (A) inactivation of 5-hydroxytryptamine
   (B) inactivation of epinephrine
   (C) inactivation of bradykinin
   (D) inactivation of prostaglandin
   (E) inactivation of norepinephrine

90. The alveolar–arterial oxygen difference ($AaDo_2$)

   (A) in normal adults is about 40 to 80 torr
   (B) can be measured directly
   (C) increases linearly with age
   (D) increases with age because of a decrease in alveolar oxygen tension
   (E) is a good screening tool for detecting ventilation/perfusion (V/Q) changes

91. Reynold's number

   (A) concerns turbulent versus laminar flow
   (B) concerns surface tension
   (C) concerns carbon dioxide diffusion
   (D) concerns oxygen transport

   (E) concerns the critical amount of humidification in the airway

92. All of the following are true of the calculation of Reynold's number EXCEPT

   (A) a value above 2000 has significance
   (B) it involves density
   (C) it involves length
   (D) it involves viscosity
   (E) it involves velocity

DIRECTIONS (Questions 93 through 181): For each of the items in this section, ONE or MORE of the numbered options is correct. Choose the answer

A if only 1, 2, and 3 are correct,
B if only 1 and 3 are correct,
C if only 2 and 4 are correct,
D if only 4 is correct,
E if all are correct.

93. Positive end-expiratory pressure (PEEP)

   (1) always improves oxygenation
   (2) increases lung volume at end-expiration [functional residual capacity (FRC)]
   (3) decreases lung compliance
   (4) increases ventilation/perfusion (V/Q) ratio

94. Physiologic dead space

   (1) is increased in areas of high ventilation/perfusion (V/Q) ratio
   (2) is increased in old age
   (3) is increased in zone 1 of the lung
   (4) is increased after administration of atropine

95. The following anesthetic agents have been shown to cause bronchodilation

   (1) halothane
   (2) ether
   (3) isoflurane
   (4) enflurane

96. The work of breathing

   (1) involves both resistive and elastic work
   (2) is expended mostly in expiration
   (3) to overcome elastic forces is increased when breathing is deep and slow
   (4) to overcome resistive forces is decreased when breathing is fast and shallow

97. Carbon dioxide is transported

   (1) in physical solution
   (2) as carbonic acid
   (3) as bicarbonate
   (4) as carbaminohemoglobin

98. The respiratory pattern seen with various levels of anesthesia with halothane includes

    (1) irregular respirations at light (less than minimal alveolar concentration) levels
    (2) faster, more shallow respirations at moderate levels
    (3) jerky, gasping respirations at deep levels
    (4) a rocking-boat pattern at deep levels due to the loss of diaphragmatic movement

99. A decrease in functional residual capacity (FRC) under anesthesia may be due to

    (1) the supine position
    (2) increased intraabdominal pressure
    (3) a cephalad shift in the diaphragm
    (4) bronchial dilation

100. Hypoxic pulmonary vasoconstriction is decreased by

    (1) mitral stenosis
    (2) intravascular volume overload
    (3) hypothermia
    (4) inhalational anesthetics

101. Increased dead space ventilation may occur during anesthesia due to

    (1) deliberate hypotension
    (2) short rapid ventilations
    (3) pulmonary embolus
    (4) decreased airway pressure

102. Vital capacity includes

    (1) tidal volume
    (2) inspiratory reserve volume
    (3) expiratory reserve volume
    (4) functional residual capacity (FRC)

103. Hypoxemia may occur under anesthesia because of

    (1) blood loss
    (2) depressed myocardial function
    (3) shunting
    (4) airway obstruction

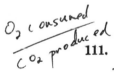

$$\frac{O_2 \text{ consumed}}{CO_2 \text{ produced}}$$

104. In the patient with an intrapulmonary shunt

    (1) decreased cardiac output will increase Po_2
    (2) increased oxygen consumption will decrease oxygen content
    (3) decreased cardiac output will increase oxygen content
    (4) decreased cardiac output will decrease oxygen content

105. Pathways in the lung for collateral ventilation include

    (1) the intraalveolar pores of Kohn
    (2) connections between respiratory bronchioles and terminal bronchioles
    (3) interlobar connections
    (4) interbronchial connections

106. A patient with hypercapnia will have

    (1) decreased levels of epinephrine
    (2) increased levels of norepinephrine
    (3) respiratory alkalosis
    (4) increased plasma potassium

107. The patient who is hyperventilated to a Pco_2 of 20 torr under anesthesia will have

    (1) increased cerebral blood flow
    (2) increased ionized calcium
    (3) increased oxygen delivery to the tissues
    (4) increased ventilation/perfusion (V/Q) mismatch due to inhibition of hypoxic pulmonary vasoconstriction

108. Pulse oximeter readings

    (1) are not affected by low perfusion states
    (2) of 90% correspond to a Po_2 of 60 torr
    (3) are equally reliable with oxyhemoglobin, carboxyhemoglobin, and methemoglobin
    (4) may be inaccurate due to light interference

109. Specific effects of anesthesia on control of breathing include

    (1) decreased response to carbon dioxide
    (2) decreased response to hypoxemia
    (3) decreased response to metabolic acidemia
    (4) decreased response to added airway resistance

110. Factors leading to pulmonary edema include

    (1) increased capillary pressure
    (2) decreased oncotic pressure
    (3) lymphatic insufficiency
    (4) increased capillary permeability

111. The respiratory quotient

    (1) depends on the CO_2 output
    (2) is independent of the metabolic substrate
    (3) depends on the O_2 uptake
    (4) is always 0.8

112. Positive end-expiratory pressure (PEEP) improves oxygenation by

    (1) prevention of airway closure
    (2) prevention of air trapping
    (3) improving diffusion of gases in the alveoli
    (4) decreasing cardiac output

SUMMARY OF DIRECTIONS				
A	**B**	**C**	**D**	**E**
1, 2, 3 only	1, 3 only	2, 4 only	4 only	All are correct

113. Positive end-expiratory pressure (PEEP) usually

    (1) increases functional residual capacity (FRC)
    (2) decreases compliance
    (3) decreases work of breathing
    (4) decreases lung volume

114. In the technique of one-lung anesthesia, the method used to ventilate the dependent lung is important. It is true that

    (1) hyperventilation of the dependent lung may inhibit hypoxic pulmonary vasoconstriction
    (2) high airway pressure to the dependent lung may be harmful
    (3) high inspired oxygen concentration may lead to absorption atelectasis
    (4) high inspired oxygen concentration may lead to vasoconstriction

115. Body position may have an effect on functional residual capacity (FRC). You would expect

    (1) a marked reduction in the supine position
    (2) a marked reduction in the head-down position
    (3) a moderate reduction in the lateral position
    (4) a small change in the prone position

116. When assessing the hypoxemic patient, causes that may be important are

    (1) hypoventilation
    (2) physiologic shunt
    (3) ventilation/perfusion (V/Q) mismatch
    (4) abnormal diffusion

117. Therapy directed at the hypoxemic patient in the postoperative period may include

    (1) supplemental oxygen
    (2) improving alveolar ventilation
    (3) prevention of atelectasis
    (4) administration of carbon dioxide to stimulate ventilation

118. In the lateral decubitus position, the lung relationships

    (1) are the same as in the semirecumbent position; ie, the apex is in zone 1 and the bases are in zone 3
    (2) ventilation is highest at the apex
    (3) perfusion is greater in the upright lung
    (4) perfusion is greater in the dependent lung

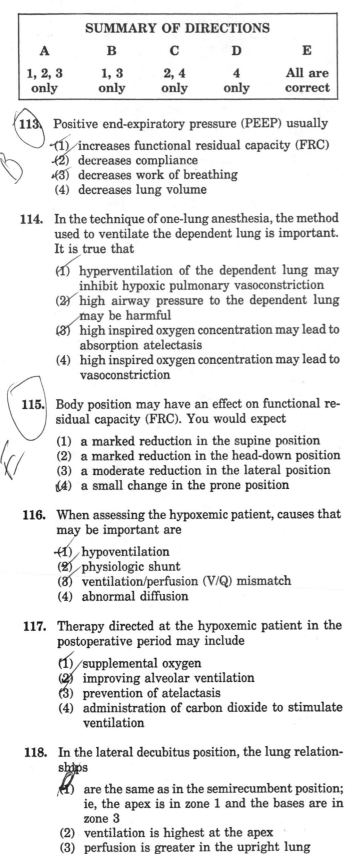

119. Oxygen toxicity of the lung

    (1) is not a significant problem in the patient with normal lungs if the alveolar oxygen tension is kept below 350 torr
    (2) is more apt to occur in critically ill patients
    (3) is not reason to withhold 100% oxygen if needed
    (4) is more apt to occur if the F_{IO_2} is over 0.5

120. An appropriate level of positive end-expiratory pressure (PEEP) in the patient with acute lung injury

    (1) must take into consideration the oxygen content
    (2) must take into consideration the patient's perfusion
    (3) must take into consideration the patient's oxygen tension
    (4) must take into consideration the patient's risk of barotrauma

121. The adult trachea is

    (1) 15 cm in length
    (2) about the size of the patient's index finger in diameter
    (3) in the midline of the neck
    (4) bifurcates at the level of the 3rd thoracic vertebra

122. The right lung

    (1) is the smaller of the two
    (2) has three lobes
    (3) has a single fissure
    (4) contains the middle lobe

123. Shunt pathways include

    (1) those through atelectatic areas
    (2) those through the bronchial circulation
    (3) a patent foramen ovale
    (4) the thebesian veins

124. Total pulmonary compliance

    (1) is measured by dividing pressure by volume
    (2) involves the lung only
    (3) involves the measurement of time
    (4) is increased by surfactant

125. Airway resistance

    (1) is a dynamic measurement
    (2) is measured by dividing volume per second by pressure
    (3) depends on the caliber of the airway
    (4) is independent of the pattern of air flow, ie, whether it is laminar or turbulent

126. The relationship between closing capacity (CC) and functional residual capacity (FRC)

    (1) is unimportant
    (2) is such that anything that increases FRC relative to CC results in areas of low ventilation/ perfusion (V/Q)
    (3) is such that anything that decreases CC relative to FRC results in areas of low V/Q
    (4) is such that if the closing volume is below the tidal volume, lung units stay open and no shunting occurs

127. Dead space to tidal volume ratio (VDS/VT)

    (1) is a measure of ventilatory efficiency
    (2) is normally under 0.30
    (3) is increased in the patient with chronic lung disease
    (4) increases require increased minute volumes to maintain the same P_{CO_2}

128. During anesthesia, the diaphragm assumes a more cephalad position because of

    (1) paralysis from muscle relaxants
    (2) decreased functional residual capacity (FRC)
    (3) surgical retraction
    (4) spontaneous ventilation

129. Hypercarbia occurring under anesthesia may be due to

    (1) increased dead space ventilation
    (2) exhaustion of soda lime
    (3) pulmonary embolism
    (4) hypoventilation

130. Forced exhaled vital capacity

    (1) is a measure of restrictive disease
    (2) is a measure of inspiratory reserve volume
    (3) is affected by restrictive disease in the first second
    (4) may vary with patient cooperation

131. The medullary chemoreceptors are maximally stimulated by

    (1) low oxygen tension
    (2) reflex activity from the diaphragm
    (3) carbon dioxide
    (4) hydrogen ion

132. In a mixture of gases (such as air)

    (1) each gas obeys Dalton's law
    (2) each gas contributes a partial pressure that is proportional to its solubility
    (3) each gas contributes a partial pressure that is proportional to its relative concentration in the mixture

    (4) the total pressure is equal to the sum of the gases divided by the number of gases

133. The composition of alveolar gases differs from that of inhaled gas because

    (1) oxygen is being absorbed from the alveoli
    (2) carbon dioxide is being added to the alveoli
    (3) water vapor is being added
    (4) nitrogen is taken up by the alveolar capillaries

134. Assuming a constant rate of carbon dioxide formation, alveolar ventilation responds to change in carbon dioxide and hydrogen ion concentration in a manner that

    (1) carbon dioxide is inversely proportional to ventilation
    (2) doubling ventilation will lead to respiratory alkalosis
    (3) reducing ventilation to one fourth of normal will lead to a profound respiratory acidosis
    (4) alveolar ventilation only responds to endogenous CO_2

135. The pulmonary arterial circulation

    (1) is related directly to cardiac output; ie, the higher the cardiac output, the higher the pulmonary artery pressure
    (2) is related to cardiac output in a way that makes zone 3 extend higher into the lung when the cardiac output is higher
    (3) has a passive relationship to cardiac output
    (4) distribution is primarily related to gravity

Questions 136 through 139

A 26-year-old black man is admitted to the emergency room with first-, second-, and third-degree burns of his chest, face, and arms. He is alert but in severe pain. His respirations are shallow and rapid. Arterial blood gases are obtained on room air, and the results are: pH 7.48, P_{CO_2} 30, P_{O_2} 78.

136. This patient's laboratory results demonstrate

    (1) an uncompensated respiratory acidosis
    (2) a respiratory alkalosis
    (3) an oxygen tension that is normal
    (4) an oxygen tension that is low but that does not require immediate treatment

137. The patient's pulmonary status

    (1) will likely deteriorate over the ensuing 24 hours
    (2) should be observed carefully for a least 24 hours
    (3) is dependent to a degree on the type of burn
    (4) will always require a tracheostomy

SUMMARY OF DIRECTIONS				
A	B	C	D	E
1, 2, 3 only	1, 3 only	2, 4 only	4 only	All are correct

138. His oxygenation may be adversely affected by

(1) pulmonary edema
(2) sickle cell disease
(3) carbon monoxide poisoning
(4) alkalosis

139. The patient's shallow, rapid respirations

(1) move air more efficiently
(2) are due to increased compliance
(3) allow him to oxygenate better with little effort
(4) magnify the effect of dead space on total ventilation

Questions 140 through 148

A 75-year-old woman undergoes an exploration and removal of her right kidney and adrenal gland for a large tumor. The procedure is performed in the left lateral decubitus position, with flexion of the table and use of the kidney rest. The patient is intubated, and ventilation is controlled. Anesthesia is maintained with halothane, nitrous oxide, oxygen, and D-tubocurarine.

140. The blood pressure, initially 136/80, falls to 80/40 after positioning and incision. This may be due to

(1) poor ventilation
(2) poor cardiac output
(3) halothane anesthesia
(4) blood loss

141. The initial response(s) to this situation is (are)

(1) listen to the chest to ascertain good ventilation
(2) decrease halothane concentration
(3) lower kidney rest
(4) check for blood loss

142. After blood pressure is restored and exploration proceeds, there is a rise in blood pressure to 180/100 and multiple ectopic ventricular beats on the electrocardiogram. This may be due to

(1) poor ventilation
(2) pneumothorax
(3) hormone released from the adrenal tumor
(4) hypocapnia

143. The step(s) to be taken in this situation is (are)

(1) shut off halothane
(2) shut off nitrous oxide

(3) inject 10 ml of 4% lidocaine
(4) inform surgeon of the difficulty

144. The operation is completed, and the patient is transported to the recovery room. At this time

(1) the patient is in more danger from poor ventilation than when in the operating room
(2) bronchopulmonary secretions are of little consequence
(3) narcotics should be used with caution
(4) coughing is to be avoided and preventive measures taken

145. The patient, on arrival in the recovery room, was breathing spontaneously, with a tidal volume of 350 ml and a respiratory rate of 10 per minute, and she was barely arousable. With these data we can assume

(1) that the patient is able to ventilate sufficiently
(2) that extubation is possible
(3) that the patient does not need supplemental oxygen
(4) nothing; more data are needed

146. Assisted ventilation is initiated with a Bennett MA1 ventilator. After 15 minutes of ventilation, the patient begins to fight the ventilator. At this time, the

(1) patient should be extubated
(2) endotracheal tube should be checked
(3) patient should be sedated
(4) patient should be examined and the lungs auscultated

147. The endotracheal position is noted by the following: examining the patient, the numerical markings on the tube, and the chest x-ray. Which of the following is (are) consistent with the proper position?

(1) the left side is ventilated better than the right side
(2) the tip of the tube is 30 cm from the upper front teeth
(3) the tip of the tube overlies the 6th thoracic vertebra
(4) both sides ventilate equally

148. Causes of this patient's restlessness may be

(1) discomfort from the endotracheal tube
(2) hypoxia
(3) gastric distention
(4) pain

149. In describing air flow through a tube

(1) Henry's law is important
(2) radius is a crucial factor

(3) tube length is the important factor
(4) viscosity is more important than density

150. A 34-year-old woman with myasthenia gravis is ventilated with 100% oxygen. This may cause

(1) injury to her lungs
(2) Po_2 values in excess of 760 torr
(3) absorption atelectasis
(4) retrolental fibroplasia

151. After induction of anesthesia with halothane, you would expect

(1) tidal volume to increase as the depth of anesthesia increases
(2) a decrease in tidal volume
(3) a decrease in respiratory rate as depth increases
(4) a tachypnea that may also be due to hypoxemia

152. The factors that influence arterial oxygen tension under anesthesia include

(1) inspired oxygen concentration
(2) barometric pressure
(3) alveolar oxygen tension
(4) age

153. Assuming a normal oxyhemoglobin dissociation curve position

(1) a Po_2 of 90 torr will give a saturation of 96.5%
(2) a Po_2 of 90 torr will give a dissolved oxygen of 0.27 ml O_2/100 ml blood
(3) a Po_2 of 90 torr will give a combined oxygen of 19.80 ml/100 ml blood
(4) a Po_2 of 30 torr will give an oxygen saturation of 30%

154. A 12-year-old boy with muscular dystrophy is scheduled to have an operation to correct scoliosis. Evaluation of this patient should

(1) include x-ray to determine the amount of curvature
(2) include pulmonary function testing
(3) help predict the possible postanesthesia problems
(4) not proceed if vital capacity is under 35% of that predicted

155. Factors that increase P_{50} of hemoglobin include

(1) increased temperature
(2) decreased DPG
(3) increased hydrogen ion concentration
(4) methemoglobin

156. The factors that influence late postoperative hypoxemia include

(1) type of anesthesia

(2) atelectasis
(3) analgesics
(4) age and sex

157. Mixed venous oxygen tension is

(1) normally 60 torr
(2) a guide for determining tissue hypoxia
(3) independent of metabolic conditions and body temperature
(4) best sampled from the pulmonary artery

158. A patient with an endotracheal tube in place has a suction catheter inserted to clear secretions. During the procedure, an arrhythmia is noted. This may be

(1) due to carbon dioxide accumulation
(2) due to hypoxia
(3) of no consequence
(4) prevented in many cases by hyperventilating with 100% oxygen before suctioning

159. The pulmonary vascular system

(1) has no alpha or beta receptors
(2) is well endowed with smooth muscle
(3) has no connections to autonomic ganglia
(4) responds to norepinephrine by vasoconstriction

160. Mucociliary flow will be altered during halothane anesthesia in response to

(1) concentration of halothane
(2) airway humidity
(3) body temperature
(4) FIo_2

161. Neurogenic pulmonary edema

(1) may follow head injury
(2) is not associated with hypoxemia
(3) is resistant to treatment unless intracranial pressure is reduced
(4) develops only in a denervated lung

162. Closing capacity is

(1) the lung volume at which the onset of airway closure is detected
(2) increased in obesity
(3) related to closing volume
(4) functionally related to functional residual capacity (FRC)

163. Transpulmonary pressure

(1) measures intralung pressure
(2) is always a positive value
(3) is a gradient between the airway opening and the alveolar pressure
(4) is the result of a number of factors, including airflow resistance, compliance, and tissue inertia

SUMMARY OF DIRECTIONS				
A	B	C	D	E
1, 2, 3 only	1, 3 only	2, 4 only	4 only	All are correct

164. Deliberate hypotensive technique may affect pulmonary gas exchange by increasing

    (1) respiratory dead space
    (2) the $AaDo_2$ gradient
    (3) ventilation/perfusion inequality
    (4) shunting

165. In interpreting pulmonary function tests, it is important to remember that

    (1) vital capacity measurement is not related to speed
    (2) spirometric tests fail to detect early disease in small airways
    (3) maximal breathing capacity is dependent on cooperation
    (4) the FEV_1 will detect restrictive disease

166. The calculated shunt fraction (Qs/Qt)

    (1) may change with changes in pulmonary and cardiac function
    (2) increases with atelectasis
    (3) will not be corrected with 100% oxygen
    (4) increases in patients with pulmonary embolus

167. Airway resistance

    (1) decreases with maximal inspiration
    (2) increases with parasympathetic stimulation
    (3) increases with acetylcholine
    (4) increases with inhalation of smoke

168. An apneic patient is treated with doxapram at the end of the surgical procedure. This drug

    (1) may reverse the effect of muscle relaxants
    (2) is metabolized rapidly when given intravenously
    (3) has a prolonged effect due to peripheral receptor stimulation
    (4) has a central effect

Questions 169 and 170

A patient with chronic obstructive lung disease is admitted with the following arterial blood gases: pH 7.10, Pco_2 92, and Po_2 52. She is in acute respiratory distress.

169. Her treatement should consist of

    (1) oxygen by face mask at 10 L/minute
    (2) intubation and hyperventilation
    (3) sodium bicarbonate, 90 mEq intravenously
    (4) low-flow oxygen and treatment of the underlying cause of the crisis

170. The patient's course later requires intubation and artificial ventilation: Pco_2 is lowered precipitously to 35 torr, and the patient has a cardiac arrest. The factor(s) contributing to this is (are)

    (1) increased blood bicarbonate
    (2) rapid mobilization of CO_2 from body stores
    (3) slow mobilization of bicarbonate
    (4) body chloride ion depletion

171. The immediate preoperative preparation of a patient with asthma includes

    (1) bronchodilators
    (2) corticosteroids
    (3) high fluid intake
    (4) cromolyn sodium

172. Alpha$_1$-antitrypsin deficiency is

    (1) associated with early-onset of emphysema
    (2) nonfamilial
    (3) determined by serum assay
    (4) due to a lack of an enzyme produced by the lung

173. Oxygen should be administered in the recovery room

    (1) only to those who have had general anesthesia
    (2) only to those with cyanosis
    (3) without mist to avoid excess secretions
    (4) by mask if the patient is breathing through the mouth

174. A patient who arrives in the recovery room after a general anesthetic should be

    (1) allowed to awaken without disturbance
    (2) encouraged to lie on the back for easier access to the airway
    (3) given narcotics liberally to prevent pain
    (4) closely observed for respiratory depression

175. A 14-gauge catheter is inserted through the cricothyroid membrane and attached to a wall oxygen source in such a way that oxygen can be delivered intermittently. With this technique

    (1) pneumothorax is inevitable
    (2) adequate oxygenation is possible
    (3) gastric dilatation is a hazard
    (4) pulmonary aspiration is minimized

176. Bronchitis refers to a disease that

    (1) is a nonneoplastic disorder of the structure or function of the bronchi resulting from infectious or noninfectious irritation

(2) may include hypertrophy of the mucus-secreting apparatus

(3) must last at least 3 months to be termed *chronic*

(4) includes abnormal enlargement of the air spaces (~~emphysema~~

Questions 177 through 180

A 35-year-old man is admitted to the emergency room following an automobile accident. It is noted that there is a contusion over the anterior thorax, he is tachypneic, and he has a scaphoid abdomen. Auscultation reveals poor breath sounds on the left side. Chest x-ray shows a large air cavity in the left side of the thorax. Blood pressure is 80/60, and heart rate is 120 per minute.

177. Diagnoses that must be considered include

    (1) ruptured spleen
    (2) pneumothorax
    (3) diaphragmatic hernia
    (4) cardiac contusion

178. A diagnosis of diaphragmatic hernia is made, and the patient is transported to the operating room. In transport, the patient becomes apneic and is bagged with a bag and mask unit. You would expect

    (1) the patient's condition to deteriorate
    (2) compliance to decrease

(3) a shift of the mediastinum
(4) more effective ventilation

179. As soon as the patient reaches the operating room, he should

    (1) be intubated
    (2) have a nasogastric tube inserted
    (3) be stabilized
    (4) have a thoracotomy to relieve pressure

180. When this patient is intubated, he should

    (1) be allowed to breathe spontaneously until stabilized
    (2) be ventilated with high-volume, controlled ventilation
    (3) have slow induction with anesthetic agent and oxygen
    (4) be allowed to breathe a mixture of nitrous oxide and oxygen

181. Acute respiratory insufficiency will manifest itself by

    (1) hypoxia
    (2) dyspnea
    (3) hypercapnia
    (4) hypotension

$$\frac{124}{181}$$

Answers and Explanations

1. **(B)** Pleural pressure increases 0.25 cm H_2O every centimeter down the lung. Thus, it is lowest at the apex and highest at the base. The pleural pressure is related to body position in that in different positions, different areas will be dependent. *(1:1117; 75:892)*

2. **(D)** The LaPlace law states that the pressure within an elastic sphere is directly proportional to the tension of the wall and inversely proportional to the radius of the curvature. In this case, the sphere is the alveolus. Alveoli are lined with a film of surfactant, which exerts a surface tension. The surfactant lends stability to the alveoli by decreasing the surface tension as the radius of the alveolus becomes smaller. Without this ability to vary surface tension, small alveoli would empty into large alveoli and alveolar stability would be lost. *(1:1141; 32:34)*

3. **(D)** Surfactant is a substance containing dipalmitoyl lecithin produced by the type II alveolar epithelial cells of the lung. The substance is important in adults as well as newborns. *(1:1142; 15:710)*

4. **(D)** The FRC is composed of expiratory reserve volume and residual volume. Tidal volume plus inspiratory reserve volume comprise the inspiratory capacity. The other options are not designated capacities. *(1:1129; 75:899)*

5. **(C)** The maximum volume of air inhaled from the end-inspiratory level is referred to as the inspiratory reserve volume. *(1:1129; 75:899)*

6. **(C)** The FRC measurement is possible by body plethysmography. Another technique is the use of helium dilution. Spirometry, direct measurement, x-ray, and esophageal balloon are not used for measurement of FRC. *(1:1127; 75:900)*

7. **(A)** At FRC, there is no pressure difference between the alveoli and atmosphere. The total pulmonary vascular resistance is at its lowest at FRC. Further ventilation is possible, since FRC is the volume that exists at the end of a normal tidal volume. *(1:1121; 75:899)*

8. **(D)** The cilia of the respiratory tract move a double layer of mucus toward the larynx. There is an inner layer of thin mucus and an outer layer of thick mucus, which is able to trap particulate matter or microorganisms. The cilia are part of the columnar cells lining the trachea. Body temperature does have an effect on ciliary motility. *(1:1152; 2:4)*

9. **(A)** All of the factors cited except for an increase in the caliber of the airways will lead to increased airway resistance. The supine position will cause increased resistance due to decreased lung volume. The presence of an endotracheal tube increases resistance, and this may be aggravated by secretions and kinking. *(1:1148; 9:85)*

10. **(B)** The bronchial tree divides into right and left bronchi, the left bronchus being narrower and longer. Foreign bodies are more apt to go to the right side. The trachea moves during respiration and with movement of the head. It is lined with pseudostratified columnar epithelium. The rings of cartilage do not completely encircle the trachea. *(2:16–24; 15:709)*

11. **(E)** The larynx lies at the level of the 3rd–6th cervical vertebrae, and in the adult, the narrowest portion is at the level of the vocal cords. The larynx is supplied by the recurrent laryngeal nerve and the superior learyngeal nerve. It lies within the thyroid cartilage. The wide margin of the cricoid cartilage is posterior. *(1:524; 2:12)*

12. **(D)** Humidification of inhaled gases is at its optimum with the patient breathing through the nose. Atropine will dry out secretions. Endotracheal tubes and tracheostomies bypass the humidification process of the nose. A closed system will keep humidity in the system. *(1:83; 8:144; 15:718)*

13. **(A)** The principal muscle of respiration is the diaphragm. The other muscles, although involved, do not exert nearly the influence of the diaphragm. The diaphragm can account for the entire amount of inspired air during quiet respiration, and in a maximum breathing effort, it can still account for 60%. *(2:44; 6:4; 8:145)*

14. **(B)** The dependent areas are better ventilated, since the alveoli in the dependent areas expand more per unit pressure change than do nondependent alveoli. *(1:1119; 75:892)*

15. **(A)** Inspiratory force is a measurement of reserve of ventilatory effort. It is a simple method that does not depend on patient cooperation. Therefore, it is particularly useful in the unconscious or anesthetized patient. A pressure in excess of 20 cm H_2O below atmospheric pressure is considered minimum to show adequate reserve. *(3:51–52; 75:1409)*

16. **(C)** Patients with pickwickian syndrome demonstrate a decreased expiratory reserve volume and higher intraabdominal pressure when supine. These patients have alveolar *hypo*ventilation and increased work of breathing, and one would expect this to improve after weight loss. *(1:261; 75:1118)*

17. **(B)** Primary alveolar hypoventilation has been described with all of the disease states except hyperthyroidism. It has been seen with advanced myxedema, or hypothyroidism. *(4:106; 55:24)*

18. **(E)** All of the options do contribute to physiologic shunt except nonperfused alveoli, which produce increased dead space. *(3:12; 75:896)*

19. **(D)** Insufflation of oxygen to the unventilated lung will decrease the shunt and attenuate the desaturation. This implies that some alveoli are in continuity with the proximal airways. Shunting does occur in the unventilated lung. CO_2 removal is not usually a problem. *(1:1414; 37:511)*

20. **(D)** After bilateral carotid endarterectomy, a patient will be more susceptible to hypoxemia because of denervation of the carotid body. The patient will not respond to hypoxemia with hyperventilation. In addition, the resting P_{CO_2} is elevated, and the response to small doses of narcotics may be accentuated. Hypertension is not a constant finding in these patients. *(1:1636; 38:823)*

21. **(E)** Adequacy of alveolar ventilation is obtained by measuring the carbon dioxide tension. Oxygen values may be affected by ventilation, but the measure of ventilation is carbon dioxide. *(1:1138; 75:894)*

22. **(B)** The measure of oxygen tension requires the Clark electrode. This measurement is affected by temperature. The Severinghaus electrode is used for the measure of carbon dioxide. The Severinghaus electrode uses the Henderson-Hasselbalch equation to relate pH to carbon dioxide. *(1:86; 75:677)*

23. **(C)** Anesthesia usually causes a decrease in FRC, which leads to hypoxemia. All of the other options can lead to hypoxemia: hypoventilation by decreased FRC and increased shunt, hyperventilation by shift of the oxyhemoglobin dissociation curve and decreased cardiac output, supine position by decreased ventilation and decreased FRC, and increased airway pressure by change in the ventilation–perfusion relationships. *(1:1147; 75:1411)*

24. **(A)** When venous admixture and oxygen remain constant, a decrease in cardiac output will decrease arterial oxygen. This is because the blood passing through the shunt circuit will be more desaturated due to the decreased cardiac output. This leads to more desaturation in the tissues. Urinary output usually decreases with decreased cardiac output. *(1:1153, 1931; 10:2)*

25. **(C)** Patients who are hyperventilated for long periods of time have their carbon dioxide stores depleted. Postoperatively, these patients hypoventilate in an effort to restore their carbon dioxide and, in so doing, may become hypoxemic if not given supplemental oxygen. *(1:1159, 1930; 45:467–469)*

26. **(A)** The carbon dioxide retention is due primarily to V/Q abnormalities. There is evidence that carbon dioxide retainers and those who are able to eliminate carbon dioxide have similar minute ventilations. *(1:2221; 44:1232–1235)*

27. **(A)** Tracheal mucus flow and, necessarily, ciliary activity are impeded by deviation from ambient oxygen tension. Tracheal mucus flow is increased in patients with obstructive lung disease. Tracheal mucus flow is an important cleansing mechanism. Mucus flow and ciliary activity are depressed by cigarette smoke. *(1:683; 75:881)*

28. **(C)** Closing volume is increased in the small baby and in the elderly. Measurement of closing volume will detect changes in the small airways before they would become apparent by spirometry. *(1:2070; 2:58)*

29. **(D)** A high concentration of oxygen may be harmful to many organ systems. It is especially harmful to the patient with obstructive lung disease who is functioning on a hypoxic drive to ventilation. *(1:2224; 75:1412)*

30. (C) The medullary centers located in the pons and medulla respond primarily to hydrogen ion concentration. Although this is related to the level of carbon dioxide, the primary stimulant is hydrogen ion. Chronic hypercapnia depresses the centers. *(4:17–18; 34:27; 75:885)*

31. (C) The peripheral chemoreceptors are primarily responsible for the hypoxic drive to respiration. They are shut off at very high oxygen tensions. The peripheral chemoreceptors respond to changes in oxygen tension, not content. *(4:17; 6:2; 75:885)*

32. (A) Compliance refers to a change in volume per unit change in pressure. Compliance is the reciprocal of elastance. No time units are involved, since it is a static measurement. *(1:2341; 75:711)*

33. (B) Vital capacity is decreased when the exposure is more than 12 hours. All of the other options are true. *(1:1157; 2:136)*

34. (D) Obviously, all the factors have to be taken into consideration, but in evaluating the patient, it is important to note the rate of change that is occurring and the consequences of continued hypoventilation. For this reason, it is difficult to give a set number of values that are acceptable; it is more important that the patient be watched in the context of the disease. *(7:2; 40:43)*

35. (A) Oxygen toxicity develops after 12 hours of exposure to 100% oxygen. Once can breathe 25% oxygen for an indefinite period of time. There are some patients who need 100% oxygen, and, in those patients, it should be used as long as needed. One should take such steps as are available to decrease the concentration needed. *(1:1157; 75:1412)*

36. (D) General anesthesia leads to an alteration of chest wall mechanics, resulting in decreased FRC. Breathing at the lower lung volume may also affect the lung mechanics, leading to increased elastic recoil and decreased compliance. *(9:86; 42:674)*

37. (B) The curve is shifted to the right with acidosis. The other options are correct. Appreciation of oxygen saturation shifts has important implications in the care of critically ill patients. *(1:1338; 75:679)*

38. (B) The patient with restrictive disease will have a decrease in FVC. The FEV_1 may be decreased also, but the FEV_1/FVC% usually is normal. *(1:2055; 32:44)*

39. (B) This patient represents a common situation. In view of his cervical cord injury and his other sites of trauma, treatment of the respiratory failure is of utmost importance. Evaluating this patient in view of his history, his deterioration, and the fact that

his ventilation is already compromised, the treatment of choice is to intubate and ventilate him. *(1:2271; 75:1461)*

40. (D) This patient is not functioning on a hypoxic drive; therefore, 40% oxygen should not contribute to his respiratory depression. The other options are all possible. *(1:2271; 75:1460)*

41. (A) This patient lacks any ability to clear his airway because he has a high cervical lesion. His lesion is not high enough to predispose to aspiration. Shock from blood loss and pulmonary oxygen toxicity, if it occurs as a result of high oxygen concentrations needed in his treatment, will contribute to his respiratory failure. *(1:2271; 75:1460)*

42. (E) This patient has a normal oxygen tension, a normal inspiratory capacity, a high P_{CO_2}, a normal vital capacity, and abnormal O_2 saturation. *(34:218; 75:906)*

43. (A) To correct the patient's high P_{CO_2} level, either the tidal volume could be increased or the dead space should be decreased. Assuming the tidal volume to be correct and normal, the alternative is to decrease the dead space. *(34:218)*

44. (B) Hysteresis is present when the path of deformation on application of a force differs from the path taken when the force is withdrawn. This is seen in the inflation–volume curves and is due to the presence of alveolar stability, which is possible because of surfactant and its effect on surface tension. *(4:23; 8:155)*

45. (B) The curve for saline is also shifted to the left, showing that less pressure is needed to inflate and deflate the lung under saline. When air is involved and surfactant is present, air spaces will remain open, and the curve differs as shown. *(4:23; 8:155)*

46. (C) All of the factors cited are presumptive evidence of ventilation. The only good measure of those listed is the analysis of blood gases, especially carbon dioxide. *(1:428; 8:208)*

47. (D) Pulmonary vascular resistance is the result of cardiac output, the state of vasomotion, and pressure. A change in cardiac output will be followed by changes in the radius of the vessels to allow maintenance of normal pressure. The resistance is equal to pressure divided by flow. *(1:1120; 75:1412)*

48. (E) Hypoxic pulmonary vasoconstriction causes diversion of blood flow from hypoxic to nonhypoxic lung tissue. In the usual circumstance, blood is diverted to areas where flow is decreased, eg, to the apices. This causes a decrease in the dead space/tidal volume ratio. *(1:1121; 75:1412)*

49. **(A)** During anesthesia, exhalation becomes more active, resulting in more work. The work of breathing involves both elastic and resistance work. The optimum rate is about 15 breaths per minute. In the patient with restrictive disease, short shallow breaths decrease the amount of work. *(1:1125–1127; 32:382)*

50. **(B)** Closing volume measurement requires nitrogen washout or the use of a tracer gas. Its measurement is not possible by spirometry. The other values are available by spirometry. *(1:1129; 75:900)*

51. **(D)** Anatomic dead space increases with increased lung volume. The normal dead space is 1 ml/pound of body weight. Equipment dead space may greatly increase the amount of dead space, and that is why it is so important to consider dead space in dealing with small children *(1:1132; 32:59)*

52. **(B)** P_{50} is the Po_2 level on the oxyhemoglobin dissociation curve at which hemoglobin is 50% saturated. The normal value is 27 torr and may change with the other factors that cause a shift in the oxyhemoglobin dissociation curve. *(1:1135; 75:679)*

53. **(E)** Carboxyhemoglobin is involved in the transport of carbon monoxide. The other options are intimately involved in the transport of carbon dioxide. *(1:1138: 75:670)*

54. **(D)** The Bohr effect describes the effect of carbon dioxide on the uptake of oxygen. Option B describes the Haldane effect. Carbonic anhydrase, hydrogen ion, and catalytic enzymes are not involved. *(1:1139; 2:106; 9:78)*

55. **(D)** Hypercapnia may result from rebreathing of CO_2 while using an Ayre T-piece with low flows. The other options all cause a decreased carbon dioxide tension. *(1:1155; 9:94; 75:973, 1409)*

56. **(D)** In zone 1, the alveolar pressure is higher than the arterial or venous pressure; therefore, these areas act as dead space units. *(1:1116; 75:893)*

57. **(E)** In zone 2, the blood flow is dependent on arterial pressure and the alveolar pressure. These change with the status of ventilation. Venous pressure is still not a determinant of blood flow in this zone. *(1:1116; 75:893)*

58. **(A)** In zone 3, blood flow is determined by the arteriovenous difference. Dead space is low, since the units are being perfused, alveolar pressure is not high, and the venous pressure is lower than arterial but higher than alveolar pressure. *(1:1116; 75:893)*

59. **(C)** Henry's law states that the amount of a given gas that will dissolve in a liquid is directly proportional to the pressure of the gas. *(34:159; 51:238)*

60. **(B)** Boyle's law states that the volume of a gas at a constant temperature is inversely proportional to the pressure. *(57:98; 75:102)*

61. **(B)** The main buffer in the body is the bicarbonate system. It is not the only system; the other options involve the other buffering systems. *(1:1294–1295; 8:254)*

62. **(A)** Hemoglobin is the primary noncarbonic buffer. It is an important buffer and can work in the carbonic and noncarbonic systems. Hemoglobin is a weaker acid than carbonic acid. Hemoglobin exists within the red cell as a potassium salt. *(1:1294; 8:256)*

63. **(D)** Analysis of arterial blood gases is the most reliable method of documenting hypoxemia. Detection of cyanosis, respiratory responses, and circulatory responses are all subjective and may not be accurate. The pulse oximeter has improved the detection of hypoxemia with a faster response than transcutaneous oxygen readings. *(1:1931; 75:1410)*

64. **(A)** An increased FRC should improve oxygenation. The other options may all contribute to hypoxemia. *(1:1930–1931; 75:1410)*

65. **(D)** Hypoventilation in the recovery room is more common after intravenous anesthesia technique than after inhalation technique. It may or may not respond to narcotic reversal, depending on the anesthesia technique employed. The patient with hypoventilation may be hypotensive. The best way to document the hypoventilaton is the use of arterial blood gases. *(1:1933–1934; 75:1406)*

66. **(B)** The time for nitrogen elimination is dependent on the volume of the breaths and the underlying lung condition. Patients with lung disease will eliminate the nitrogen more slowly, as will smokers and the elderly. *(1:2067; 2:83, 137)*

67. **(A)** Chemoreceptor stimulation leads to an increased ventilatory effort. Many rely on bradycardia as the only sign of hypoxemia, but the response is a complex one. *(1:424)*

68. **(D)** Carbon dioxide tension rises under apneic ventilation and may contribute to the problems seen. It will rise more quickly in one in whom there is lung disease. All arrhythmias are not due to hypoxemia but may be due to increased catecholamines. These in turn may be increased due to increased carbon dioxide. Pulse oximetry has been of definite benefit in these procedures. *(1:1867–1868; 9:297; 75:929)*

69. (C) Boyle's law relates volume and pressure. The gas laws are of importance because of the pressure relationships in the lungs and in the anesthesia equipment. *(51:98; 75:102)*

70. (E) Charles' law relates volume directly to temperature. *(32:114; 75:102)*

71. (D) Graham's law relates diffusion of a gas inversely to the square root of its molecular weight. *(32:250; 75:888)*

72. (E) Carboxyhemoglobin is not usually involved in the transport of oxygen. The other factors are important. *(1:1137; 2:105)*

73. (B) The Haldane effect refers to the shift in the CO_2 dissociation curve caused by altered levels of oxygen. Low Po_2 shifts the curve so that the blood is able to pick up more CO_2. *(1:1139; 2:108; 9:78)*

74. (C) The V/Q ratio is higher at the apex. The blood flow and ventilation are greatest at the base. The Po_2 is higher at the apex. *(1:1119; 8:201)*

75. (D) Shunting refers to blood that goes through the lung without being oxygenated. It is perfusion in excess of ventilation. Ventilation in excess of perfusion is dead space or wasted ventilation. *(53:53; 75:893)*

76. (A) The cuff of an endotracheal tube should be inflated enough to prevent aspiration and still allow capillary flow in the underlying trachea. A pressure of 20 torr will allow this in a high-volume, thin-walled cuff. *(1:533; 32:273)*

77. (A) When patients breathe an increased Fio_2, there is an increased amount of shunt present due to absorption atelectasis. The lung units with low V/Q ratios have a greater tendency to collapse. *(1:1151; 9:90)*

78. (A) The Bohr equation is used to calculate dead space. It requires measurement of expired carbon dioxide and alveolar carbon dioxide. It does not require mixed venous CO_2 or O_2 measurement. *(2:53; 53:19)*

79. (D) Bronchoconstriction that has been attributed to thiopental administration is probably due to light planes of anesthesia at the time of airway manipulation. *(1:806; 75:235)*

80. (D) Compliance becomes better as one moves down the lung. The alveoli become smaller, and pleural pressure increases. Ventilation of the alveoli increases due to increased compliance. *(1:1117–1118; 75:892)*

81. (C) The internal laryngeal branch is almost entirely sensory. The other nerves are almost entirely motor. *(2:13; 75:543)*

82. (B) The musculature of the bronchioles encircles them. The musculature becomes thinner as it is more distal, but it is relatively thicker in relation to the diameter of the bronchiole. The musculature is important in maintaining the size of the bronchiolar lumen. The elastic fibers are embedded in the musculature. *(2:20–21)*

83. (A) The Hering-Breuer reflex is now thought to have little importance in the adult human. The reflex is depressed by barbiturates. *(2:24; 53:120)*

84. (D) There is a difference in the cord position depending on the extent of nerve damage. If the nerve is completely sectioned bilaterally, the cords will be open in the midposition. If there is partial damage, the cords may be closed in the midline. *(2:14–15; 75:1068)*

85. (E) The slope of the response curve is an index of the patient's sensitivity to carbon dioxide. The slope and position may change. Increased work leads to a flatter slope. Anesthetics differ in their effect on the curve. *(1:692: 2:34; 53:122)*

86. (E) Nitrous oxide, in 50% concentrations does not depress the response to CO_2. The other options all have an effect on the response. *(1:692; 2:34; 53:120)*

87. (E) The diaphragm has a central tendon and is innervated by the phrenic nerve, which arises from cervical nerves 3, 4, and 5, but principally the 4th. There is controversy about the extent of diaphragmatic movement in tidal ventilation. Some references state that there is an excursion of only 1 to 1.5 cm, whereas others state that the excursion is 10 cm. *(2:44; 8:145; 53:86)*

88. (D) The circulation to the lung is of two systems, but the bronchial system is expendable, as is seen in lung transplants. The pressure in the pulmonary circuit is low relative to the left side. The arterial branches follow the airway branching. *(9:29; 53:8)*

89. (B) The metabolic functions of the lung include the inactivation of many substances but not epinephrine. *(2:29; 53:49)*

90. (D) The $AaDo_2$ increases linearly with age. In adults, the normal value is about 25. The increase is due to changes in arterial oxygen tension not the alveolar oxygen tension. It is not a good tool for measuring V/Q changes, since it is difficult to measure alveolar oxygen tension. *(1:2065; 2:96)*

91. **(A)** Reynold's number is a value determined by a calculation involving density, velocity, radius, and viscosity. A value above 2000 means that flow probably will be turbulent. *(8:140; 53:101)*

92. **(C)** See answer to Question 91. *(8:140; 53:101)*

93. **(C)** PEEP does increase FRC and V/Q ratios. It may not improve oxygenation, and it increases lung compliance. *(1:1414; 75:1412)*

94. **(E)** All the options are correct. Dead space is increased in zone 1 and that is an area of high V/Q ratio. It is known to be increased after administration of atropine. *(2:53; 8:673, 894)*

95. **(E)** All of the agents listed have been shown to cause bronchodilation. *(1:668; 8:142)*

96. **(B)** The work of breathing involves both elastic and resistive work. If breathing is deep and slow, more effort is expended in overcoming elastic work. Most of the breathing effort is expended in inspiration. *(1:1125; 8:46)*

97. **(E)** All the options are correct. Carbaminohemoglobin is the form that CO_2 takes in the red cell. *(1:1138; 9:77)*

98. **(A)** The first three options are true. The reason for the rocking-boat type of ventilation is that the diaphragm is the only muscle available. It is not lost with deep anesthesia, as are the intercostals. *(1:1143; 75:299, 300)*

99. **(A)** A decrease in FRC results from the supine position, with the resultant increased intraabdominal pressure and cephalad shift of the diaphragm. The airways have a tendency to narrow. *(1:1147–1148; 9:85)*

100. **(E)** All of the options are true. The vessels must constrict against the pressure inside, and anything that increases pressure in the pulmonary circulation will decrease hypoxic pulmonary vasoconstriction. The first three options all increase intravascular pressure. It is also known that anesthetic agents reduce hypoxic pulmonary vasoconstriction. *(1:1153; 9:53)*

101. **(A)** Increased dead space may result from hypotension, short, rapid ventilation, and pulmonary embolus. Increased airway pressure leads to increased dead space. *(1:1155; 8:224)*

102. **(A)** Vital capacity includes tidal volume and inspiratory and expiratory reserve volumes but not all of FRC. FRC includes residual volume. *(2:50; 8:129)*

103. **(E)** All of the factors cited may be involved in causing hypoxemia. Blood loss, cardiac output, and shunting are involved in oxygen transport, and airway obstruction is involved in ventilaton. *(1:1153; 10:2)*

104. **(C)** Increased oxygen consumption will decrease oxygen content, as will decreased cardiac output. If the cardiac output is low, more oxygen will be extracted as the blood moves through the tissues. *(1:1137; 10:2)*

105. **(E)** All of the options are correct, although it is not known how significant the role of collateral ventilation is. *(1:1142; 9:29)*

106. **(C)** The patient with hypercapnia has increased catecholamines, respiratory acidosis, and increased plasma potassium. The potassium comes from the liver and other tissues. *(1:1158; 9:97)*

107. **(D)** Hypocapnia leads to decreased cerebral blood flow, decreased ionized calcium, and decreased oxygen delivery to the tissues. There is an inhibition of hypoxic pulmonary vasoconstriction leading to V/Q mismatch. *(1:1159; 9:99)*

108. **(C)** Pulse oximetry is affected by perfusion and by light interference. The oximeter may give a reading with various hemoglobins, but one must remember that a reading of 100% with carboxyhemoglobin (in burn patients) does not mean that the patient is adequately oxygenated. *(10:4; 75:119)*

109. **(A)** The anesthetized patient has decreased ability to respond to increased CO_2, low oxygen, and metabolic acidemia. The ability to respond to added airway resistance is not lost. *(11:3–4)*

110. **(E)** All of these factors may lead to pulmonary edema in the awake patient or under anesthesia. It is important to know the reason for the pulmonary edema so that treatment is directed accordingly. *(8:188; 12:5)*

111. **(B)** Respiratory quotient is the rate of CO_2 output divided by the rate of O_2 uptake. It may vary with the metabolic substrate and, therefore, will not always be 0.8. *(1:1138; 32:552)*

112. **(A)** The first three options are correct and are beneficial effects of PEEP. One of the side effects that we strive to avoid is decreased cardiac output. *(32:408; 75:1412)*

113. **(B)** PEEP increases FRC and decreases the work of breathing. Compliance is increased, and the lung volume is increased. *(1:2217; 75:1412)*

114. **(A)** The ventilation of the dependent lung in one-lung anesthesia techniques is important. The first three options are all methods to increase oxygenation but may, in themselves, be harmful. The fourth option is not true, since the high F_{IO_2} may cause vasodilation. *(1:1412; 75:922)*

115. **(E)** All of the options are true. The prone position is described in Miller's text to be associated with a small change. In Martin's text on positioning, it is apparent that if one is to have only small changes, one must be sure the patient is well positioned. This requires careful placement of rolls under the body so that no pressure is placed on the abdomen. *(1:1152; 16:207)*

116. **(A)** Hypoventilation, shunt, and V/Q mismatch are problems that are of most importance. Abnormal diffusion is of rare importance and is associated with lung diseases, such as sarcoidosis. *(9:83; 13:3)*

117. **(A)** Supplemental oxygen and maneuvers to improve ventilation and prevent atelectasis are important. The use of carbon dioxide is not a current treatment. *(13:5; 75:1410)*

118. **(D)** In the lateral position, lung relationships change. The perfusion is now greater in the dependent lung. *(1:1389; 9:106)*

119. **(E)** If a patient's alveolar oxygen tension is kept below 350 torr, no problem should occur. Oxygen toxicity does occur more often in the patient who is critically ill. The risk of oxygen toxicity should not make one withhold necessary oxygen. If the F_{IO_2} is over 0.5, there is an increased risk of oxygen toxicity. *(9:97; 14:4)*

120. **(A)** The patient's oxygenation and cardiac output must be taken into account when deciding on the amount of PEEP that is appropriate. Shapiro does not believe that the risk of barotrauma should prevent one from using the PEEP that is necessary in acute lung injury. *(14:6; 75:1461)*

121. **(A)** The trachea is a midline structure about 15 cm in length and about the diameter of a person's index finger. It bifurcates at the level of the 5th thoracic vertebra. *(9:23–24; 75:880)*

122. **(C)** The right lobe is the larger of the two. It has three lobes and two fissures and contains the middle lobe. *(9:25; 75:879)*

123. **(E)** All of these pathways may cause shunting. In the postoperative period, only the atelectasis may be treated in an effort to improve oxygenation. *(9:54–56; 75:896)*

124. **(D)** Total pulmonary compliance is volume divided by pressure. It involves the lung and the chest wall. There is no time unit in the calculation. It is increased by surfactant. *(9:57; 75:889)*

125. **(B)** Airway resistance is a dynamic measurement obtained by dividing pressure by flow. It is dependent on the caliber of the airway and on the pattern of flow. *(9:58; 32:36)*

126. **(D)** The FRC/closing capacity relationship is important in determining if the airway will remain open. If CC falls below tidal volume, the airways remain open as in the normal situation. If the CC falls within tidal volume, the airways will be open part of the time, and areas of low V/Q will result. If the CC is above the FRC, the airways will remain closed, resulting in atelectasis. *(1:1131; 9:67)*

127. **(E)** All of the options are correct. V_D/V_T ratio is a measure of wasted ventilation. If the percentage of tidal volume that is wasted goes up, one must compensate by increasing minute ventilation. *(9:68–70; 75:896)*

128. **(A)** Spontaneous ventilation does not predispose to cephalad position of the diaphragm. The other options do predispose to more cephalad movement. *(8:148; 9:86)*

129. **(E)** All of these statements can cause hypercarbia. In the patient in whom hypercarbia occurs, various causes must be sought. *(9:94; 75:1409)*

130. **(D)** The forced vital capacity is affected primarily by obstructive lung disease and has the greatest impact in the first second. The results vary with patient cooperation. It is not a measure of inspiratory reserve volume. *(8:208; 15:713; 32:42)*

131. **(D)** The primary stimulus is hydrogen ion. Carbon dioxide reacts with water to form hydrogen ion; thus, CO_2 is involved, but the direct stimulus is hydrogen ion. *(15:715; 75:885)*

132. **(B)** Each gas contributes to the total pressure in an amount that is proportional to its concentration. Dalton's law states that each gas exerts the same pressure that it would if it alone occupied the container. *(15:721; 51:61)*

133. **(A)** The composition of alveolar gas differs by the first three options. Nitrogen remains constant, since an equilibrium is established. *(15:722; 53:52)*

134. **(A)** Carbon dioxide is inversely proportional to ventilation; ie, the higher the ventilation, the lower the CO_2. Ventilation will increase in response to endogenous or exogenous CO_2. *(8:173; 15:736)*

135. **(E)** Zone 3 extends higher into the lung because the arterial pressure increases, shifting the relationship with alveolar and venous pressure. The distribution is determined by gravity, with the lower segments getting more of the blood. *(9:40; 32:56)*

136. **(C)** The patient has a respiratory alkalosis. His oxygen tension is low. Calculation of his expected P_{O_2} using the alveolar air equation shows his oxygen tension should be over 100 torr. Although the patient's oxygenation seems to be stable it is important to follow this type of patient because there may be increasing difficulty in the subsequent hours. It is also important to consider that this patient may have compromised his oxygenation as a result of carbon dioxide poisoning. *(53:71; 57:2–3)*

137. **(A)** Patients who have flame burns are at greater risk from smoke and flame damage to the lungs than are those who have another type of burn, eg, a chemical burn or scald. The patient may need a tracheostomy in the future, but it is not necessary at this point. *(58:3; 59:451)*

138. **(E)** His oxygenation will be affected by pulmonary edema, should it occur, sickle cell disease, should it be present, carbon monoxide poisoning, and alkalosis. The alkalosis will affect oxygenation by shifting the oxyhemoglobin dissociation curve to the left, causing an increased affinity of hemoglobin for oxygen. *(58:4; 75:1370)*

139. **(D)** Rapid, shallow respirations magnify the effect of dead space ventilation on total ventilation. As the tidal volume decreases, dead space, which is fixed, becomes a larger percentage, and there is a decrease in the actual alveolar ventilation. *(34:14)*

140. **(A)** The circumstances cited may be due to poor ventilation because the patient has been placed in an unphysiologic position. Cardiac output may drop as a result of compression of the vena cava, and halothane anesthesia may cause cardiac depression. Blood loss should not be a problem at this stage of the procedure. *(1:1390; 16:246)*

141. **(A)** After positioning a patient, it is important to confirm that good ventilation is present. If the pressure is down, decreasing the amount of halogenated agent being delivered is prudent. The kidney rest should be lowered to rule out caval compression. Checking for blood loss should not be necessary. *(1:1390; 16:247)*

142. **(A)** The surgical approach to the kidney sometimes causes a pneumothorax, which should be watched for. This can cause hypoventilation, and the resulting hypercapnia could account for the hypertension and ectopic beats. In addition, any procedure involving the kidney should suggest that the tumor involved may be a hormone-releasing tumor, such as a pheochromocytoma. *(1:1159; 16:1390)*

143. **(C)** The surgeon should be informed of the difficulty encountered. With an arrhythmia, the patient should be kept anesthetized with the halothane. If the arrhythmia continues, switching to another agent may be prudent. The nitrous oxide should be discontinued to allow maximum oxygen and to avoid an enlarging air space if there is a pneumothorax. The injection of 10 ml of 4% lidocaine represents an overdose. *(1:639: 61:61–65)*

144. **(B)** Once the operation is completed, the patient is transported to the recovery room where constant vigilance is necessary to avoid hypoventilation. At this time, the patient's secretions may be a problem and should be removed by coughing, if possible. Therefore, narcotics should be used judiciously. *(1:1926, 1938; 62:180–181)*

145. **(D)** Ventilatory adequacy depends on the size of the patient. The minute volume cited here may be sufficient for a small patient but would be woefully inadequate for a larger patient. Therefore more data are needed. *(3:44–46; 75:1412)*

146. **(C)** The recovery room patient and all patients who are restless when on ventilators should have a thorough examination before a decision is made about treatment or extubation. The restlessness may reflect tracheal irritation, respiratory embarrassment secondary to malfunction of the ventilator, or hypoxia. *(1:1938; 39:146)*

147. **(D)** The equal ventilation of both sides is consistent with proper tube placement, although it does not guarantee it. The other choices are incorrect. Unequal ventilation obviously demonstrates poor tube placement. The distance from the lips to the carina in a female is about 25 cm. Therefore, the tube distance of 30 cm from the upper teeth is excessive. The carina lies at the level of the 5th thoracic vertebra. Therefore, the tube placement by chest x-ray also is incorrect. *(1:532; 9:24)*

148. **(E)** There are many causes of restlessness that should be sought, since they may be treated easily. A kink in a urinary catheter may be relieved, gastric distention may be relieved by a nasogastric tube, and so on. The assumption should not be made that the problem is the endotracheal tube. *(1:1938; 75:1410)*

149. **(C)** Air flow through a tube is dependent on the radius and length of the tube, the radius being more important. Viscosity is more important than density. *(1:89; 53:99)*

150. (B) Patients breathing 100% oxygen are at risk of developing pulmonary toxicity. They can also develop absorption atelectasis secondary to the oxygen being breathed in the absence of an inert gas. Obviously, Po_2 values are not present in excess of atmospheric pressure, and retrolental fibroplasia is not a concern in an adult. (*1:1157; 53:134*)

151. (C) Ventilation under anesthesia is characterized by a decrease in tidal volume as the depth of anesthesia increases. The decrease in tidal volume is compensated for by an increase in respiratory rate. Two things are important to note: (1) the rate is a compensatory adjustment, and therefore if the tachypnea is treated with a narcotic, the patient may hypoventilate because he or she will then be left with a lowered tidal volume, uncompensated, and (2) the tachypnea may also be due to hypoxia, and this must be guarded against. (*1:1143; 75:299*)

152. (E) All of these factors are important in providing the proper amount of oxygen to the anesthetized patient. Since oxygen is so important and changes so subtle, monitoring the oxygenation of the anesthetized patient is becoming a standard of care. (*10:2; 53:52*)

153. (A) The first three statements are true, but the fourth is false; a Po_2 of 30 torr gives a saturation of 60%. (*1:1135; 34:184*)

154. (A) Patients with scoliosis present many intraoperative problems. The references speak to timing the surgery to occur at a time most conducive to good ventilatory care. If vital capacity is < 35%, surgery is not precluded, but postoperative complications and ventilation must be discussed. (*1:2072; 64:649*)

155. (B) Increased body temperature and increased hydrogen ion concentration both shift the oxyhemoglobin dissociation curve to the right, thereby increasing the P_{50}. Methemoglobin is a hemoglobin molecule in which the iron is in the ferric state and is unable to combine with oxygen. (*1:1135; 2:104; 34:192*)

156. (E) All of these factors will be important in the patient's postoperative course. (*1:1931; 66:196*)

157. (C) Mixed venous oxygen is usually about 40 torr. It is best sampled from the pulmonary artery. Since mixed venous oxygen reflects oxygen usage by the body, it can be an indicator of tissue hypoxia. In the reference cited (67), mixed venous oxygen tension was a better indicator of hyperlactatemia and death than either arterial Po_2 or cardiac output. (*1:1175; 67:570–574*)

158. (C) Arrhythmias occurring during suctioning are of clinical significance. For this reason, patients should always be hyperventilated with 100% oxygen before suctioning. The suctioning process should be efficient and swift. (*1:2182; 32:248*)

159. (D) The pulmonary vascular system is not well enveloped in smooth muscle but has rich connections in the autonomic nervous system and has many alpha and beta receptors. Injection of norepinephrine will lead to vasoconstriction. (*8:158; 68:1*)

160. (E) Mucociliary flow is altered under anesthesia in normal conditions. In the presence of an upper respiratory infection, the body's ability to respond to the infection may be further hampered by an anesthetic. (*1:683; 8:144*)

161. (B) Neurogenic pulmonary edema may follow head injury or other cause of increased intracranial pressure. It is resistant to treatment unless the pressure is reduced. It will lead to hypoxemia. It is known that it will not develop in a denervated lung. (*32:474; 52:193; 70:94–95*)

162. (E) All of the options are true of closing capacity. It is intimately related to FRC. It is increased in obesity. (*1:1130; 8:211; 75:1117*)

163. (C) Transpulmonary pressure is the pressure gradient across the lung measured as the pressure difference between the airway opening and the pleural surface. (*1:1126; 72:125*)

164. (A) In reference 1 cited at the end of this explanation, deliberate hypotension was carried out with sodium nitroprusside and halothane. No shunt was noted in these studies. Miller cites one article in which shunt was increased. (*1:1964; 75:673*)

165. (A) Statements 1, 2, and 3 are basic to understanding pulmonary function tests. Small airways disease will not be detected by spirometry. The FEV_1 detects obstructive disease. (*1:2053–2056; 75:900*)

166. (A) Pulmonary embolus increases dead space. Shunt fraction will vary with changes in cardiac output and pulmonary changes. Therefore, if one is monitoring a patient with shunt fractions, this must be taken into account. (*1:2162; 53:54*)

167. (E) All of these options are true. The resistance decreases with inspiration because the airways dilate. (*8:141–142; 34:127*)

168. (C) Doxapram is a central respiratory stimulant that is metabolized rapidly. It has no effect on muscle relaxants. It should not be used routinely after thiopental administration. (*15:518*)

169. **(D)** Patients who have respiratory acidosis, hypercarbia, and hypoxia can be treated initially with low-flow oxygen and treatment of the underlying cause of the crisis. This demands very close observation in the event that intubation and ventilation become necessary. *(1:2224; 32:512)*

170. **(E)** Patients who are chronically hypercarbic develop a compensatory higher bicarbonate. The chloride is depleted by diuretics and other agents. With hyperventilation, there is rapid mobilization of CO_2 from the body stores and relatively slow mobilization of bicarbonate. This leaves the patient with central nervous system alkalosis, which may lead to cardiac arrest. *(1:1307; 78:993–996)*

171. **(A)** Cromolyn has no place in the immediate preparation, since it does not relieve bronchospasm. It would be helpful in the long-term preparation. *(4:124; 110:2)*

172. **(B)** Alpha$_1$-antitrypsin deficiency is familial and is determined by serum assay. The assay measures the level of a protective enzyme produced in the liver that acts to prevent autodigestion of lung tissue by the proteolytic enzymes of phagocytic cells. *(79:1243; 118:837)*

173. **(D)** Most patients recovering from an anesthetic are in need of supplemental oxygen. One must not wait for the onset of cyanosis before administration of oxygen. The oxygen should be administered in a mist to help the patient mobilize secretions. Although there are some studies showing that a nasal catheter is sufficient, oxygen is better administered by mask if the patient is breathing through the mouth. *(75:1412; 80:27)*

174. **(D)** Even in the recovery room, the patient can be started on a stir-up regimen to help him or her handle secretions. Narcotics should be used carefully in an amount that will treat the pain but still allow the patient to breathe deeply and mobilize secretions. *(1:1925, 1938; 80:25)*

175. **(C)** This describes a method of emergency ventilation that can be used to ventilate a patient adequately. If there is no obstruction above, there is sufficient air leak to prevent pressure buildup and pneumothorax. Gastric dilatation does not occur, since the air will be vented to the atmosphere. Pulmonary aspiration is minimized because the flow is sufficient to blow the secretions out of the larynx. *(1:1875; 81:38–40)*

176. **(A)** The first three choices are included in the definition of bronchitis; the last refers to emphysema. *(31:585; 32:505)*

177. **(E)** All of these diagnoses must be considered. In the patient with anterior chest injury, cardiac contusion must be considered. *(17:1–5; 82:109)*

178. **(A)** Ventilating a patient by means of a bag and mask unit may result in gastric distention, thereby decreasing effective ventilation. The patient's condition will deteriorate, and with a shift of the mediastinum, cardiac arrest may occur. Statement 4, although correct for the short term, obviously will increase the problem over the long term. *(17:5; 82:112–113)*

179. **(A)** Treatment of this patient includes endotracheal intubation to ensure ventilation, insertion of a nasogastric tube to decompress the stomach and thereby decrease the amount of air in the thorax, and stabilization in general. Only after stabilization has occurred should the patient have a thoracotomy to relieve the pressure. *(9:394; 82:112)*

180. **(B)** Patients who have entrapped bowel in their thorax do not do well with high ventilatory pressures and volumes. The large intrathoracic pressure further compromises the entrapped viscera. Nitrous oxide should be avoided because of the diffusion into air-containing spaces. The patient, once intubated, should have a careful induction of anesthesia to avoid problems with cardiovascular instability. *(82:112)*

181. **(E)** All of these may be seen in the patient with acute respiratory insufficiency. *(3:28; 32:332)*

CHAPTER 2

Circulation
Review

Our ability to understand and to monitor the parameters of cardiovascular function has allowed us to undertake many procedures that were not possible in the past. These advances have led to improvement in the conduct of anesthesia not only for cardiovascular procedures but for many other procedures as well.

The heart is a four-chambered pump with its own intricate blood supply and conduction system.

The coronary circulation derives from the base of the aorta and is supplied by two main vessels, the right and left coronary arteries. There are few anastomoses between the two vessels. The vessels lie on the surface of the heart. The left coronary vessel divides into the circumflex artery and the left anterior descending artery. These vessels supply the anterior aspect of the left ventricle. The right coronary artery supplies the right ventricle and the more posterior portions of the left ventricle.

The predominant flow is during diastole, since little flow can occur during systole. The heart muscle extracts much of the available oxygen, leaving the venous blood with a saturation of about 25%. The venous runoff from the coronary circulation is into the coronary sinus. A small amount of blood returns directly into the left ventricle via the thebesian veins. This contributes to shunt.

The coronary blood flow responds to pressure forces as well as to humoral influences. The pressure component of most importance is the diastolic pressure, since most of the flow occurs during diastole. Other influences include low oxygen tension, carbon dioxide, and hydrogen ions.

The neural control of the heart is via the autonomic nervous system. The atria are abundantly supplied by both sympathetic and parasympathetic nerves, whereas the ventricles are supplied principally by the sympathetic system.

The cardiac cycle is now better understood. The heartbeat is generated by the pacemaker cells and transmitted through the conduction system. The pacemaker cells reside in the sinoatrial node, and the conduction system consists of the interconnecting pathways to the atrioventricular node and then the His-Purkinje system. An appreciation of the drug effects on these systems, especially the autonomic agonists and antagonists, has helped treat disorders in conduction. In addition, artificial pacemakers have been developed to pace the heart when that is needed. Pacers have a code that designates the method of pacing, the chamber being paced, and how the pacer is programmed. These can be determined preoperatively. Mapping of the conduction system allows pinpointing of the site of conduction block. In addition, the mechanism of many arrhythmias is known. All of this allows us to choose agents and techniques that are best suited to the patient.

A major advance in the physiologic control of the patient came with the development of the flow-directed pulmonary catheter. Principles, such as the Frank-Starling mechanism, could now be put into clinical use. This mechanism, in essence, states that the stroke volume will increase with increasing venous return. The pulmonary artery catheter can be equipped with a thermistor that allows cardiac output or oxygen saturation to be measured. With the flow-directed catheter, the patient can be treated with volume while the pressure responses are measured. A series of response curves (Figure 2–1) can be drawn to show the response before and after therapeutic interventions.

Certain relationships have been established: pulmonary capillary wedge pressure (PCWP) reflects left atrial pressure (LAP), which reflects left ventricular end-diastolic volume (LVEDV), which reflects left ventricular end-diastolic pressure (LVEDP).

In spite of all the advances, we do not have a good measure of ventricular contractility. The rate of pressure change with time (dP/dt) is a reflection of contractility, as is the rate of shortening of ventricular muscle. Another problem is the lack of a good, safe method of measuring

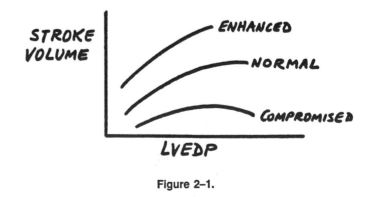

Figure 2–1.

LVEDP. New methods, eg, echocardiography, are being developed but are not in widespread clinical use.

The pulmonary artery catheter has gained widespread use, and its indications should be well known. It has not supplanted the use of other monitors, central venous pressure, arterial pressure, and electrocardiography.

An appreciation of myocardial oxygen balance has contributed to anesthesia techniques that do not stress the heart already at risk. The importance of increases in heart rate in increasing oxygen demand is well known. The former idea of "keeping them light and keeping them alive" has succumbed to modern knowledge.

The cardiovascular effects of drugs are more appreciated now, and with the advent of potent narcotics, cardiovascular procedures are much safer.

Questions

DIRECTIONS (Questions 1 through 85): Each of the numbered items or incomplete statements in this section is followed by answers or by completions of the statement. Select the <u>ONE</u> lettered answer or completion that is <u>BEST</u> in each case.

1. Myocardial oxygen demand may be decreased by

    (A) tachycardia
    (B) decreased preload
    (C) increased afterload
    (D) increased contractility
    (E) increased wall tension

2. Coronary perfusion pressure (CPP) is increased as a result of

    (A) increased diastolic blood pressure (DBP)
    (B) increased left ventricular end-diastolic pressure (LVEDP)
    (C) systolic hypertension
    (D) tachycardia
    (E) hypocapnia

3. Baroreceptor reflex activity is

    (A) unimportant as a circulatory regulator
    (B) responsive to oxygen content
    (C) located primarily in the carotid body
    (D) inversely proportional to age
    (E) responsive to CO_2 concentration

4. At a constant stroke volume, cardiac output is

    $CO = HR \times SV$

    (A) proportional to resistance
    (B) a linear function of heart rate
    (C) dependent on blood volume
    (D) related to potassium concentration
    (E) inversely proportional to arterial blood pressure

5. The intrinsic rhythmicity of the sinoatrial node is affected by the metabolism of the pacemaker cells themselves and may be increased by

    (A) digitalis
    (B) hypothyroidism
    (C) increased body temperature
    (D) hyperkalemia
    (E) calcium

6. Heart rate is controlled primarily by

    (A) drugs
    (B) environmental influence
    (C) blood pressure fluctuations
    (D) the adrenergic system
    (E) the parasympathetic system

7. Stroke volume is primarily a function of

    (A) the extent of myocardial fiber shortening
    (B) heart rate
    (C) peripheral resistance
    (D) arterial oxygen content
    (E) serum potassium level

8. Afterload of the left ventricle is

    (A) related only to the aortic valve
    (B) dependent on the distensibility of the large arteries
    (C) best measured by estimating the mean arterial pressure
    (D) increased by vasodilators
    (E) unrelated to ventricular size

9. The intrinsic rate of the sinoatrial node is

    (A) 20 to 40 beats per minute
    (B) 40 to 60 beats per minute
    (C) 70 to 80 beats per minute
    (D) 80 to 100 beats per minute
    (E) 100 to 120 beats per minute

10. Slow diastolic depolarization (phase 4) is

    (A) a property of all cardiac muscle
    (B) due to potassium flux
    (C) the process underlying intrinsic rhythmicity in pacemaker cells
    (D) more pronounced in the bundle of His than in the sinoatrial node
    (E) unrelated to rhythmicity

11. Cardiac output will be decreased by

    (A) raising the heart rate from 50 to 72 beats per minute
    (B) increased preload
    (C) decreased afterload
    (D) myocardial disease
    (E) digitalis

    $CO = HR \times SV$
    $SV = EDV - ESV$

12. Observation of the direct blood pressure display can give the following information

    (A) relative strength of left ventricular contraction
    (B) estimate of stroke volume
    (C) estimate of systemic vascular resistance (SVR)
    (D) heart rate
    (E) all of the above

    $SVR = \dfrac{MAP - CVP \times 80}{C.O.}$

13. Heart rate is responsive to all of the following EXCEPT

    (A) chemoreceptors
    (B) body temperature
    (C) impulses from cranial centers
    (D) vascular reflexes
    (E) Hering-Breuer reflex

14. The second heart sound coincides with all of the following EXCEPT

    (A) closing of the aortic valve
    (B) isometric relaxation of myocardial fibers
    (C) closure of the mitral valve
    (D) the T wave of the electrocardiogram
    (E) closure of the pulmonic valve

15. As a flow-directed catheter is inserted, you would expect to observe all of the following EXCEPT

    (A) a right atrial pressure of 15 mm Hg
    (B) a right ventricular systolic pressure of 30 mm Hg
    (C) a pulmonary artery pressure of 20 mm Hg
    (D) a pulmonary artery diastolic pressure higher than right ventricular diastolic pressure
    (E) a wedge pressure of 12 mm Hg

16. The cardiac conduction system includes all of the following EXCEPT

    (A) the sinoatrial node
    (B) atrial conduction pathways
    (C) right bundle branch
    (D) left bundle branch
    (E) coronary sinus

17. The standard electrocardiogram records the correct electrical potentials when leads are placed such that

    (A) lead I reads left arm–left leg
    (B) lead I reads right arm–right leg
    (C) lead II reads right arm–left leg
    (D) lead III reads right arm–left leg
    (E) lead II reads right arm–left arm

18. Calcium ion

    (A) decreases myocardial contractile force
    (B) decreases duration of systole
    (C) decreases vascular tone
    (D) decreases ventricular automaticity
    (E) enters the cardiac cell, causing excitation

19. Electrocardiographic monitoring is indicated during anesthesia to detect all of the following EXCEPT

    (A) efficacy of pump function
    (B) arrhythmias
    (C) ischemia
    (D) electrolyte disturbance
    (E) pacemaker function

20. Blood volume measurement is based on

    (A) the Fick principle
    (B) change in body temperature
    (C) oxygen consumption
    (D) a technique using an injection of glucose
    (E) the dilution effect

21. dP/dt is a measure of

    (A) myocardial oxygen demand
    (B) rate of change of ventricular pressure with time
    (C) right atrial pressure
    (D) renal perfusion
    (E) blood pressure

Questions 22 through 24

Please refer to the following figure:

22. The graph shown relates left ventricular stroke work to left ventricular end-diastolic pressure. Left ventricular end-diastolic pressure is most closely approximated by

    (A) arterial blood pressure

(B) central venous pressure
(C) pulmonary artery systolic pressure
(D) pulmonary capillary wedge pressure
(E) right atrial pressure

23. The curves marked 3 and 4 in the graph shown could be seen in patients

(A) with increased contractility
(B) on digitalis or epinephrine
(C) who are in heart failure
(D) who have been treated with glucagon
(E) who respond to increased left ventricular end-diastolic pressure (LVEDP) with increased stroke work

24. If the patient's response is noted to be represented by point A on curve 4 in the graph shown, administration of an inotropic agent may

(A) shift him to the normal curve
(B) take him to point B or C
(C) take him to point B only
(D) have no effect
(E) shift him to curve 2

25. Echocardiography uses

(A) x-ray technology
(B) ultrasound technique
(C) tomographic technology
(D) measurement of electrical potentials to measure cardiac structures
(E) fluoroscopy

26. The coronary circulation responds to hyperventilation with

(A) no change
(B) an increase in flow
(C) a decrease in flow
(D) a transient increase followed by an intense vasodilatation
(E) intense vasoconstriction

27. Myocardial oxygen consumption is most closely tied to

(A) heart rate
(B) blood viscosity
(C) cardiac output
(D) stroke volume
(E) F_{IO_2}

28. The systemic circulation is under control of

(A) an isolated center in the medulla
(B) the heart
(C) the cerebral cortex
(D) a complex, diffuse, and flexible integrative mechanism
(E) the muscular wall of the vessels

29. Venous pressure in the median basilic vein of the arm is

(A) equal to right atrial pressure
(B) above right atrial pressure
(C) below right atrial pressure
(D) not related to blood volume
(E) independent of arm position

30. Venous tone is

(A) constant and unvarying
(B) under both neural and hormonal control
(C) unresponsive to CO_2
(D) unresponsive to oxygen tension
(E) equal in superficial veins and venae cavae

31. The microcirculation

(A) is under the control of the autonomic nervous system
(B) contains no musculature
(C) is always open
(D) consists only of capillaries
(E) contains at least 20% of the blood volume

32. If the recorded blood pressure is 160/100, the mean pressure is

(A) 110 mm Hg
(B) 120 mm Hg
(C) 130 mm Hg
(D) 140 mm Hg
(E) 150 mm Hg

$MAP = DBP + 2/3 DBP$
$MAP = 1/3 SBP + 2/3 DBP$
$MAP = DBP + 1/3 DBP$
$100 + 1/3 \cdot 60 \quad PP$

33. To assure an accurate indirect blood pressure measurement

(A) the average width of the inflatable bladder for an adult should be 12 to 14 cm
(B) the length of the bladder should be sufficient to encircle the arm
(C) the length of the bladder is more important than the width
(D) the inflatable bladder need not be over the artery
(E) the manometer must read near zero to start

34. The presence of a bubble in an arterial line

(A) is not significant if it is small
(B) leads to an artificially high reading
(C) affects only the diastolic pressure
(D) leads to a damping of the tracing
(E) has a greater effect on the mean blood pressure

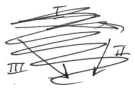

35. Under normal circumstances, the plasma protein osmotic pressure is

   (A) 5 mm Hg
   (B) 10 mm Hg
   (C) 15 mm Hg
   (D) 20 mm Hg
   (E) 25 mm Hg

36. Pulmonary edema may result from all of the following EXCEPT

   (A) altered permeability
   (B) decreased pulmonary capillary pressure
   (C) decreased oncotic pressure
   (D) increased negative airway pressure
   (E) head injury

37. Pulmonary edema in the recovery room

   (A) usually occurs as a late sign
   (B) is always associated with a rise of central venous pressure (CVP)
   (C) will be detected because of distended neck vessels
   (D) may be due to airway obstruction
   (E) usually occurs without wheezing being present

38. The microcirculation, under shock conditions, is the site of all of the following EXCEPT

   (A) vasodilatation
   (B) sludging of blood
   (C) decreased viscosity of blood
   (D) hypercoagulability of blood
   (E) hypoxia

39. The microcirculation

   (A) is devoid of any sphincter control
   (B) has no vasomotion
   (C) has precapillary sphincters that are sensitive to humoral factors
   (D) has precapillary sphincters that are under neurogenic influence
   (E) has no postcapillary sphincters

40. Measurement of systolic time intervals

   (A) is an invasive technique
   (B) is a noninvasive technique
   (C) requires an arterial line and a pulmonary artery catheter
   (D) is performed with a slow-speed recorder of ECG
   (E) is a measure of the duration of contraction

41. Measurement of systolic time intervals can be used to detect all of the following EXCEPT

   (A) right atrial enlargement
   (B) mitral stenosis
   (C) hypertension

   (D) myocardial infarction
   (E) aortic valvular disease

42. Treatment of cardiogenic pulmonary edema may include the reduction of preload. This may include all of the following EXCEPT

   (A) rotating tourniquets
   (B) intravenous morphine
   (C) phlebotomy
   (D) administration of dopamine
   (E) diuretics

43. The drug of choice to increase myocardial contractility in pulmonary edema is

   (A) oxygen
   (B) digitalis
   (C) morphine
   (D) furosemide
   (E) nitroglycerin

44. Mechanisms by which patients in heart failure compensate for low cardiac output include all of the following EXCEPT

   (A) increased sympathetic drive to the heart
   (B) myocardial hypertrophy
   (C) renal loss of salt and decreased blood volume
   (D) secondary hyperaldosteronism
   (E) increased ventricular filling pressure

45. The Frank-Starling mechanism refers to the relationship of

   (A) the left and right ventricles
   (B) the left and right atria
   (C) preload and stroke volume
   (D) afterload and ventricular volume
   (E) stroke volume and afterload

46. Noninvasive methods for measurement of cardiac contractility include

   (A) systolic time intervals
   (B) Walton-Brodie strain gauge
   (C) catheter tip flowmeters
   (D) angiography
   (E) determination of dP/dt

47. If the size of the ventricle increases

   (A) wall tension needed to pump the same amount of blood is less
   (B) less oxygen is needed to pump blood
   (C) the heart becomes more efficient
   (D) wall tension will increase proportionally with the radius
   (E) wall tension will be proportional to wall thickness

48. Coronary blood flow

(A) is independent of the systolic pressure
(B) is not affected by humoral agents
(C) is increased by a slow heart rate
(D) is increased by a fast heart rate
(E) occurs almost entirely in systole

49. Pulmonary artery pressure

(A) increases passively with increases of cardiac output
(B) remains constant with change of cardiac output
(C) is not important to pulmonary vascular resistance
(D) is not dependent on the radius of the vessels
(E) depends entirely on cardiac output

50. Hypertension

(A) should always be controlled with medication preoperatively
(B) is a problem only if the systolic is over 180 torr
(C) in general, does not pose a risk to the patient for anesthesia
(D) is always accompanied by increased cardiac output
(E) medications should be continued preoperatively

51. The transplanted heart

(A) has an abnormal Frank-Starling mechanism
(B) responds as does an innervated heart to atropine
(C) has intact alpha and beta receptors
(D) has a normal appearing electrocardiogram
(E) does not increase cardiac output with increased preload

52. Signs and symptoms associated with an increased incidence of postoperative congestive heart failure include all of the following EXCEPT

(A) New York Heart Association functional class II
(B) previous pulmonary edema
(C) presence of an S 3 gallop
(D) jugular venous distention
(E) signs of left heart failure

53. The patient with congestive heart failure may have symptoms due to the presence of low cardiac output. These include all of the following EXCEPT

(A) memory loss
(B) weakness
(C) fatigue
(D) confusion
(E) anxiety

54. Effects of halogenated hydrocarbons on the healthy heart include

(A) halothane produces a dose-related decrease in left ventricular function
(B) halothane produces a significant decrease in vascular resistance
(C) enflurane increases ventricular function
(D) enflurane decreases heart rate
(E) isoflurane causes peripheral vasoconstriction

55. Hypotension noted on initiation of cardiopulmonary bypass may be due to all of the following EXCEPT

(A) hemodilution
(B) decreased catecholamines
(C) aortic stenosis
(D) persistent systemic to pulmonary shunt
(E) aortic dissection

56. Myocardial preservation during cardiopulmonary bypass may include all of the following EXCEPT

(A) maintaining the ventricle in a distended state
(B) cardioplegia
(C) cold irrigations
(D) avoidance of ventricular fibrillation
(E) maintaining the heart at a low temperature

57. The addition of nitrous oxide to isoflurane during cardiopulmonary bypass

(A) increases myocardial contractility
(B) decreases the risk of air embolism
(C) has no physiologic effect
(D) promotes blood flow to the ischemic areas
(E) decreases myocardial contractility in ischemic areas

58. You are called to see your patient in the recovery room because of elevated blood pressure readings. Your approach should be

(A) treat the blood pressure with small doses of an antihypertensive medication
(B) do nothing, but wait to see if the hypertension is a transient problem associated with emergence from anesthesia
(C) examine the patient for evidence of hypoxia or hypercarbia
(D) recheck the blood pressure yourself to make sure the cuff is the correct size
(E) arrange a cardiology consultation

59. Appropriate drug therapy for the patient in Question 58 would be

(A) initiation of treatment with a diuretic
(B) starting an infusion of nitroprusside
(C) use of diazoxide
(D) starting a ganglionic blocking agent
(E) starting a calcium channel blocking agent

60. The patient with an arrhythmia is at increased risk for anesthesia. Those arrhythmias presenting the LEAST risk are

    (A) multifocal PVCs
    (B) R-on-T disturbances
    (C) complete heart block
    (D) isolated atrial rhythms
    (E) bundle branch block

61. Cardiovascular changes that occur with advancing age are

    (A) decreasing blood pressure
    (B) increase in cardiovascular reserve
    (C) loss of elasticity of the vascular tree
    (D) increased number of myofibrils
    (E) increase in cardiac output

62. The right ventricle

    (A) has little function in the adult patient
    (B) is very easily cooled in the patient undergoing cardiopulmonary bypass
    (C) can overcome pulmonary vascular resistance very effectively, and, therefore, is not of concern in terminating cardiopulmonary bypass
    (D) is more likely to be injured by intracoronary air than is the left ventricle during cardiopulmonary bypass
    (E) is unaffected by PEEP

63. Systemic hypertension

    (A) is usually due to an increased cardiac output
    (B) can usually be attributed to a single cause
    (C) is not a reason to cancel a surgical procedure unless the diastolic pressure is over 120 torr
    (D) by definition is a pressure greater than 160/95
    (E) that is well treated still presents great risk during an operative procedure

64. A cause of systemic hypertension that is amenable to surgical correction is

    (A) essential hypertension
    (B) secondary aldosteronism
    (C) renal parenchymal disease
    (D) pheochromocytoma
    (E) long-standing renal artery stenosis

65. Allen's test

    (A) is used to assess adequacy of radial artery perfusion
    (B) has little predictive value
    (C) is positive if good flow occurs
    (D) is negative if good flow occurs
    (E) is independent of hand position

66. Blood pressure may be measured noninvasively by

    (A) the Dinamap, which uses an ultrasound technique
    (B) the Infrasonde, which uses ultrasound technique
    (C) the Doppler, which uses a laser method
    (D) the Arteriosonde, which uses the Doppler effect
    (E) the Penaz method using palpation of the pulse distal to the cuff

67. Central venous pressure (CVP) monitoring

    (A) can give valuable information concerning the left side of the heart
    (B) is not useful for estimating blood volume
    (C) is most successfully accomplished by the internal jugular approach
    (D) is of little value in the patient in shock
    (E) is valuable as a single reading

68. Central venous pressure (CVP) monitoring is indicated in all the following procedures EXCEPT

    (A) a surgical procedure in which there is an unusual position, eg, head-down position
    (B) patients in shock
    (C) hyperalimentation
    (D) intravenous administration of vasopressors
    (E) procedures in which large volume shifts may occur

69. Methods to determine cardiac output include all of the following EXCEPT

    (A) thermodilution
    (B) chest wall impedance
    (C) iodinated tracer techniques
    (D) Doppler ultrasound
    (E) the Fick principle

70. In evaluating the left ventricular performance

    (A) a central venous line usually is adequate
    (B) the ideal would be left ventricular pressure measurement
    (C) pulmonary capillary wedge pressure always reflects left ventricular end diastolic pressure
    (D) left ventricular end diastolic volume always reflects left ventricular preload
    (E) a high pulmonary capillary wedge pressure always reflects a poor ventricular performance

71. The precordial thump is indicated at the time of cardiac arrest

    (A) in all patients with arrest
    (B) only in pediatric patients
    (C) since it can do nothing but good
    (D) only in those with unmonitored arrhythmias
    (E) and should be delivered to the midpart of the sternum

72. Defibrillation is

    (A) indicated in all instances of cardiac arrest
    (B) delivered at an energy level of 400 joules in all patients
    (C) always successful if used early
    (D) the initial step in resuscitation of the unwitnessed arrest
    (E) best attempted with an energy level of 200 joules in an adult

73. Current recommendations for basic life support during resuscitation include

    (A) chest compressions at a rate of 60 per minute in the adult
    (B) a fast compression that occupies 30% of the cycle
    (C) rescue breaths that allow at least 1 second for inflation
    (D) head tilt–neck lift to open the airway
    (E) one breath between every two compressions in two-person resuscitations

74. In advanced life support

    (A) epinephrine is used primarily for its beta effect
    (B) bretylium is preferable to lidocaine because of its less severe side effects
    (C) atropine is a first-line drug used to reduce vagal tone
    (D) isoproterenol is used first for the treatment of bradycardia
    (E) sodium bicarbonate should be started immediately

75. Administration of drugs during advanced life support

    (A) may be by intramuscular injection
    (B) should preferably be by peripheral line
    (C) should be by femoral line if possible
    (D) should be via central line if possible
    (E) may be via the endotracheal tube, but only epinephrine and bicarbonate can be given by this route

76. Reproducibility of thermodilution cardiac outputs may be affected by all of the following EXCEPT

    (A) timing of injection in relation to respiration
    (B) temperature of injectate
    (C) temperature of patient
    (D) intracardiac shunts
    (E) tricuspid regurgitation

77. Factor(s) that may lead to erroneous readings of pulmonary artery pressure include

    (A) placing the transducer at the level of the angle of Louis and attaching it to the bed
    (B) doing a two-point calibration of the transducer

    (C) repositioning the catheter to avoid apposition to the vessel wall
    (D) reading pressures from a printout
    (E) failure to identify a and v waves in the tracing

78. A problem with the pulmonary artery catheter with fiberoptic bundles for the measurement of continuous mixed venous oxygen saturation is

    (A) decreased accuracy of oxygen saturation determinations
    (B) decreased accuracy of cardiac output
    (C) difficulty in calibration
    (D) expense
    (E) determination of pulmonary artery pressure is compromised

79. All of the following may be seen in the patient with hypovolemia EXCEPT

    (A) increased heart rate
    (B) wide pulse pressure
    (C) decreased urine volume
    (D) flat neck veins
    (E) pale mucous membranes

80. When monitoring the central venous pressure (CVP)

    (A) a waveform printout should be evaluated for the most accurate reading
    (B) the catheter should be placed in the right atrium
    (C) an accurate reflection of fluid status is obtained in all patients
    (D) analysis of waveforms is no better than a digital readout
    (E) a flow-directed pulmonary artery catheter should always be used, since it will give the CVP and other information

81. When using arterial pressure monitoring

    (A) it is best to use a catheter that approximates the size of the vessel to avoid pressure artifact
    (B) one should never aspirate the catheter during decannulation
    (C) a heparin flush system should be employed
    (D) the duration is not related to complications
    (E) caution is needed if using the radial artery, since it has few collaterals

82. A heart lesion associated with high pulmonary flow is

    (A) pulmonic stenosis
    (B) tetralogy of Fallot
    (C) coarctation of the aorta
    (D) ventricular septal defect
    (E) tricuspid atresia

83. A true statement in reference to sites of vessel cannulation is that

(A) chylothorax is common with right internal jugular cannulation
(B) brachial plexus trauma is common with antecubital approach for central venous cannulation
(C) pneumothorax is common with the subclavian approach
(D) Allen's test gives good evidence of collateral flow
(E) the dorsalis pedis is the artery of choice in a patient with diabetes

84. The distribution of blood flow to various organs is

(A) kidney 50%
(B) brain 3%
(C) heart 35%
(D) liver 15%
(E) skin 35%

85. The patient with aortic stenosis has

(A) a rapid downhill course once symptoms are present
(B) a large left ventricular cavity
(C) a low cardiac output with moderately slow heart rates
(D) protection against ischemia due to the large ventricle
(E) a very compliant ventricle

DIRECTIONS (Questions 86 through 169): For each of the items in this section, ONE or MORE of the numbered options is correct. Choose the answer

A if only 1, 2, and 3 are correct,
B if only 1 and 3 are correct,
C if only 2 and 4 are correct,
D if only 4 is correct,
E if all are correct.

86. Anesthetic agents may predispose the patient to intraoperative arrhythmias by

(1) a reentrant mechanism (halogenated agents)
(2) myocardial sensitization to catecholamines (halothane)
(3) blocking norepinephrine reuptake (cocaine)
(4) hypotension (ketamine)

87. Sinus bradycardia

(1) is a serious arrhythmia when seen during anesthesia
(2) is an irregular rhythm
(3) always requires treatment
(4) is characterized by a rate of 40 to 60 beats per minute

88. The tetralogy of Fallot includes

(1) atrial septal defect (ASD)
(2) ventricular septal defect (VSD)
(3) patent ductus arteriosus (PDA)
(4) pulmonary outflow obstruction

89. The preoperative electrocardiogram can be used to detect

(1) chamber enlargement
(2) ischemic heart disease
(3) electrolyte disturbances
(4) heart block

90. Cardiac output is

(1) governed solely by the heart
(2) usually 5 to 6 L/minute in a 70 kg man
(3) unaffected by blood volume
(4) the product of heart rate and stroke volume

91. Left ventricular compliance may be decreased in

(1) aortic stenosis
(2) ischemia
(3) inotrope usage
(4) the patient on vasodilators

92. Preload is affected by

(1) total blood volume
(2) increased heart rate
(3) atrial function
(4) venous tone

93. Myocardial contractility is decreased by

(1) sympathetic stimulation
(2) parasympathetic inhibition
(3) inotrope administration
(4) myocardial ischemia

94. The coronary circulation is composed of the right and left coronary arteries

(1) the right supplying the right ventricle
(2) which are remarkably constant in their configuration and areas they supply
(3) the left dividing into the left anterior descending and the circumflex
(4) both of which empty into the right ventricle

95. When inserting a central venous pressure (CVP) line

(1) air embolism may occur
(2) the tip should be placed in the right atrium
(3) use of the external jugular vein avoids many of the major complications
(4) the left side of the neck is preferred

can predispose to dig toxicity

96. Calcium administration

   (1) decreases myocardial contractility
   (2) decreases excitability
   (3) can be antagonized by calcium chelating agents, but the effects are too long for clinical use
   (4) may potentiate development of digitalis toxicity

97. The Allen test

   (1) should be performed, since only 40% of patients have a complete ulnar arch
   (2) should be done with the wrist in extension
   (3) is described as "positive" if good flow is demonstrated
   (4) should be described in terms of return of color and time

98. To obtain an accurate central venous pressure (CVP)

   (1) the catheter tip should be within the thoracic portion of the vena cava
   (2) the tip should be at the caval–atrium junction
   (3) the pressure should be demonstrated to fluctuate with respiration
   (4) one must be able to aspirate blood

99. Factors of importance when choosing the cephalic versus the basilic vein for insertion of a cental venous catheter are

   (1) the cephalic vein is usually smaller
   (2) the cephalic vein does not become progressively larger as it approaches the heart
   (3) the cephalic vein enters the axillary vein at a 90 degree angle
   (4) the basilic vein lies lateral to the cephalic vein

100. Determination of cardiac output with the thermodilution technique

   (1) requires a pulmonary artery catheter with a thermistor
   (2) uses the same principle as the dye-dilution technique
   (3) requires the use of an exact amount of fluid with a known temperature
   (4) requires the measurement of the temperature in the pulmonary artery

101. Correct intracardiac pressure value(s) include

   (1) right atrium: mean 5
   (2) right ventricle: 25/5
   (3) pulmonary artery: 23/9
   (4) wedge pressure: 10

102. The effect of hyperventilation on coronary blood flow

   (1) is to cause increased flow
   (2) leads to coronary spasm
   (3) does not respond to nitroglycerin
   (4) can be suppressed by diltiazem

103. Factors that affect myocardial ischemia are

   (1) anemia, which aggravates it
   (2) adrenergic blockade, which aggravates it
   (3) digitalis treatment in the failing heart, which alleviates it
   (4) nitroglycerin, which aggravates it

104. Cardioplegia is an important adjunct, since

   (1) oxygen consumption increases with ventricular fibrillation
   (2) oxygen consumption is reduced to one fourth with arrest
   (3) coronary resistance is reduced
   (4) myocardial oxygen consumption varies with rhythm

105. Air embolism seen with cardiopulmonary bypass

   (1) is most common after aortic valve procedures
   (2) is alleviated with the use of a ventricular vent
   (3) is alleviated by the use of an aortic vent
   (4) comes in part from air that accumulates in the pulmonary veins during bypass

106. Indications for pacemakers include

   (1) Stokes-Adams attacks
   (2) heart block
   (3) tachyarrhythmias
   (4) myocardial ischemia

107. Methods of detecting intraoperative air embolism include

   (1) mass spectrometry
   (2) end-tidal carbon dioxide determination
   (3) Doppler monitoring
   (4) measurement of end-tidal oxygen — *not good method*

108. The position of the tip of the central venous pressure (CVP) catheter can be confirmed by

   (1) electrocardiography
   (2) x-ray
   (3) pressure monitoring
   (4) Doppler monitoring while injecting 1 ml of air

109. Blood flow is affected by

   (1) pressure
   (2) protein content
   (3) hematocrit
   (4) viscosity

A	B	C	D	E
SUMMARY OF DIRECTIONS				
1, 2, 3 only	1, 3 only	2, 4 only	4 only	All are correct

110. The phlebostatic axis

(1) is located at the tip of the left ventricle
(2) is defined at the level at which a change of position will cause a pressure change of less than 1 mm Hg
(3) has no clinical importance
(4) is used for pressure references

111. The vasomotor center

(1) is located in the right temporal area of the brain
(2) is affected by the hypothalamus
(3) secretes serotonin
(4) is affected by the cerebral cortex

112. Baroreceptor structures include

(1) the walls of the large arteries of the neck and thorax
(2) the carotid sinus
(3) the aortic arch
(4) the glossopharyngeal nerve

113. The renin–angiotensin mechanism includes

(1) renin, which is in the liver
(2) converting enzyme, which is in the lung
(3) the conversion of renin substrate to angiotensin I by the converting enzyme
(4) initiation of the entire process by an elevation of the blood pressure

114. Cerebral function changes after cardiopulmonary bypass have been attributed to

(1) hypotension while on pump
(2) barbiturate administered while on pump
(3) microemboli from the pump
(4) pulmonary hypertension

115. A pacemaker with the letter code AVTPN

(1) paces the atrium
(2) senses the ventricle
(3) triggers a pacemaker spike on sensing an impulse
(4) is not programmable

116. Pacemaker threshold changes that can occur by various agents and chemical changes include

(1) an increase with stress
(2) a decrease with decrease in carbon dioxide
(3) an increase with increase in potassium
(4) an increase with hypoxia

117. Thebesian veins

(1) always drain into the left atrium
(2) are part of the pulmonary circulatory system
(3) carry oxygenated blood
(4) which empty into the left ventricle contribute to shunt

118. Cardiac index

(1) is synonymous with cardiac output
(2) is calculated by dividing the cardiac output by the patient's weight
(3) is lower in an adult than in a child
(4) is calculated to give a better comparison among patients of varying size

119. After insertion of a flow-directed pulmonary artery catheter, you note the presence of large v waves. This may be due to

(1) tricuspid atresia
(2) aortic valve stenosis
(3) aortic regurgitation
(4) mitral regurgitation

120. Coarctation of the aorta

(1) may be the cause of hypertension
(2) may be associated with congestive heart failure
(3) may be associated wit catecholamine depletion
(4) in the neonate is always associated with other heart lesions

121. Transesophageal echocardiography

(1) cannot be used in a continuous mode
(2) can only be used in the closed chest, therefore is not useful in the cardiac surgery patient
(3) gives poor delineation of the left ventricle
(4) gives good visualization of the right heart

122. Lymph

(1) is essentially interstitial fluid
(2) enters the venous circulation through the external jugular vein
(3) flow is increased by exercise
(4) from the intestine is low in fat

123. An esophageal electrocardiographic lead used intraoperatively is

(1) not practical clinically
(2) not effective in detecting P waves
(3) not as effective as lead II
(4) best for differentiating dysrhythmias

124. Factors that increase the risk of anesthesia include

(1) an S3 gallop
(2) rhythm other than sinus
(3) age >70
(4) emergency operations

125. Methods of detecting ventricular dysfunction include

(1) determination of ejection fraction
(2) wall motion studies
(3) determination of cardiac output
(4) determination of end-diastolic pressure

126. During cardipulmonary resuscitation (CPR)

(1) a central line is preferable for drug administration
(2) a femoral line is preferable to an antecubital line   → not good blood flow below diaphram
(3) lidocaine, atropine, and epinephrine may be administered via the endotracheal tube
(4) intracardiac injections should be attempted before an attempt is made to secure a central line

127. Correct drug dosage for CPR in an adult includes

(1) epinephrine, 5 to 10 ml of 1:10,000 IV
(2) sodium bicarbonate, 1 mEq/kg IV
(3) lidocaine, 1 mg/kg IV
(4) isoproterenol, 0.05 mg/kg IV   2-10 ug/min .002

128. Factors that increase cardiac output include

(1) anxiety
(2) anoxia
(3) anemia
(4) hypothyroidism   ↓ C.O.

129. The blood flow in veins

(1) in the standing position is dependent on the pressure differential between the capillaries and right atrium
(2) is independent of gravity
(3) in the upright position requires the presence of valves
(4) is independent of the autonomic nervous system

130. The baroreceptors

(1) are stretch receptors
(2) respond to absolute pressure change as well as rate of change in pressure
(3) function through the cardioinhibitory and vasomotor centers
(4) are reset by chronic hypertension

131. The arterial supply to the spinal cord includes

(1) the anterior spinal arteries
(2) the posterior spinal arteries

(3) radicular arteries
(4) artery of Adamkiewicz

132. The pericardium

(1) serves as a buffer to the heart at times of acceleration
(2) contains nerve fibers that, when stimulated, will slow the heart rate
(3) minimizes cardiac dilatation
(4) is not essential to cardiac function

133. Appropriate drug therapy in the perioperative period for the patient undergoing cardiac surgery includes

(1) stopping all propranolol preoperatively
(2) use of propranolol as part of the preoperative medication and intravenously during the procedure as needed
(3) stopping all calcium entry blockers
(4) continuing all antihypertensive agents

134. The right and left ventricles

(1) are completely independent of one another assuming the septum is intact
(2) are affected identically by a deep inspiration
(3) are not affected by septal position
(4) are each affected by the systolic pressure of the other

135. Idiopathic hypertrophic subaortic stenosis (IHSS) is

(1) treated with inotropic agents
(2) a form of primary myocardial disease
(3) always responsive to medical treatment
(4) treated with beta-blocking agents

136. Afterload will decrease after

(1) a reduction of blood viscosity
(2) the opening of an arteriovenous fistula
(3) administration of a vasodilator
(4) development of mitral regurgitation

137. Stroke volume is dependent on myocardial fiber shortening, which is determined by

(1) preload
(2) contractility of the myocardium
(3) afterload
(4) heart rate

138. Treatment of cardiac decompensation requires

(1) reduction of circulatory demands
(2) increasing myocardial contractility
(3) search for precipitating cause
(4) increasing oxygen demand   supply

SUMMARY OF DIRECTIONS				
A	B	C	D	E
1, 2, 3 only	1, 3 only	2, 4 only	4 only	All are correct

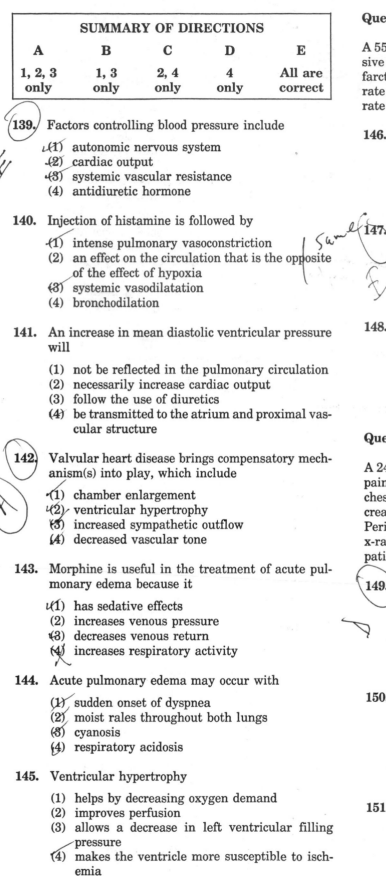

139. Factors controlling blood pressure include

   (1) autonomic nervous system
   (2) cardiac output
   (3) systemic vascular resistance
   (4) antidiuretic hormone

140. Injection of histamine is followed by

   (1) intense pulmonary vasoconstriction
   (2) an effect on the circulation that is the opposite of the effect of hypoxia
   (3) systemic vasodilatation
   (4) bronchodilation

141. An increase in mean diastolic ventricular pressure will

   (1) not be reflected in the pulmonary circulation
   (2) necessarily increase cardiac output
   (3) follow the use of diuretics
   (4) be transmitted to the atrium and proximal vascular structure

142. Valvular heart disease brings compensatory mechanism(s) into play, which include

   (1) chamber enlargement
   (2) ventricular hypertrophy
   (3) increased sympathetic outflow
   (4) decreased vascular tone

143. Morphine is useful in the treatment of acute pulmonary edema because it

   (1) has sedative effects
   (2) increases venous pressure
   (3) decreases venous return
   (4) increases respiratory activity

144. Acute pulmonary edema may occur with

   (1) sudden onset of dyspnea
   (2) moist rales throughout both lungs
   (3) cyanosis
   (4) respiratory acidosis

145. Ventricular hypertrophy

   (1) helps by decreasing oxygen demand
   (2) improves perfusion
   (3) allows a decrease in left ventricular filling pressure
   (4) makes the ventricle more susceptible to ischemia

Questions 146 and 147

A 55-year-old male is admitted with a history of hypertensive heart disease and evidence of acute myocardial infarction. Vital signs show blood pressure 170/100, heart rate 124/minute, body temperature 101°F, and respiratory rate 24 per minute.

146. Efforts to improve oxygenation should include

   (1) decreasing arterial blood pressure
   (2) decreasing body temperature
   (3) slowing heart rate
   (4) administration of oxygen

147. Blood pressure can be reduced by

   (1) diuretics
   (2) application of tourniquets
   (3) phlebotomy
   (4) administration of vasodilators

148. Cerebral symptoms occurring after cardiopulmonary bypass may be due to

   (1) cerebrovascular disease
   (2) heparin administered during bypass
   (3) hypoperfusion
   (4) protamine

Questions 149 through 152

A 24-year-old female was admitted for evaluation of chest pain. The pain was sharp and aggravated by breathing. A chest x-ray showed an enlarged heart, ECG showed decreased voltage, and there was a pericardial friction rub. Pericardiocentesis demonstrated purulent fluid. Serial x-rays showed widening of the cardiac shadow, and the patient was scheduled for a pericardial drainage.

149. You would expect to find

   (1) a water-hammer pulse
   (2) an increased cardiac output
   (3) distended neck veins that flatten in the sitting position
   (4) decreasing arterial pressure

150. A pulsus paradoxicus is a pulse that

   (1) reduces in amplitude on inspiration
   (2) shows alternate strong and weak beats
   (3) is merely an exaggeration of the normal respiratory effect on the arterial pulse
   (4) is stronger on inspiration

151. In monitoring this patient, the

   (1) arterial blood pressure is of no help
   (2) Swan-Ganz catheter is mandatory
   (3) x-ray evaluation is of utmost importance
   (4) central venous pressure will provide superior information

152. This patient is brought to the operating room for the procedure. In administering anesthesia

    (1) a thiopental induction should always be used
    (2) vasodilators should be avoided or used very cautiously
    (3) efforts should be made to increase cardiac output
    (4) cardiac depressants must be avoided or used cautiously

153. Coronary artery circulation is influenced by

    (1) oxygen saturation of the blood
    (2) cardiac output
    (3) autoregulation
    (4) adenosine

154. Myocardial oxygen consumption is

    (1) increased by propranolol
    (2) decreased by digitalis
    (3) increased by nitroglycerin
    (4) increased by isoproterenol

155. Calculation of systemic vascular resistance requires determination of

    (1) mean arterial pressure
    (2) mean central venous pressure
    (3) cardiac output
    (4) pulmonary artery pressure

156. Venous return is

    (1) the major determinant of cardiac preload
    (2) impeded by muscular contractions
    (3) increased by a decrease in right atrial pressure
    (4) impeded by the valves below the superior vena cava

157. Oxygen consumption under anesthesia

    (1) is unrelated to premedication
    (2) falls about 15%
    (3) varies with tidal volume
    (4) will fall more in a patient who is excited before induction

158. Goals for the anesthetic management of a patient with coronary artery disease are to

    (1) maintain high afterload
    (2) maintain contractility
    (3) maintain high heart rate
    (4) maintain sinus rhythm

159. The capillaries are

    (1) the site of gas exchange between blood and tissue
    (2) seldom open to full capacity
    (3) regulated by local physical and chemical agents

    (4) primarily controlled by the autonomic nervous system

160. The patient with mitral stenosis usually has

    (1) left ventricular hypertrophy
    (2) increased left atrial pressure
    (3) increased cardiac output
    (4) right ventricular hypertrophy

Questions 161 and 162

Please refer to the following figure:

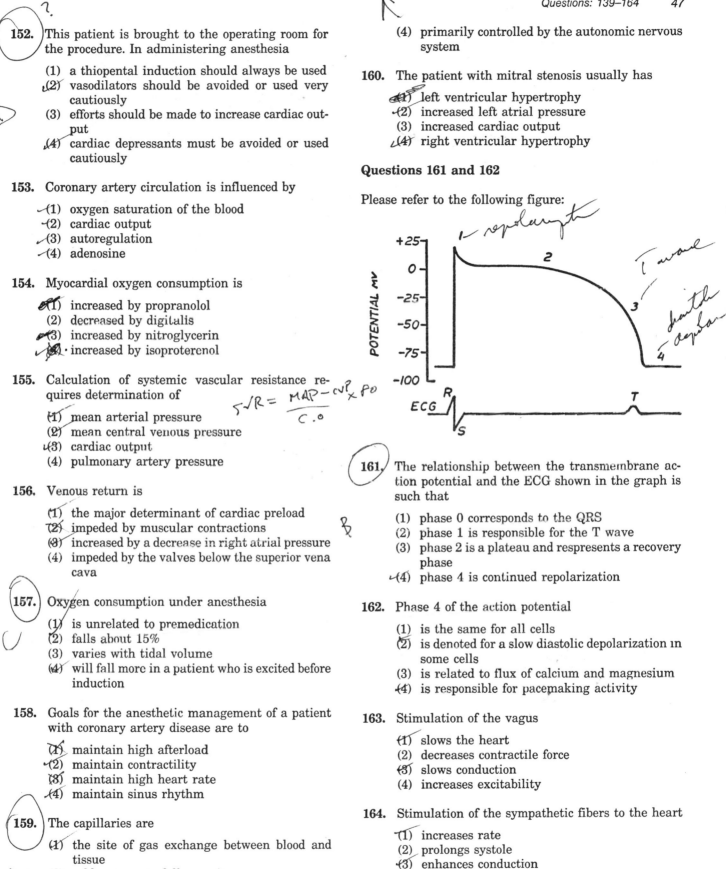

161. The relationship between the transmembrane action potential and the ECG shown in the graph is such that

    (1) phase 0 corresponds to the QRS
    (2) phase 1 is responsible for the T wave
    (3) phase 2 is a plateau and respresents a recovery phase
    (4) phase 4 is continued repolarization

162. Phase 4 of the action potential

    (1) is the same for all cells
    (2) is denoted for a slow diastolic depolarization in some cells
    (3) is related to flux of calcium and magnesium
    (4) is responsible for pacemaking activity

163. Stimulation of the vagus

    (1) slows the heart
    (2) decreases contractile force
    (3) slows conduction
    (4) increases excitability

164. Stimulation of the sympathetic fibers to the heart

    (1) increases rate
    (2) prolongs systole
    (3) enhances conduction
    (4) weakens contractions

SUMMARY OF DIRECTIONS				
A	**B**	**C**	**D**	**E**
1, 2, 3 only	1, 3 only	2, 4 only	4 only	All are correct

165. The coronary sinus

(1) represents a minor drainage system of the heart
(2) receives the entire coronary venous blood flow
(3) drains into the pulmonary artery
(4) contains blood with an oxygen saturation of less than 30%

166. The pulmonary arterial circulation

(1) arises from the aorta
(2) has an arteriole for every two bronchioles
(3) contains arterioles with thick muscular walls
(4) contains a broad capillary network

167. The bronchial arteries

(1) are part of the systemic circulation
(2) arise from the pulmonary artery
(3) drain into the azygos vein
(4) have no anastomoses with the pulmonary artery

168. Pulmonary circulation

(1) is very expansile, being able to accept large changes in cardiac output
(2) time is about 11 seconds
(3) totals about 400 to 600 ml of blood at any one time
(4) from the right ventricle equals the output from the left ventricle

169. The Valsalva maneuver

(1) decreases blood return to the right ventricle
(2) increases venous pressure in the head
(3) decreases cardiac output
(4) results in a reflex increase in heart rate

Answers and Explanations

1. **(B)** Myocardial oxygen consumption is increased by tachycardia. It causes increased demand for oxygen at the same time that it leads to decreased oxygen supply by decreasing coronary blood flow. Increased afterload leads to increased wall tension, both of which require more oxygen. Increases of contractility require more oxygen. *(1:1192,1472; 18:66)*

2. **(A)** Coronary perfusion occurs for the most part during diastole. The CPP relationship is

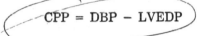

$$CPP = DBP - LVEDP$$

As DBP rises or LVEDP falls, the flow will increase. Tachycardia decreases time of perfusion, since diastole is shortened. Systolic hypertension decreases perfusion, since the ventricle contracts harder, allowing less perfusion during systole. *(1:1187; 19:176)*

3. **(C)** The baroreceptors are located principally in the carotid body. These are important to the regulation of circulation. The baroreceptors respond to pressure, not to carbon dioxide or oxygen. *(1:1781; 75:184; 85:398)*

4. **(B)** At a constant stroke volume, cardiac output is a linear function of heart rate. The other factors are important in the generation of cardiac output, but they are taken into consideration with stroke volume: resistance (afterload), arterial pressure, and blood volume (preload). Cardiac output is not directly related to potassium concentration. *(1:1167; 86:1124)*

5. **(C)** Intrinsic rhythmicity is affected by anything that affects diastolic depolarization. Increased temperature increases heart rate. Digitalis decreases rhythmicity. Hypothyroidism does not increase rhythmicity. Calcium does not alter the resting membrane potential but does alter the threshold potential. Hyperkalemia decreases rhythmicity. *(19:61; 75:959; 86:1124)*

6. **(E)** Heart rate is under the predominant influence of the parasympathetic nervous system. Drugs of various categories have an influence, as do environmental influences. The adrenergic system does have a definite influence, but it is not the main factor. Blood pressure fluctuations can influence the heart rate, but it is through the baroreceptors, mediated by the vagus. *(1:1167; 86:1126)*

7. **(A)** Stroke volume is related to myocardial fiber shortening. Heart rate and peripheral resistance do not have a direct effect on stroke volume. Serum potassium and arterial oxygen saturation are not factors in regulation of stroke volume. *(1:1167; 86:1127)*

8. **(B)** Afterload is dependent on the distensibility of the arteries into which the ventricle ejects the blood. The best measure of afterload is the systemic vascular resistance (SVR). The calculation of SVR takes mean blood pressure into account. Afterload involves the aortic valve but not solely. Vasodilators decrease afterload. Ventricular size is related to afterload but is not an important consideration. *(1:1170)*

9. **(C)** The intrinsic rate of the sinoatrial node is 70 to 80 beats per minute. Since it has a faster rate, it is the dominant pacemaker. As you progress down the conduction system, the rates are slower. The atrioventricular node, eg, has an intrinsic rate of 40 to 60 beats per minute. *(15:688; 56:169)*

10. **(C)** The process of slow diastolic depolarization is a property of pacemaker cells and is the process causing intrinsic rhythmicity. The process is due to calcium changes. The higher the pacemaker, the more pronounced is the process. Therefore, it is seen less in the His bundle. *(8:5; 75:959)*

11. **(D)** Myocardial disease will decrease cardiac output. Rate increases will increase output assuming

that the stroke volume is constant. An increase in preload or a decrease in afterload will increase output. Digitalis, through an increase in contractility, will increase output. *(1:1116; 15:659)*

12. **(E)** Observation of the direct display of arterial pressure will give all of the information cited. However, Barash disputes whether one can accurately assess changes in SVR. *(1:435; 15:641; 57:20)*

13. **(E)** Heart rate is responsive to all of the factors listed except the Hering-Breuer reflex. The neural influences are predominant, with sympathetic influences increasing the rate and parasympathetic influences decreasing the rate. *(1:1167; 75:964)*

14. **(C)** At the time of the second heart sound, the mitral valve is opening. The closing of the aortic and pulmonic valves, isometric relaxation, and the T waves are all coincident. *(15:680,685; 19:7)*

15. **(A)** The drawing in reference 75 shows the typical tracing familiar to anyone who has inserted a flow-directed catheter. The right atrial pressure is about 5 mm Hg. The step-up in diastolic pressure shows the entry into the pulmonary artery. *(20:129; 21:68; 75:574)*

16. **(E)** The conduction system includes the sinoatrial node, the principal pacemaker. The impulse is transmitted through the atrial conduction pathways to the atrioventricular node and then to the bundle of His before dividing into the right and left branch bundles. The coronary sinus is not involved in impulse conduction but receives the venous drainage of the heart. *(15:688; 19:60–61)*

17. **(C)** The correct lead placement is right arm–left leg in lead II. The other leads are right arm–left arm in lead I and left arm–left leg in lead III. *(8:20; 22:422)*

18. **(E)** Excitation of the cardiac cell membrane and depolarization are accompanied by calcium entering the cell. Calcium ions increase myocardial contractile force, prolongs duration of systole, increases vascular tone, and increases ventricular automaticity. *(1:1171; 75:1501)*

19. **(A)** The ECG cannot detect efficacy of pump function. The ECG may show a normal sinus rhythm during electromechanical dissociation when the pump is not working effectively at all. The tracing can be observed for changes in electrolyte disturbance, especially calcium and potassium. Ischemia is detected by changes in the tracing. Pacemaker function is checked by observing the tracing. Arrhythmias are detected by the ECG. *(1:466; 19:55)*

20. **(E)** Blood volume determination uses the dilution effect. This test is not often performed, since its accuracy has been questioned. In general, a measured volume of a tracer is injected and allowed to circulate. A blood sample is then obtained, and the concentration of the tracer is determined. This allows a calculation of the blood volume. Questions of the completeness of circulation and other technical problems led to its disuse. *(22:114)*

21. **(B)** dP/dt is a measure of ventricular contractile force over time. *(56:163; 75:964)*

22. **(D)** Pulmonary capillary wedge pressure approximates left ventricular end-diastolic pressure. By measuring changes in cardiac output and pressures, a ventricular function curve can be drawn and therapeutic interventions evaluated. Measuring pressures on the right side of the heart will not give the information needed on the left side. Therefore, central venous pressure gives the worst approximation of left side function. *(1:444,1186; 19:14)*

23. **(C)** The curves are representative of patients who are not responding to increases in LVEDP with increases in stroke volume. These do not show any effect of increased contractility or any effect of inotropic intervention. In a given patient, inotrope administration may be the next logical step. *(1:1170; 19:14; 75:576)*

24. **(B)** A patient on such a low curve may respond to an administered inotropic agent by advancing to point B, but the patient may also react adversely and fall even farther down on the curve. This would be represented by point C. Other interventions would then be needed. It is doubtful that such a patient would advance to the normal curve or curve 2. *(1:1177; 19:14)*

25. **(B)** Echocardiography uses an ultrasound technique. These sound waves, above the audible range, are reflected from various structures in the heart and recorded. Tomography is not involved. *(1:1183; 75:108)*

26. **(C)** Coronary circulation reacts to carbon dioxide in a manner similar to cerebral circulation. Although this may be salutary in the instance of head trauma, in the patient with chest pain and ischemia, hyperventilation may lead to further decrease of coronary flow. The decrease is not an intense vasoconstriction. *(1:1192; 21:229)*

27. **(A)** Myocardial oxygen consumption is closely and directly related to cardiac rate over wide ranges. The rate–pressure product is also closely related to

myocardial oxygen consumption. An increase in stroke volume does not cause as much of an increase in oxygen as an increase in pressure. *(1:1192; 19:182)*

28. **(D)** The heart, the medullary center, the cerebral cortex, and the muscular walls of the blood vessels all play a part in the regulation of systemic circulation. There are other influences, including humoral influences, but the more correct answer is that there is a complex integrated mechanism for the control. *(1:1165; 15:648)*

29. **(B)** Since blood flow to the heart runs along pressure gradients in the upper extremities, the blood in the basilic vein runs from a site of higher pressure to a site of lower pressure, the right atrium. In the lower extremities, blood flow is assisted by valves and muscular activity. *(75:974; 113:52,99)*

30. **(B)** Venous tone varies with a number of factors. Humoral factors, such as sympathetic stimulation, can affect the venous bed. In addition, temperature-regulating mechanisms are involved. Oxygen and carbon dioxide tensions play a role in the regulation of venous tone. Changes in tone contributes to regulation of capacitance and the ability to respond to changes in blood pressure and changes in cardiac output. *(75:974; 113:197)*

31. **(A)** The microcirculatory beds are not always open but in a constantly changing state of flow. This flow is regulated by the autonomic nervous system and local factors, including the state of oxygenation. The amount of muscular investment varies with the specific structure, being higher in arteriole than in metarteriole and even less in the venules. The capillary beds, although small, hold a great amount of the blood volume at any one time. *(56:231; 113:59)*

32. **(B)** Various formulas are given for calculation of the mean pressure. In the references cited, the calculation gives a mean pressure of 120 torr.

MAP = systolic pressure + 2/3 (diastolic pressure)
(1:100; 113:88)   or $DBP + \frac{1}{3} PP$

33. **(A)** The width of the inflatable bladder must encircle only one-half the arm. In the average adult, the width of 12 to 14 cm is appropriate. In the person who is not average, spurious readings may result if a standard adult cuff is used. This is particularly true in the child, and the need for an assortment of cuffs is apparent. The manometer should be calibrated on a routine basis to ascertain that the manometer is giving true readings. The reading should always start *at* zero. *(1:102; 118:1215)*

34. **(D)** The pressure wave form may be affected by the presence of even small bubbles. The bubble, being very compliant, leads to a damping of the trace and a reading that hovers around the mean. In the reference, there is a drawing of the effects of the overdamping and underdamping of the wave form. Both systolic and diastolic pressure will be affected. *(1:100)*

35. **(E)** The plasma oncotic pressure is important in maintaining the fluid balance in the capillaries. The balance between the driving pressure and the oncotic pressure prevents tissue edema. The delicate balance can be disturbed by either increases or decreases in pressure or increases or decreases in oncotic pressure. *(22:617; 101:243)*

36. **(B)** As discussed in Question 35, pulmonary edema results from an increase in pulmonary capillary pressure. Pulmonary edema may also result from neurologic injury. Negative airway pressure pulmonary edema has been reported in the patient with airway obstruction who is breathing against a closed glottis or an occluded endotracheal tube. *(1:2216; 101:295)*

37. **(D)** The patient who develops pulmonary edema in the recovery room usually does so within the first hour. Distended neck veins or increased CVP many be absent, but the patient is usually wheezing. An occluded endotracheal tube may be the problem. *(1:1929)*

38. **(C)** The shock patient has vasodilatation. Sludging of blood is common due to an increased viscosity and hypercoagulability of the blood. Local hypoxia is present. *(56:329; 74:549)*

39. **(C)** The precapillary sphincters are sensitive to humoral factors. The sphincters regulate the flow through the capillary bed, the opening and closing of which is termed "vasomotion." Postcapillary sphincters also are present. *(56:329; 113:59)*

40. **(B)** Systolic time interval measurement is a noninvasive technique. It does not require an arterial line or a pulmonary artery line but does require a high-speed recorder. Simultaneous recordings are made of the phonocardiogram, ECG, and carotid pulse tracings. *(19:17; 74:54)*

41. **(A)** Systolic time intervals are a measure of the function of the left side of the heart. Cardiac function can be evaluated in the patient with mitral stenosis, hypertension, myocardial infarction, or aortic valvular disease, but the right atrium cannot be assessed. *(19:17; 74:55)*

42. (D) Dopamine is an inotropic agent. It does not decrease preload. The other options are all aimed at decreasing preload: rotating tourniquets by limiting the blood return, morphine by dilating the capacitance vessels, phlebotomy by decreasing the blood volume, and diuretics by decreasing blood volume. *(1:2217; 103:499)*

43. (B) The drug of choice to improve contractility is an inotropic agent. Digitalis is the only appropriate choice. Oxygen should be administered to improve oxygenation. Furosemide may be required to decrease venous return. Morphine may be appropriate to provide decreased venous return and provide sedation. Nitroglycerin may be appropriate to improve myocardial flow and to decrease afterload. *(1:2217; 103:500)*

44. (C) The failing heart attempts to compensate by salt retention and increasing blood volume. Myocardial hypertrophy occurs, and there is an increased sympathetic outflow to improve output. Ventricular filling pressure increases as the heart decompensates. *(1:1477, 1520; 24:2)*

45. (C) The Frank-Starling "law of the heart" is the underlying principle in the use of ventricular function curves. It relates preload and stroke volume. As more volume is presented, more output will occur, assuming that the heart is normal. *(1:1176; 113:149)*

46. (B) The Walton-Brodie strain gauge is a device that is sutured to the ventricle to measure contractility. It is obviously of limited clinical value. The other options are noninvasive and are of varying clinical usefulness. *(1:1180; 19:16)*

47. (D) As the size of the ventricle increases, the radius increases, and the wall tension increases. The law of LaPlace states that more tension is needed to generate the same pressure as the radius increases. This makes the heart more inefficient and requires more oxygen to pump blood. *(1:1169; 19:181)*

48. (C) Coronary perfusion is improved by slow heart rates, since most of perfusion occurs during diastole. The coronary flow is not independent of systolic pressure, since areas of the subendocardium are poorly perfused during systole. *(1:1187; 113:156)*

49. (A) As the cardiac output increases, pulmonary artery pressure increases. Other factors also are involved in pulmonary artery pressure, eg, the radius of the vessels. Vasoconstriction and vasodilatation of the pulmonary vessels occur with changes of cardiac output to regulate pulmonary vascular resistance. *(1:1120)*

50. (A) There is obviously controversy over the value of pretreatment of the hypertensive patient, as evidenced by the number of studies that have addressed the problem. Hypertension does pose a risk for the patient under anesthesia. The level of control is subject to dispute. Most people today will continue the antihypertensive regimen into the perioperative period. The cardiac output is not increased in all hypertensive patients. *(1:281; 113:92)*

51. (C) The transplanted heart has intact alpha and beta receptors. The Frank-Starling effect is intact. Atropine will not have any effect, nor will any other parasympathetically mediated drugs. The electrocardiogram is different in that it shows two P waves, the donor P wave being associated with the QRS and the P wave recipient being dissociated from the QRS. *(23:2; 75:619)*

52. (A) The increased incidence of postoperative congestive heart failure is seen in the patient with a NYHA functional class IV. Patients with less severe heart disease have not had increased problems. The remaining options are all associated with signs of heart failure and should be sought and corrected in the preoperative period. *(1:369; 24:1)*

53. (E) The anxiety seen in patients with congestive heart failure is due to increased sympathetic activity. The increased sympathetic activity is a compensatory mechanism, and it is not directly related to the low flow state, as are the other options. Memory loss, weakness, fatigue, and confusion are directly caused by low output. *(1:1521; 24:1)*

54. (A) Halothane produces a dose-related decrease in left ventricular function. It does not produce a decrease in peripheral vascular resistance. Enflurane also is associated with a decrease in ventricular function. Enflurane is associated with an increased heart rate, as is isoflurane. Isoflurane is associated with peripheral vasodilatation. *(19:104; 25:1)*

55. (C) Hypotension persisting after initiation of bypass may be a sign of aortic insufficiency. The initial hemodilution may cause decreased catecholamines and decreased viscosity. These should be transient. If persistent, one must look for other problems, eg, a persistent shunt or aortic dissection. *(1:1501; 19:346; 28:1)*

56. (A) Allowing the ventricle to overdistend can be detrimental, and most centers use a ventricular vent to decompress it. The ventricle should be kept in a nonbeating state and kept cold to lower oxygen consumption. Fibrillation should be avoided, since the oxygen cost is great. *(1:1503; 28:4)*

57. (E) Nathan found that nitrous oxide led to decreased mechanical function in areas of ischemia. This work was done in dogs. Other studies have shown that nitrous oxide may induce ischemia in an area supplied by a stenotic vessel. These studies make one question the use of nitrous oxide in a patient with ischemia. There is also an added risk of air embolus. Nitrous oxide is not innocuous. *(1:1497; 29:407)*

58. (C) The recovery room patient with hypertension should be examined to rule out hypoxia or hypercarbia. If present, these must be treated, and that takes precedence over other considerations. After you have ruled out those problems, you can proceed with a methodical assessment of the problem: retake the pressure, and if it is not life threatening, you may want to watch it or treat it with a drug. In some cases, a consultation may be in order. *(1:1936; 30:4)*

59. (A) If the patient requires treatment, a nitroprusside infusion may be initiated to begin therapy. Diazoxide may be needed if the hypertension is malignant, but it must be administered as a bolus. After control is established, longer-acting drugs may be needed and can be started at that time. *(1:1936; 30:5)*

60. (D) Isolated atrial rhythms are the least risk to the patient about to be anesthetized. Other rhythms, eg, multifocal PVCs, R-on-T disturbances, complete heart block, and bundle branch block require delineation before the patient is given an elective anesthetic, since they may be life threatening. *(1:368; 30:1)*

61. (C) The vascular tree becomes less elastic with age. Blood pressure rises with age, which may be a reflection of the loss of elasticity. The number of myofibrils decreases, and the cardiac output decreases. The cardiovascular reserve decreases as a reflection of the other changes. *(1:1802; 35:1)*

62. (D) Right ventricular function is receiving much more attention and the interdependence of the two ventricles is being appreciated to a greater degree. The right ventricle is always functional. Blood flow occurs during systole and diastole. Since there is good collateral flow, it is harder to cool the right ventricle. Pulmonary vascular resistance is hard to overcome, since the ventricle muscle is not as well developed. PEEP will be transmitted to the right ventricle, decreasing venous return. *(1:1376; 36:7)*

63. (D) The patient with hypertension presents a problem to the anesthesiologist. Should we proceed or delay the procedure? The patient with long-standing hypertension can be evaluated in regard to adequacy of treatment and control. Newly discovered hypertension should be evaluated to find a cause. Primary hypertension has many contributing factors. The cardiac output usually is normal. If the blood pressure is >110 torr diastolic, better control should be established. Once the patient is well controlled, the risk, though still present, is decreased. *(1:278; 39:2)*

64. (D) Pheochromocytoma is amenable to surgical correction. Other causes of secondary hypertension, secondary aldosteronism and renal parenchymal disease, may not be amenable. The patient with renal artery stenosis may be treated surgically if the condition is diagnosed early. If later, surgery may be of no help. *(1:278; 39:2)*

65. (B) Allen's test is used to assess the adequacy of ulnar artery flow when cannulating the radial artery. Studies have shown poor correlation with subsequent problems. The reason for this is that many of the problems are embolic in nature and will not be ascertained at the time of the Allen test. In addition to the lack of data showing correlation, there is confusion as to what is "positive" or "negative." It is better to describe the result of the test. Since the position of the wrist is important, one must ascertain that the wrist is not hyperextended when performing the test. *(1:435; 57:20; 75:566)*

66. (E) The Penaz method uses palpation of the pulse distal to the cuff as the method of detecting blood pressure. The Dinamap uses oscillation of the cuff pressure as its principle; the Infrasonde uses auscultation of the Korotkoff sounds, the Arteriosonde uses blood flow detection as the blood flows beneath the cuff. *(60:2; 75:566)*

67. (C) The most successful approach to the cannulation for CVP monitoring is the internal jugular site. CVP is still useful and gives information about the right side of the heart. It gives little data applicable to the left side if there is any ventricular disparity. The trend of CVP is more valuable than a single reading. Valuable data can be obtained from the patient in shock. *(1:439; 60:3)*

68. (A) CVP is not indicated because the patient is in an abnormal position. It is indicated in the patient in shock. Hyperalimentation, inotropic drugs, and irritating solutions should be infused through a deep line. When doing a procedure where large fluid shifts are expected, CVP is very useful and should be used. *(1:439; 60:3)*

69. (C) Iodinated tracers are not used for cardiac output determinations. The other options are used, some with more frequency than others. The Thermodilution method is the most prominent. *(1:104; 60:3)*

70. **(B)** The ideal measurement of left ventricular performance would be a left ventricular pressure measurement. Lacking this, we rely on relationships that are usually operational. In each given case, the validity of the data must be established. The central venous pressure (CVP) is not a good determinant of left-sided function. The pulmonary capillary wedge pressure gives an approximation of left atrial pressure. This relationship may not be true if there is high airway pressure. The left atrial pressure is an approximation of left ventricular end diastolic pressure. If the mitral valve is not intact, that relationship may not be true. *(1:1169; 57:20)*

71. **(E)** The precordial thump is administered to the midpart of the sternum with the fleshy part of the fist from a distance of about 8 to 12 inches. It is recommended in monitored situations. It is not recommended in children. Indiscriminate use may lead to worse arrhythmias. *(1:2125; 63:3)*

72. **(E)** The current recommendation is to attempt defibrillation with an energy level of 200 joules in an adult. If that is unsuccessful, a second attempt is made with 200 to 300 joules; if that is unsuccessful, a third attempt with 360 joules is made. It is not always indicated, and it is not always successful. *(1:2127; 63:3)*

73. **(C)** The current recommendation is that there be at least 1 second for each inhalation. The chest compressions should be at a rate of 80 to 100 per minute in an adult, and there should be a pause between every 5 compressions for a breath. The head tilt–neck lift is no longer recommended and has been supplanted by the head tilt–chin lift method. The compressions should occupy 50 to 60% of the cycle. *(1:2114; 63:1)*

74. **(C)** Atropine is the first-line drug for reducing vagal tone. Epinephrine is used for its alpha effect. Lidocaine is preferred over bretylium because of lidocaine's fewer side effects. Isoproterenol is not used first in cases of bradycardia. *(1:2128; 63:3)*

75. **(D)** Drug administration should be by central line if possible. If no central line is available, a peripheral line can be used. Femoral lines are not favored, since circulation below the diaphragm is not as good. If no access is available, the endotracheal tube may be used for administration of epinephrine, atropine, and lidocaine. Sodium bicarbonate cannot be used via the endotracheal route. *(1:2128; 63:2)*

76. **(C)** The hypothermic patient may produce potential problems but reference 65 cites work that shows that it is usually not a source of concern. Timing at the same phase of the respiratory cycle contributes to reproducibility. The temperature of the injectate must be accurate, since it is critical to the calculation. Intracardiac shunts and tricuspid regurgitation both contribute to mixing, which renders the measurement invalid. *(1:454; 65:2)*

77. **(E)** If the a and v waves are not identified in the tracing, an artificially high left ventricular filling pressure may be interpreted. Placing the transducer at the angle of Louis is appropriate. A two-point calibration of the transducer should be done. Repositioning the catheter is needed to demonstrate free flow and accurate pressure readings. The most accurate estimation of the pressures can be obtained from a readout on paper. *(65:3)*

78. **(D)** Continuous saturation monitoring of the mixed venous blood is a valuable tool if the patient's total pathophysiology is taken into consideration. It is accurate and easily calibrated. One problem, albeit a small one, is that these catheters cost about twice the amount of the standard thermodilution catheter. *(65:4)*

79. **(B)** In hypovolemic states, the pulse pressure is narrowed. Heart rate is increased to maintain cardiac output, and the neck veins are flat. Urine volume is decreased to preserve volume. The mucous membranes are pale, reflecting lower blood flow to peripheral areas. *(68:1)*

80. **(A)** The most accurate interpretation of CVP is by analysis of waveform. The catheter should not be placed in the right atrium, since perforation may occur. CVP gives an indication of fluid status but is not accurate in all patients. Patients with disparate ventricular function should be monitored by pulmonary artery catheter. It is not necessary to use a flow-directed catheter in every patient. Some can be monitored by CVP alone, and the extra risk is not warranted. *(1:440; 68:2)*

81. **(C)** A heparin flush system is indicated in pressure monitoring. When decannulating the vessel, gentle aspiration is advised to aspirate any clots or debris that may be present. The arterial catheter should be the smallest that is compatible with the need, and it should be removed as soon as possible, since the complication rate rises with the time of placement. The radial artery is a favorite site, since it has good collateral. *(1:435; 69:1)*

82. **(D)** Ventricular septal defect is associated with high pulmonary flow. The options of pulmonic stenosis, tetralogy of Fallot, and tricuspid atresia are associated with decreased blood flow to the pulmonary circuit. Coarctation of the aorta is not associated with a change in pulmonary flow. *(19:264)*

83. **(E)** Pneumothorax is a common problem with subclavian cannulation. Chylothorax is a complication of left internal jugular cannulation. There should be no brachial plexus trauma with the antecubital approach. Allen's test is not a foolproof method to determine the patency of the ulnar arch. The dorsalis pedis artery should be avoided in the patient with diabetes or peripheral vascular disease. *(1:436; 69:3)*

84. **(D)** The correct amounts of blood flow to the various organs are: kidney 25%, brain 15%, heart 5%, liver 15%, and skin 35%. *(113:5)*

85. **(A)** The patient with aortic stenosis has a rapid course once angina, syncope, and congestive heart failure occur. The size of the ventricular muscle mass increases, but the cavity size does not change. The increased size also renders the muscle more prone to ischemia. Fast heart rates will cause a low cardiac output, since ventricular filling will be compromised. In addition, coronary perfusion will suffer. Low heart rates can also be devastating, since the stroke volume is fixed. The most common problem is that of tachycardia. *(19:233; 71:1)*

86. **(A)** There are various mechanisms for the causation of arrhythmias during anesthesia. Halothane and enflurane cause arrhythmias by reentrant pathways. Halothane will cause sensitization to catecholamines. Both cocaine and ketamine are known to block the reuptake of norepinephrine. Ketamine does not cause hypotension but is usually associated with increases in blood pressure. *(1:472; 75:202,391)*

87. **(D)** Sinus bradycardia is characterized by rates of 40 to 60 beats per minute. There are many causes of bradycardia, and most do not require treatment. An exception to this general statement is the bradycardia occurring in the newborn. Any rate under 100 in the newborn is bradycardia and treatment is appropriate, since the newborn has a rate-dependent cardiac output. Sinus bradycardia is regular. Another point is that the cause must be established; if the bradycardia occurs in a patient with a sick sinus, treatment may be appropriate. *(1:477,501)*

88. **(C)** The tetralogy of Fallot includes a VSD, pulmonary outflow obstruction, overriding of the aorta, and right ventricular hypertrophy. An ASD or PDA is not part of the complex. *(19:267; 75:1233)*

89. **(E)** The preoperative ECG can be used for the detection of all the options. Chamber enlargement is readily seen in the tracing, as are some electrolyte disturbances, especially changes in calcium and potassium. Heart block is seen, as are ischemic changes. *(1:466; 19:55)*

90. **(C)** Cardiac output is a measurement of many components of the circulatory system. The typical output is 5 to 6 L/minute in an adult. Output is affected by blood volume. Cardiac output is the product of heart rate and stroke volume. *(1:1166; 19:12)*

91. **(A)** Left ventricular compliance is decreased in the patient with aortic stenosis or ischemia and in the patient receiving inotropes. It is increased in the patient on vasodilators. The typical aortic stenosis patient has a normal-sized cavity with a large myocardial mass. Small increases in fluid lead to a large increase in pressure. *(1:1168; 75:911)*

92. **(E)** Preload is affected by all the options. Volume changes are important for preload, since the volume is the chief determinant of the amount of blood returning to the heart. Venous tone plays a part by assisting venous return. Heart rate is important, since large increases in heart decrease filling time. The atrial contribution is important to ventricular filling. *(1:1169; 19:5)*

93. **(C)** Myocardial contractility is affected by both neural and humoral factors. Parasympathetic inhibition and myocardial ischemia both decrease contractility, whereas sympathetic stimulation and inotrope administration increase contractility. *(1:1171)*

94. **(B)** There are many variations of the blood supply to the heart, but the usual configuration is for a right coronary artery supplying the right side, and a left coronary that divides into the left anterior descending and the circumflex. Most of the venous drainage empties into the coronary sinus, but there are also direct connections of the thebesian veins into all chambers. *(1:1186; 75:961)*

95. **(B)** When inserting a CVP line, air embolus may occur if the catheter is left exposed to the air when the patient creates a negative pressure in the thorax. The tip should be out of the atrium to avoid perforation of that chamber. The external jugular vein is less prone to complications than the internal. The right side of the neck is preferred because of the presence of the thoracic duct on the left. *(1:441; 73:965)*

96. **(D)** Calcium administration increases myocardial contractility and increases excitability. The effect of calcium can be antagonized by calcium chelating agents, but the effect is too short for clinical use. Calcium may predispose to digitalis toxicity. *(21:9; 75:1501)*

97. **(D)** The Allen test should be described in terms of return of flow and time to return to flow, since there

is confusion in terminology regarding "positive" and "negative." There is controversy concerning the usefulness of the test in general. Extension of the wrist can itself affect perfusion. Eighty percent of patients have a complete volar arch. *(1:435; 21:55, 56; 75:567)*

98. **(E)** A satisfactory CVP line should be in the thoracic portion of the vena cava or great veins, preferably at the caval–atrium junction. It should not be in the heart chambers. To demonstrate patency and proper placement, there should be variation of pressure with respiration and aspiration should be possible. *(1:441; 21:59)*

99. **(A)** Reasons for choosing the basilic vein in preference to the cephalic are the larger size of the basilic and a straighter shot with the basilic. The basilic vein becomes larger as it proceeds proximally. The basilic vein lies medial to the cephalic vein. *(21:59; 75:570)*

100. **(E)** Cardiac output determination with the thermodilution technique uses a dilution calculation just as does the dye-dilution technique. A thermistor measures the change in temperature in the pulmonary artery. In the dye-dilution technique, changes in dye concentration are determined. Attention to detail is important, including the injection of an exact amount with a known temperature. *(1:454; 21:70)*

101. **(E)** The values are all correct. *(21:67)*

102. **(C)** Hyperventilation decreases coronary flow and can cause spasm of the coronary arteries. This effect can be suppressed by diltiazem, and the decreased flow can be treated with nitroglycerin. *(21:229; 75:961)*

103. **(B)** Many factors affect the ischemic heart. Anemia aggravates ischemia by decreasing the amount of oxygen available. Adrenergic blockade alleviates ischemia by decreasing oxygen demand. Digitalis will increase oxygen demand, but it increases the pumping function of the heart, making it more efficient. This relieves some of the ischemia. Nitroglycerin increases blood flow, which alleviates the ischemia. *(1:1194; 21:304)*

104. **(E)** Cardioplegia has improved the success rate of cardiac procedures, since it provides a relaxed heart. This factor leads to a decrease in oxygen consumption and coronary resistance. Oxygen consumption is about doubled with ventricular fibrillation. *(1:1504; 21:308)*

105. **(E)** Air embolism is a factor in many procedures but is most problematic in procedures on the aortic valve. Vents that are placed in the ventricle and aorta allow the air to escape. Some air accumulates in the pulmonary veins. This air can be evacuated by expansion of the lungs while the vents are still in place. *(21:322; 28:6)*

106. **(A)** Pacemakers are indicated for rhythm disturbances. Stokes-Adams attacks occur from episodes of bradycardia. Heart block and tachyarrhythmias are also rhythm disturbances that are amenable to pacing. Myocardial ischemia, as an isolated entity, is not an indication for pacing. *(21:413; 75:424)*

107. **(E)** All the options are methods of detecting air embolism. Measurement of end-tidal oxygen is not a good method. In the presence of air embolism, end-tidal oxygen will rise. Doppler monitoring will detect small amounts of air. Mass spectrometry measures levels of nitrogen. End-tidal carbon dioxide, which decreases with air embolism, is sensitive but requires some decrease in pulmonary blood flow before a change is noted. The esophageal stethoscope is not sensitive. *(1:1585; 20:282)*

108. **(A)** The position of the tip of the CVP catheter can be detected by the injection of 1 ml of air, but that is a dangerous method, since it can cause an air embolus. Carbon dioxide should be used. Electrocardiography can be used, looking for large P waves as the catheter is advanced. X-ray with contrast medium in the catheter is very useful. Pressure monitoring on insertion, similar to that used when inserting a pulmonary artery catheter, also is helpful. *(20:126)*

109. **(E)** Blood flow is affected by viscosity and driving force (pressure). Higher pressure increases flow. Higher viscosity decreases flow. Viscosity is increased by increased concentration of plasma proteins and elevation of hematocrit. *(56:207)*

110. **(C)** The phlebostatic axis is a reference for measuring pressures. It is the level of the heart at which there is little pressure change with change of position. It is of obvious clinical importance, since monitors must have a good reference level. The site is at the lower aspect of the atrium. *(56:224)*

111. **(C)** The vasomotor center, located in the reticular formation of the medulla and lower pons, receives input from the cortex and the hypothalamus. It secretes norepinephrine. *(56:239)*

112. **(E)** All of the structures are involved with baroreceptor activity. The carotid sinus is the most important structure involved, but baroreceptors are also present in the arch of the aorta and the wall of the great vessels of the neck. Impulses are carried to the vasomotor center by the glossopharyngeal nerve. *(8:71; 56:247; 75:184)*

113. (D) The renin–angiotensin system includes renin, which is secreted by the kidney. Renin acts on plasma angiotensinogen to form angiotensin I, which is converted to angiotensin II by converting enzyme in the lung. The entire process is set into motion by decreased blood volume. *(1:263; 56:254)*

114. (B) Postbypass neurologic changes have been attributed to hypotension and decreased perfusion while on the pump. Others have postulated that debris caused by the pump may be at fault. Attempts to improve the outcome have led to the use of barbiturates during bypass. The pulmonary artery pressure should have no direct effect. *(21:317)*

115. (A) There is a standard code for pacemakers:

1st letter:	The chamber paced
2nd letter:	The chamber sensed
3rd letter:	Mode of response
4th letter:	Programmable features
5th letter:	Dysrhythmia treatment

When treating a patient who has a pacemaker, it is important to know what kind of pacer is involved. *(1:292–293; 19:196)*

116. (C) The pacemaker threshold can respond to many bodily changes, including decreased threshold with stress. This may be related to hyperventilation and decrease in carbon dioxide, which also decreases the threshold. Increased potassium values cause a lowered threshold. Hypoxia increases the threshold. *(19:98)*

117. (D) Thebesian veins form part of the venous drainage system of the heart. The veins carry desaturated blood, and they empty into any chamber. They are part of the coronary circulatory system. Since they carry desaturated blood, they increase shunt when they empty into the left side of the heart. *(15:683; 113:155)*

118. (D) Cardiac index is an attempt to match data from various sized patients. It is calculated by dividing the patient's cardiac output by the surface area. Thus, when comparing two patients of varying size, comparison can be done on the basis of surface area. Cardiac index in an adult is about 3.5 L/minute/m^2, and in a 2-year-old, it is about 2.1 L/minute/m^2. *(1:2327; 19:12)*

119. (D) The presence of large v waves is due to some influence affecting left atrial filling. Large v waves may show evidence of mitral regurgitation. Aortic valve and tricuspid valve abnormalities should not be reflected in the measurements. It would be very difficult to insert a pulmonary artery catheter into a patient with tricuspid atresia. *(65:4)*

120. (A) Coarctation of the aorta can be the cause of hypertension. In the infant, it may be associated with congestive heart failure due to left ventricular failure. Catecholamine depletion may occur in the infant with ventricular obstruction. Coarctation of the aorta may occur as an isolated lesion in the newborn. *(1:1550; 19:263)*

121. (D) Transesophageal echocardiography is not in wide clinical use but has the advantage of being able to delineate the left ventricle very well. The right ventricular structures are also well seen. It can be used in a continuous mode. With the esophageal location, monitoring can take place with the chest open or closed. *(1:1184)*

122. (B) Lymph is essentially interstitial fluid. The flow is increased by exercise. The lymph flowing from the intestine is high in fat. Lymph is returned to the systemic circulation via the thoracic duct. *(15:668)*

123. (D) The esophageal ECG lead is the best for differentiating dysrhythmias, since it gives good P wave visualization. It is better than lead II for looking at P waves. It is not difficult to use in a clinical situation. *(1:468; 19:56)*

124. (E) The reference cites the Goldman study, which showed a correlation between all the factors listed and increased risk of anesthesia. There is not complete agreement among anesthesiologists concerning the implications of the Goldman study, but it has stimulated many studies on outcome. *(1:369)*

125. (E) Ventricular dysfunction may be detected by the several methods outlined. Ejection fraction is a relatively better predictor of survival. If the ejection fraction is <40%, there is a worse prognosis. One of the problems is that there is no good, early method of evaluating ventricular dysfunction. *(33:3)*

126. (B) Injection of medications at the time of cardiac arrest usually is problematic. If a deep line is in place, it should be used. If no line is in place, an antecubital line should be attempted first. This will allow drug administration and not interrupt resuscitation procedures. If no line is available, lidocaine, atropine, and epinephrine can be administered through the endotracheal tube. *(63:2)*

127. (A) Correct dosage at the time of arrest is mandatory knowledge of all anesthesia providers. The doses for lidocaine, epinephrine, and sodium bicarbonate are correct. The dose for isoproterenol is incorrect, since that drug is always administered by infusion, not by bolus. The infusion is titrated to effect. *(1:2126; 75:1497,1503)*

128. (A) Factors that increase cardiac output include anxiety by liberation of catecholamines. Early anoxia increases output by the same mechanism; later, if anoxia persists, the output will fall. Anemia leads to an increase as a compensatory mechanism to make up for the low oxygen-carrying capacity of the blood. Hypothyroidism leads to a decreased output. (8:45)

129. (B) Blood flow in the supine position depends on the pressure difference between the site and the atrium. In the upright position other factors are involved, eg, valves, muscular contractions, and venous tone. This is apparent in the patient with varicose veins in whom the valves function poorly. Blood flow cannot occur efficiently, and stasis occurs in the lower extremities. (8:68)

130. (E) Baroreceptors are essentially stretch receptors. They respond to actual pressure and rate of change of the pressure. Through connections to the cardioinhibitory and vasomotor centers, the receptors are able to regulate cardiac output. In the patient with chronic hypertension, the baroreceptors are reset to ignore the baseline pressure and respond only to pressures above that level. (8:71; 75:184)

131. (E) The blood supply to the spinal cord is tenuous at best. There are anterior and posterior arteries that are branches of the vertebral arteries. In addition, there are radicular arteries at several levels, which supply the cord. The largest radicular artery is the artery of Adamkiewicz. These arteries are not constant, and low perfusion pressure or ligation of a large artery may jeopardize the perfusion of the cord. (2:860; 75:949)

132. (E) The pericardium is not necessary for life, as is evidenced in the many patients who function after open heart surgery without one. The function of the pericardium is to buffer the heart from sudden movement, provide lubrication between the myocardium and adjacent structures, and minimize cardiac dilatation. (75:954)

133. (C) Propranolol should be continued into the perioperative period. It is helpful in the patient who has been receiving this drug to give a dose with the premedication and to administer doses as needed during the procedure. Calcium entry blocking agents should also be continued into the perioperative period. Antihypertensive drugs should be continued. If clonidine is one of the drugs, it is important that its usage be resumed in the postoperative period to avoid rebound hypertension. (1:1467)

134. (D) There is an interdependence of the two ventricles, and changes in the pressures on one side will have an effect on the other. The interventricular septum can shift with changes in pressure and compromise the other side. In normal inspiration, right ventricular end-diastolic volume increases, while that of the left ventricle decreases. (36:2; 75:967)

135. (C) IHSS is a form of primary myocardial disease in which there is hypertrophy of the muscle cells. This may occur in an asymmetric fashion. Contraction leads to obliteration of the ventricular cavity, and diastolic filling also is impaired. Inotropic agents cause increased functional obstruction of the outflow tract and should be avoided. Beta-blocking agents can be employed. Medical treatment is not always successful. (1:1485; 19:304)

136. (E) Afterload will decrease in any situation where less pressure is demanded of the left ventricle. Decreases in blood viscosity will decrease afterload. An arteriovenous fistula will shunt blood from the arterial side. Vasodilators make the arterial bed more expansile. Mitral regurgitation decreases the force necessary to pump blood from the left ventricle. (87:87)

137. (A) Preload, contractility, and afterload are important for determination of stroke volume. Stroke volume and heart rate are the determinants of cardiac output. (19:5; 86:1127)

138. (A) The patient with decompensated heart disease requires measures to reduce circulatory demand while simultaneously increasing the heart's contractility. If a cause can be determined, it should be eliminated when possible. Decreasing oxygen demand is another goal of treatment. (1:1521; 103:499)

139. (E) Systemic blood pressure is controlled by many factors. The autonomic nervous system is important in both regulating tone and heart rate and force of contraction. Changes in cardiac output also will affect blood pressure. As systemic vascular resistance increases, blood pressure will increase. Antidiuretic hormone will affect blood pressure by its effect on blood volume. (75:971)

140. (B) Histamine injection causes pulmonary vasoconstriction and systemic vasodilatation. There is also bronchoconstriction. The effect seen on the circulation is the same, in general, as that seen with hypoxia. (8:159; 15:375)

141. (D) An increase in mean diastolic ventricular pressure is usually reflected in the pulmonary circulation, assuming the mitral valve is competent. The increases may not have an effect on cardiac output depending on where the patient is on the Starling curve—an increase may lead to decompensation.

Treatment with diuretic leads to a decrease in volume. The increase usually is transmitted to the atrium and proximal vascular structures. *(119:205)*

142. **(A)** Mechanisms of compensation for valvular disease include chamber enlargement and ventricular hypertrophy. These are efforts to increase the contractile force. In addition, there is increased sympathetic outflow, which increases vascular tone. *(1:1477; 75:984)*

143. **(B)** Morphine has beneficial effects in the patient with acute pulmonary edema. These include its sedative effects and venous dilatation. There will be an increase in venous pressure with its administration and a decrease in respiratory activity. *(19:114; 103:499)*

144. **(E)** Acute pulmonary edema can occur with all of the options. Treatment is aimed at the cause and oxygenation of the patient. Positive pressure ventilation may be necessary. *(74:554)*

145. **(D)** Ventricular hypertrophy presents additional problems to an already injured heart. Hypertrophy increases oxygen demand. Perfusion is decreased, since diastolic pressure is decreased. The enlargement of the chamber requires an increased filling pressure. The ventricle becomes more susceptible to ischemia even in the absence of coronary artery disease. *(75:985)*

146. **(E)** This patient has the typical list of problems. One must do what is possible to limit the inequities of myocardial oxygen supply and demand. Lowering the pressure will decrease demand, as will lowering the temperature and heart rate. Administration of oxygen will increase the supply. *(1:1192)*

147. **(E)** Blood pressure can be lowered by diuretics. This is a slower method, even with the use of loop diuretics. Rotating tourniquets can decrease effective blood volume and is strictly a temporizing method. When the tourniquets are removed, the volume is still present. Phlebotomy is another method but is fraught with the hazard of taking off too much and thereby decreasing oxygen-carrying capacity and causing hypotension. Vasodilators are easy to start and monitor. Titration is important. *(74:555)*

148. **(B)** Cerebral symptoms occurring after cardiopulmonary bypass have been attributed to the presence of cerebrovascular disease and hypoperfusion while on the pump. There are probably other factors involved, eg, emboli of debris or air. Heparin and protamine have not been indicted. *(19:382; 75:999)*

149. **(D)** A water-hammer pulse is seen in the patient with aortic insufficiency. The patient with pericardial effusion will have a pulsus paradoxicus. The cardiac output is decreased. The neck veins are distended and stay distended in the supine position, since little drainage can occur. Blood pressure will decrease. *(1:1487; 75:425)*

150. **(A)** Pulsus paradoxicus is an exaggeration of the normal variation in the pulse with inspiration. The pulse reduces in amplitude on inspiration. In the exaggerated state of pericardial effusion, the pulse may show alternate strong and weak beats. *(15:642; 19:296)*

151. **(D)** Monitoring this patient does not require a pulmonary artery catheter. The right side of the heart should be monitored, and this can be done with a central venous catheter. An arterial line would be helpful. X-ray, once the diagnosis is established, is of little value. *(19:11,297; 122:451)*

152. **(D)** The anesthetic management of the patient with pericardial effusion is very demanding. One must maintain the cardiac output that is present. There is very little to do to improve it. Any vasodilator may cause circulatory collapse. Cardiodepressants must be avoided. Some believe that ketamine is the drug of choice. *(19:296; 75:425)*

153. **(E)** Coronary circulation is influenced by oxygen saturation and by cardiac output. The coronary flow is autoregulated to maintain flow in the pressure range of 50 to 120 torr. Autoregulation is through oxygen levels, but functions through the action of adenosine as an intermediary. *(1:1190; 75:962)*

154. **(D)** Myocardial oxygen consumption is increased by isoproterenol, due in part to increased rate and in part to increased pressure. Consumption is increased by digitalis and decreased by nitroglycerin. *(1:1194; 75:981)*

155. **(A)** The calculation requires mean arterial pressure, mean central venous pressure, and cardiac output. Pulmonary pressure is not needed. *(75:963)*

156. **(B)** Venous return is the chief determinant of preload. As the right atrial pressure increases, return will fall. Muscular contractions, especially in the lower extremities, aid in venous return. The venous valves also assist in venous return. *(15:643; 75:974)*

157. **(C)** Oxygen consumption under anesthesia will fall about 15%. It will fall more in the patient who is excited before going to sleep, since that patient has a higher consumption. The fall in consumption is not affected by premedication or tidal volume. *(75:302)*

158. (C) Goals for anesthetic management of the patient with coronary artery disease include maintaining contractility and maintaining sinus rhythm. One wants to avoid a high afterload and a high heart rate. These factors apply to the patient for cardiac or noncardiac surgery. *(75:982)*

159. (A) The capillary bed is the site of gas and nutrient exchange between blood and tissues. The bed is seldom open to full capacity but is regulated by the metarterioles and precapillary sphincters. Local physical and chemical factors play a role in the flow through the capillary bed, but capillaries themselves are not regulated by the autonomic nervous system. *(15:664)*

160. (C) The mitral stenosis patient usually has increased left atrial pressure because of poor outflow from the atrium. The right ventricle is enlarged, and the left ventricle is not enlarged. Cardiac output is decreased due to the decreased left ventricular preload. *(75:989)*

161. (B) Depolarization of the cardiac muscle cell (phase 0) corresponds to the QRS. Phase 1 is the beginning of the repolarization. Phase 2 is a plateau and represents a recovery phase. Phase 3 is repolarization and is responsible for the T wave. Phase 4 is diastolic depolarization in the automatic cell. In the nonpacemaker cell, phase 4 restores resting membrane potential pending another depolarization. *(1:501; 75:592)*

162. (C) Phase 4 of the action potential is responsible for pacemaking activity in some cells. The changes are due to fluxes of sodium and potassium. Diastolic depolarization is seen in pacemaker cells only. *(75:959)*

163. (B) Stimulation of the vagus slows the heart but does not affect contractility, since the vagus does not affect the ventricle directly. Vagal stimulation slows conduction and decreases excitability. *(75:171)*

164. (B) Stimulation of the sympathetic fibers to the heart increases the rate and enhances the conduction. The sympathetic fibers are more directed to the ventricle. Systole is decreased, and the contractions are strengthened. *(75:171)*

165. (D) The coronary sinus receives blood that is very desaturated, having passed through the myocardial tissues that extract most of the oxygen. The sinus is the major venous drainage system of the heart. It receives about 75% of the coronary blood flow. The blood from the coronary sinus drains into the right atrium. *(15:683)*

166. (D) The pulmonary arterial circulation is derived from the pulmonary artery arising from the right ventricle. The arterioles accompany each bronchiole and are invested with thin muscle coats. There is a broad capillary network. *(15:673)*

167. (B) The bronchial arteries are part of the systemic circulation, although they are rich in anastomoses with the pulmonary artery. The bronchial arteries arise from the aorta. They drain into the azygos vein. *(15:672; 75:951)*

168. (E) The pulmonary circulation from the right side of the heart is very expansile, being able to absorb large increases in blood due to increases in cardiac output. The circulation time in the pulmonary circuit is about 11 seconds. The pulmonary circuit holds about 400 to 600 ml at any one time. *(15:673)*

169. (A) The Valsalva maneuver causes a decrease of blood return to the right ventricle due to increased intrathoracic pressure. This also leads to an increased venous pressure in the head. Cardiac output falls during the pressure increase. There is a reflex decrease in heart rate. *(75:969)*

CHAPTER 3

The Nervous and Excretory Systems: Fluids, Electrolytes, and Temperature Regulation
Review

Know

The basic unit of the nervous system is the neuron, which has a cell body, an axon, and one or more dendrites (Figure 3–1). The axon may be very long. In some cases, the axon is myelinated, the myelin sheath being interrupted at the nodes of Ranvier. Postganglionic fibers in the autonomic nervous system are not myelinated.

Nerve impulses pass along the axons by way of a self-propagating process that involves the development of an action potential and the propagation of the impulse. The action potential is all or none once the threshold is reached. Propagation involves ion fluxes just as in muscle transmission.

Nerve fibers vary in type and function:

TYPE	FUNCTION	DIAMETER (μm)
A alpha	Somatic motor	6–20
beta	Touch and pressure	6–20
gamma	Muscle spindles	3–6
delta	Pain, touch, temperature	1–4
B	Preganglionic	3
C Dorsal root	Pain, temperature, touch	0.4–1.2
Postganglionic	Vasomotor, visceromotor	0.4–1.2

The brain is composed of gray matter (cell bodies) and white matter (nerve tracts). It is divided into lobes and special areas of function (Figure 3–2). The frontal lobe is an association area. The temporal lobe contains the auditory areas; the parietal lobe contains the central gyrus with its important areas of motor (precentral) and sensory (postcentral) function. The occipital lobe is important for visual function.

The two hemispheres are connected in the midline by the corpus callosum. This is made up of fibers that originate in one hemisphere and terminate in the other.

The basal ganglia lie deep within the cerebral hemispheres. They are composed of the caudate nucleus, the putamen, globus pallidus, the subthalamic nucleus, and the substantia nigra. This area is important in motor function. Parkinson's disease has its origin in this area.

The cerebellum sits at the base of the brain in the midline. It is responsible for coordination of motor activity.

The brainstem contains the medulla oblongata and the pons. These two areas contain many of the fiber tracts and the centers that regulate bodily functions, such as respiration. This area also contains the reticular activating system, which is a diffuse area of excitatory and inhibitory tracts that modulate the inputs from above and below. The reticular activating system is responsible for maintaining the conscious, alert state. Lesions in any of these areas may have serious consequences.

The electroencephalogram (EEG) is the display of electrical activity within the brain. Various waveforms and activity patterns have been described:

Alpha waves have a frequency of 8 to 13 cycles per second. These waves are typical in the awake, resting state.

B   13–30/2.
A   8–13 /r
T   4–7 /~
D   ∠4

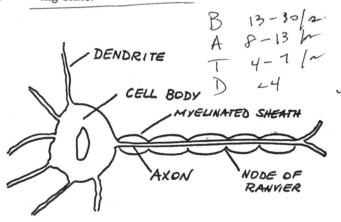
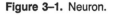

DENDRITE
CELL BODY
MYELINATED SHEATH
AXON
NODE OF RANVIER

Figure 3–1. Neuron.

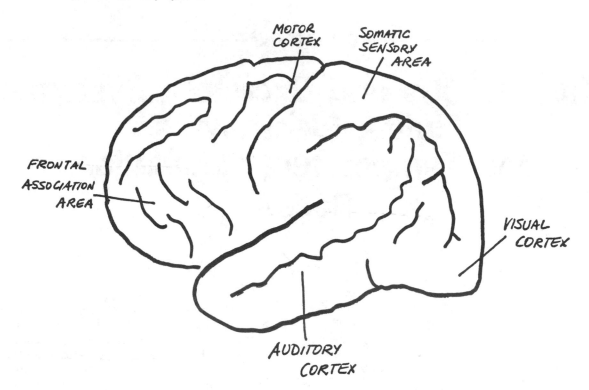

Figure 3–2. Cerebral Cortex.

Beta waves are seen with mental stimulation. The frequency is 13 to 30 per second.

Theta waves are seen most commonly in children. The frequency is 4 to 7 per second.

Delta waves have a frequency of <4 cycles per second and are seen in deep sleep.

Recent methods of monitoring the EEG by computer applications have been marketed. These monitors process the information received and present it in a more usable format. This eventually may make it feasible to monitor the depth of anesthesia in each patient. At the present time, the use is mostly limited to anesthesia for carotid endarterectomy and cardiopulmonary bypass.

The spinal cord extends from the medulla oblongata to the lower edge of the first lumbar vertebra (Figure 3–3). It is composed of gray and white matter. The gray matter contains the cells of neurons. The white matter contains the tracts to and from the brain.

The cerebrospinal fluid (CSF) is formed by the choroid plexus in the ventricles of the brain. It is formed by an active transport process (66%) and passive filtration (33%). This fluid is important as a buffer against increases in intracranial pressure, and it acts as a cushion against sudden movements. The total volume is 100 to 150 ml, but the turnover is rapid, the total formation being at a rate of 0.35 ml/min.

The specific gravity of CSF is 1.003 to 1.009. The pH is 7.33. The bicarbonate level is about equal to plasma, but the P_{CO_2} is higher.

Pain is an unpleasant sensation and is divided into two types, somatic pain and visceral pain. Somatic pain is localized to the skin, muscle, tendons, and so on. Its origin is readily identified. Visceral pain, on the other hand, is vague, and its location cannot be pinpointed. It may be associated with nausea and may be referred to other areas.

There are several theories about the cause and pathways of pain. In general, most believe that the dorsal horn is involved and that there are facilitory and inhibitory pathways involved. There is, in addition, an overlay from the cortex. Transmitter substances, substance P, and enkephalins may be involved. There is a great deal of research into the cause and relief of pain at the present time.

RENAL FUNCTION

The functional unit of the kidney is the nephron. This unit is composed of the glomerulus, the proximal convoluted tubules, the loop of Henle, and the distal convoluted tubule. These empty into the collecting ducts. As the ascending loop of Henle approaches the glomerulus, there is an area in which the cells are more closely packed, the macula densa. This area is the site of the cells that contain renin. Renin is released at the time of hypotension to maintain renal blood flow.

Filtration is accomplished by the pressure generated by the heart. This causes enough pressure to force water and crystalloids across the cell membrane. Proteins and

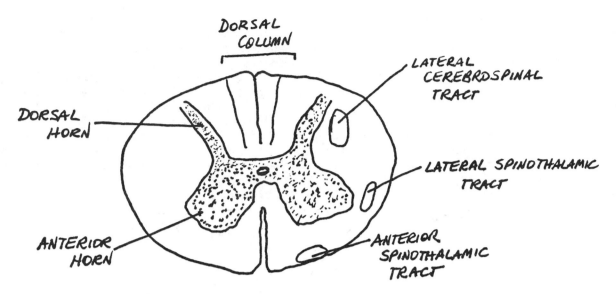

Figure 3–3. Spinal Cord.

substances with a larger molecular weight are retained as long as the membrane is intact.

Most of the sodium that is filtered is reabsorbed by the kidney as the sodium passes through the tubular system. Some of the sodium is reabsorbed as a result of the countercurrent mechanism in the loops of Henle, and some is the result of the action of antidiuretic hormone on the distal collecting tubules. The final osmolality of the urine is governed by the action of antidiuretic hormone.

FLUIDS AND ELECTROLYTES

Body homeostasis is dependent on the rigid control of the fluid volume and electrolyte composition. Total body water constitutes about 60% of the total body weight.

Distribution of the electrolytes varies with the compartment being discussed. As can be seen in Figure 3–4, sodium is the most important extracellular ion, and potassium is the important intracellular ion. The compartments must be maintained in the proper volume, concentration, and composition.

Extracellular volume is subject to change by variation in intake and variation in losses. Most of the increases in intake are due to overaggressive fluid therapy. Increased losses are due to fluid shifts at the time of illness or to overt loss from vomiting, diarrhea, or diuresis. Intracellular volume changes usually follow extracellular changes and may not be as apparent. Intracellular volume changes require more time for correction.

The composition and concentration of the body fluids are under the control of the kidney. The volume and composition of urine that is excreted vary with the bodily needs and is under the control of antidiuretic hormones. This allows the body to retain what is necessary for stability

Rapid changes in the acid-base balance of the body are prevented by an elaborate buffering system, which includes bicarbonate, hemoglobin, proteins, and phosphate. Any challenge is immediately reacted to by this system to maintain homeostasis. The body is able to do a remarkable job if the kidneys are intact and glomerular filtration is maintained. During periods of shock, cardiac

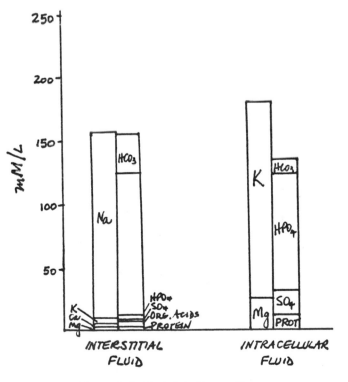

Figure 3–4. Electrolyte Composition.

output is not maintained, and homeostatic mechanisms are stressed

TEMPERATURE REGULATION

The body maintains the temperature in a narrow range that may vary throughout the day. This diurnal variation is lowest in the morning and highest during times of activity. Temperature control is maintained by the hypothalamus

There are various mechanisms that come into play at times of cold: shivering, hunger, involuntary activity, cutaneous vasoconstriction, and curling up to maintain heat. These factors either generate heat or decrease heat loss. Methods to remove heat include vasodilatation, sweating, increased respiration, inertia, and anorexia.

In the patient under anesthesia, the body temperature will tend to reach the ambient temperature. Muscle relaxants prevent shivering, major cavities may be exposed, vessels may dilate, and cold fluids may be administered. This places the patient at risk for hypothermia.

There is a set point at which the temperature is maintained. At times of illness or under drug therapy, eg, salicylates, the set point will change. This is regulated by the hypothalamus.

Questions

DIRECTIONS (Questions 1 through 51): Each of the numbered items or incomplete statements in this section is followed by answers or by completions of the statement. Select the ONE lettered answer or completion that is BEST in each case.

1. Body temperature may change intraoperatively because of all the following EXCEPT

   (A) exposure
   (B) intravenous fluids
   (C) muscle relaxants
   (D) humidification
   (E) oxygen concentration

2. Heat production in the body is decreased by

   (A) shivering
   (B) hunger
   (C) activity
   (D) secretion of epinephrine
   (E) anorexia

3. The temperature-regulating mechanism is in the

   (A) forebrain
   (B) pons
   (C) thalamus
   (D) hypothalamus
   (E) cerebellum

4. The stimulus for the temperature-regulatory center is

   (A) the epinephrine level of the blood
   (B) a hormone released from muscle cells
   (C) the temperature of the blood perfusing the center
   (D) the cerebral cortical input
   (E) the afferents from piloerector muscles

5. Total body water in an adult constitutes

   (A) 20% of body weight
   (B) 30% of body weight
   (C) 40% of body weight
   (D) 50% of body weight
   (E) 60% of body weight

6. If 1 g molecular weight of a nonionized substance is dissolved in 1 L of solution, the concentration is

   (A) 1 osmolar
   (B) 1 osmolal
   (C) 1 milliequivalent
   (D) 1 molar
   (E) 1 equivalent

7. The principal intracellular ion is

   (A) Na_+
   (B) K_+
   (C) Cl_-
   (D) HCO_3
   (E) Mg^{++}

8. Magnesium

   (A) concentration is related to irritability of nervous tissue
   (B) concentration is low intracellularly
   (C) is not excreted in the urine
   (D) is not present in bile
   (E) is not present in gastric juice

9. Ringer's lactate contains all of the following ions EXCEPT

   (A) sodium
   (B) potassium
   (C) chloride
   (D) calcium
   (E) bicarbonate

10. The circulation to the kidney

   (A) is autoregulated over a blood pressure range of 80 to 180 torr
   (B) is not regulated by neural factors
   (C) is innervated by sympathetic nerves originating in T2–T3
   (D) is not affected by epinephrine
   (E) is constricted by prostaglandin E_2

11. The glomerulus contains

    (A) an artery, a vein, and a tubule
    (B) only a tuft of capillaries
    (C) a nephron
    (D) an ascending limb and a descending limb
    (E) the macula densa

12. The countercurrent mechanism of the kidney involves

    (A) the nephron and the glomerulus
    (B) the arteries and veins
    (C) a collecting duct and a distal tubule
    (D) the loops of Henle and the vasa recta
    (E) the proximal tubule and the distal tubule

13. Hydrogen ion (H^+)

    (A) is secreted by the proximal and distal renal tubules
    (B) is not actively transported across the renal tubular cell
    (C) is exchanged for bicarbonate
    (D) is not related to the movement of other ions
    (E) movement is unrelated to HCO_3^- in the kidney

14. The liver biotransforms drugs to compounds that can be more easily excreted by the kidneys. This involves all of the following EXCEPT

    (A) oxidation
    (B) auto-oxidation
    (C) reduction
    (D) conjugation
    (E) hydrolysis

15. Glucuronyl transferase

    (A) is important in renal clearance of nitrogen
    (B) is needed to convert bilirubin to water-insoluble bilirubin glucuronide
    (C) is produced in the smooth endoplasmic reticulum
    (D) production is decreased after barbiturate administration
    (E) is important only for the conjugation of bilirubin

16. The enterohepatic circulation

    (A) describes the storage of bile in the gallbladder
    (B) is most important for the reabsorption of bile salts
    (C) is unimportant in the liver metabolism of drugs
    (D) allows all the reabsorbed substances to avoid the systemic circulation
    (E) is possible only with conjugated compounds

17. Jaundice may result from all of the following EXCEPT

    (A) excessive production of bilirubin
    (B) increased uptake of bilirubin into hepatic cells
    (C) intrahepatic obstruction of ducts
    (D) disturbed intracellular binding of bilirubin
    (E) disturbed secretion of bilirubin into the canaliculi

18. The liver receives its blood supply from

    (A) a branch of the aorta only
    (B) the portal vein only
    (C) both the aortic branch and the portal vein
    (D) vessels that run in the center of the lobules
    (E) the hepatic artery, which drains completely into the portal vein

19. The condition referred to as meralgia paresthetica is caused by entrapment of the

    (A) peroneal nerve
    (B) sciatic nerve
    (C) lateral femoral cutaneous nerve
    (D) median nerve
    (E) posterior tibial nerve

20. The total volume of cerebrospinal fluid (CSF) in the adult is

    (A) 10 to 20 ml
    (B) 20 to 40 ml
    (C) 40 to 60 ml
    (D) 60 to 100 ml
    (E) 120 to 150 ml

21. Cerebrospinal fluid (CSF) is

    (A) a true secretion
    (B) produced in the lumbar area
    (C) formed in the cerebellum
    (D) produced in the cerebral cortex
    (E) produced in the pons

22. The sciatic nerve is formed by all of the following EXCEPT the

    (A) third lumbar root
    (B) fourth lumbar root
    (C) fifth lumbar root
    (D) first sacral root
    (E) second sacral root

23. The normal cerebrospinal fluid (CSF) pressure (recumbent) is

    (A) 20 cm water
    (B) 20 mm water
    (C) 110 mm water
    (D) 110 cm water
    (E) 50 mm water

24. Absorption of cerebrospinal fluid (CSF) takes place through

   (A) ependymal cells
   (B) arachnoid villi
   (C) the pia mater
   (D) the foramen of Monro
   (E) the foramen of Magendie

25. Cerebrospinal fluid (CSF) flows through all of the following EXCEPT the

   (A) choroid plexus
   (B) cerebral ventricle
   (C) lateral ventricle
   (D) subarachnoid space
   (E) epidural space

26. The specific gravity of cerebrospinal fluid (CSF) is

   (A) 1.000 to 1.003
   (B) 1.100 to 1.200
   (C) 1.003 to 1.009
   (D) 1.200 to 1.300
   (E) under 1.000

27. A large nerve fiber associated with transmission of deep touch and temperature is the

   (A) A-alpha fiber
   (B) A-beta fiber
   (C) A-gamma fiber
   (D) B fiber
   (E) C fiber

28. A small preganglionic autonomic nerve fiber is the

   (A) A-alpha fiber
   (B) A-beta fiber
   (C) A-gamma fiber
   (D) B fiber
   (E) C fiber

29. The smallest nerve fiber, a postganglionic fiber associated with slow conduction is the

   (A) A-alpha fiber
   (B) A-beta fiber
   (C) A-gamma fiber
   (D) B fiber
   (E) C fiber

30. A medium-sized nerve fiber that is an efferent to the muscle spindle is the

   (A) A-alpha fiber
   (B) A-beta fiber
   (C) A-gamma fiber
   (D) B fiber
   (E) C fiber

31. The largest nerve fiber, associated with fast conduction and motor function, is the

   (A) A-alpha fiber
   (B) A-beta fiber
   (C) A-gamma fiber
   (D) B fiber
   (E) C fiber

32. Hepatic blood flow

   (A) is closely regulated during surgery and anesthesia
   (B) increases with arterial hypoxemia
   (C) is decreased with sympathetic stimulation
   (D) is closely regulated by dopamine
   (E) responds slowly to bodily needs

33. The liver affects glucose metabolism by all of the following mechanisms EXCEPT

   (A) glycogen storage
   (B) gluconeogenesis
   (C) glycogenolysis
   (D) insulin production
   (E) conversion of glycerol to glucose

34. The rate-limiting factor in liver metabolism of fat is

   (A) the number of chylomicrons
   (B) acetyl-CoA
   (C) cholesterol levels
   (D) glucagon levels
   (E) glucose availability

35. Unconjugated bilirubin

   (A) is nontoxic
   (B) is secreted into the intestinal tract
   (C) is the product of white cell breakdown
   (D) is conjugated with glucuronic acid
   (E) breaks down to biliverdin

36. Ascites

   (A) follows chronic decreased portal vein pressure
   (B) follows periods of hyperalbuminemia
   (C) is usually accompanied by hypernatremia
   (D) may have a severe cardiorespiratory effect
   (E) should be removed rapidly to avoid reaccumulation

37. Broca's area is

   (A) in the dominant hemisphere
   (B) an area is the cerebellum
   (C) in the sensory cortex
   (D) in the lateral spinal tract of the cord
   (E) an area associated with speech

38. The structure connecting the two hemispheres is the

    (A) posterior commissure
    (B) massa intermedius
    (C) anterior commissure
    (D) cingulate gyrus
    (E) corpus callosum

39. The area of the brain concerned with auditory sensation is the

    (A) parietal lobe
    (B) occipital lobe
    (C) superior temporal lobe
    (D) postcentral gyrus
    (E) precentral gyrus

40. An intention tremor may follow injury or pathophysiology to the area of the

    (A) temporal cortex
    (B) cerebellum
    (C) frontal cortex
    (D) limbic system
    (E) pons

41. Parkinson's disease is associated with dysfunction of the

    (A) cerebellum
    (B) lateral ventricle
    (C) pons
    (D) basal ganglia
    (E) aqueduct of Sylvius

42. The cerebellum is primarily concerned with

    (A) coordination of muscle activity
    (B) vision
    (C) auditory sensation
    (D) olfactory sensation
    (E) respiration

43. The nerve root that supplies the skin sensation to the lateral aspect of the heel is

    (A) L4
    (B) L5
    (C) S1
    (D) S2
    (E) S3

44. The foramen of Monro connects the

    (A) lateral ventricles
    (B) 3rd ventricle to the lateral ventricle
    (C) 3rd ventricle to the 4th ventricle
    (D) 4th ventricle to the spinal arachnoid system
    (E) cisterna magna to the 4th ventricle

45. The electroencephalographic (EEG) waveform with a frequency range of 8 to 10 Hz is associated with

    (A) alpha activity
    (B) beta activity
    (C) theta activity
    (D) delta activity
    (E) gamma activity

46. The compressed spectral array (CSA) recording of the electroencephalogram (EEG)

    (A) is more accurate than a standard tracing
    (B) presents data in a format of amplitude, time, and frequency
    (C) is more accurate for determination of sudden events
    (D) requires no training for interpretation
    (E) should be in use for all neurosurgical procedures

47. Somatosensory evoked potentials (SSEP)

    (A) are disrupted by small doses of thiopental
    (B) are not affected by deep levels of halothane anesthesia
    (C) are evaluated from the standpoint of amplitude only
    (D) are rendered unreadable by neuromuscular blocking agents
    (E) are little affected by nitrous oxide

48. Magnetic resonance imaging (MRI)

    (A) gives superior anatomic resolution when compared with computed tomography (CT)
    (B) requires general anesthesia in most cases
    (C) is much faster than CT
    (D) is preferable for the diagnosis of abscess formation in patients with Harrington rods in place
    (E) uses the same anesthetic technique as CT if anesthesia is needed

49. The lateral spinal column

    (A) is made up of gray matter
    (B) is only motor
    (C) is only sensory
    (D) contains the anterior horn cells
    (E) contains ascending and descending tracts

50. The substantia gelatinosa

    (A) has the highest concentration of opioid receptors in the spinal cord
    (B) is located in the lateral columns
    (C) is part of the dorsal column
    (D) is in the motor area of the brain
    (E) is in the ventral column

51. Which of the following is NOT involved in sensory transmission?

(A) dorsal root ganglion
(B) spinothalamic tract
(C) parietal cortex
(D) ventral, posterior, and lateral nuclei of the thalamus
(E) precentral gyrus

DIRECTIONS (Questions 52 through 100): For each of the items in this section, <u>ONE</u> or <u>MORE</u> of the numbered options is correct. Choose the answer

> **A if only <u>1, 2, and 3</u> are correct,**
> **B if only <u>1 and 3</u> are correct,**
> **C if only <u>2 and 4</u> are correct,**
> **D if only <u>4</u> is correct,**
> **E if <u>all</u> are correct.**

52. Proteins synthesized in the liver include

(1) haptoglobin
(2) ceruloplasmin
(3) alpha$_1$-antitrypsin
(4) antithrombin III

53. Albumin

(1) synthesis is higher in the neonate
(2) is the major serum protein
(3) is necessary for maintenance of oncotic pressure
(4) has a half-life of 20 days

54. Facts affecting interpretation of liver function tests include

(1) albumin is a good indicator of hepatocyte function but has a long half-life
(2) coagulation factors have a short half-life, therefore reflect recent changes
(3) dye-removal tests are not specific
(4) bilirubin tests are not specific for liver function

55. Hematocrit values in patients with cirrhosis may reflect

(1) coagulation disorders
(2) increased plasma volume
(3) bleeding
(4) megaloblastic anemia

56. Inhibitory transmitters in the central nervous system include

(1) dopamine
(2) glycine
(3) serotonin
(4) gamma-aminobutyric acid (GABA)

57. The reticular formation

(1) is located in the cerebellum
(2) has inhibitory function
(3) has only sensory input
(4) has excitatory function

58. Reabsorption of sodium occurs in the

(1) proximal tubule
(2) ascending loop of Henle
(3) distal tubule
(4) collecting tubule

59. Antidiuretic hormone (ADH)

(1) is under control of osmoreceptors in the hypothalamus
(2) is from the posterior pituitary
(3) is inhibited by increased stretch of the atria. baroreceptors
(4) acts on the proximal convoluted tubule

60. The decreased urinary volume seen in patients on PEEP is due to

(1) decreased renal blood flow
(2) increased sympathetic outflow
(3) release of renin
(4) antidiuretic hormone (ADH) release

61. Drug transformation mechanisms in the liver include

(1) oxidation
(2) reduction
(3) hydrolysis
(4) conjugation

62. Extracellular buffers include

(1) hemoglobin
(2) plasma proteins
(3) bicarbonate
(4) phosphates

63. Dextrose 5% solutions should be omitted in patients

(1) for transurethral resection (TUR) of the prostate
(2) for appendectomy
(3) for intracranial procedures
(4) with diabetes

64. Extracellular fluid status

(1) is best determined by laboratory values
(2) is not important for the conduct of anesthesia
(3) is best evaluated by blood pressure determination
(4) may be reflected in heart rate

<table>
<tr><td colspan="5" align="center">SUMMARY OF DIRECTIONS</td></tr>
<tr><td>A</td><td>B</td><td>C</td><td>D</td><td>E</td></tr>
<tr><td>1, 2, 3
only</td><td>1, 3
only</td><td>2, 4
only</td><td>4
only</td><td>All are
correct</td></tr>
</table>

65. Treatment of hyperkalemia includes

(1) elimination of exogenous sources
(2) correction of cause of endogenous sources
(3) administration of glucose with insulin
(4) administration of acidifying solutions

66. Blood volume

(1) of an adult is 5 L
(2) is comprised 60% of plasma
(3) averages 70 ml/kg in an adult
(4) does not include red blood cells

67. The osmolarity of plasma

(1) is 280 m0sm/L
(2) is higher than in interstitial fluid
(3) is predominantly an effect of sodium and chloride
(4) favors shifts of fluid out of capillaries

68. An isotonic fluid

(1) exerts the same osmotic pressure as plasma
(2) should always be used for fluid therapy
(3) is 0.9% sodium chloride
(4) should not contain glucose

69. Effect(s) of vasopressin include(s)

(1) production of dilute urine
(2) antidiuresis
(3) decreased urine osmolality
(4) vasoconstriction

70. The syndrome of inappropriate antidiuretic hormone release (SIADH) includes

(1) hyponatremia
(2) low serum osmolality
(3) excessive renal secretion of sodium
(4) normal renal function

71. Magnesium

(1) is an intracellular cation
(2) is mobilized from stores in bone
(3) is needed for protein and enzyme synthesis
(4) is bound to plasma proteins

72. Parenteral nutrition

(1) with lipids can be administered by peripheral vein

(2) has a low incidence of phlebitis if the dextrose concentration is kept below 5%
(3) uses lipids as an important source of calories
(4) uses protein as a calorie source

73. The blood supply to the liver is by two vessels, the hepatic artery and the portal vein. These vessels differ in that

(1) 60% of the blood supply comes from the hepatic artery
(2) the portal vein provides 50% of the oxygen supply
(3) the portal vein blood is more fully saturated than the hepatic artery
(4) the portal vein supplies the bulk of the nutrients to the liver

74. Clotting factor(s) that is (are) vitamin K dependent is (are)

(1) factor I
(2) factor VII
(3) factor V
(4) factor X

75. Autoregulation of the hepatic blood flow

(1) involves the hepatic artery
(2) involves the portal vein
(3) is via the sympathetic nervous system
(4) is via the parasympathetic nervous system

76. During hypotension from hemorrhage

(1) the hepatic vessels dilate to accept increased flow
(2) the sympathetic nervous system output increases
(3) anesthetic agents may assist with compensation
(4) the liver may squeeze 350 to 500 ml of blood into the circulation

77. A typical nerve cell has

(1) numerous dendrites that branch out
(2) three or four axons to conduct impulses
(3) a dendritic zone that is a receptor membrane
(4) a myelin sheath that covers the entire cell

78. Cerebrospinal fluid (CSF) is formed

(1) by ultrafiltration through the choroid plexus
(2) by a process requiring energy
(3) according to need, increasing greatly if needed
(4) in an amount of about 12 ml per day under normal conditions

79. Acid-base studies of cerebrospinal fluid (CSF) show

(1) a pH of 7.32
(2) a P_{CO_2} of 36

(3) that the pH level is quickly changed by alteration of blood P_{CO_2}

(4) a bicarbonate of 55

80. A typical reflex arc includes

(1) a sense organ
(2) an afferent neuron
(3) an efferent neuron
(4) one or more synapses in a central integrating station

81. The electroencephalogram (EEG)

(1) alone is sufficient for the diagnosis of brain death, because a flat line is synonymous with death
(2) will reflect increased cortical activity with hypercapnia
(3) is not useful in the diagnosis of convulsive disorder
(4) will not be affected by hysterical fits

82. The reticular activating system (RAS)

(1) is a specific area with a specific pathway system
(2) is located in the cerebral cortex
(3) has input from the spinal cord only
(4) produces the conscious, alert state that makes perception possible

83. Transmitter substance(s) that is (are) present in the central nervous system include

(1) acetylcholine
(2) dopamine
(3) serotonin
(4) vasopressin

84. The act of vomiting is an integrated activity that includes

(1) activation of the vomiting center in the cerebral cortex
(2) the closing of the glottis
(3) the closure of esophageal and gastric cardiac sphincters
(4) activation of the chemoreceptor trigger zone in the area postrema

85. A cirrhotic patient

(1) cannot produce normal amounts of protein as a result of hepatocyte dysfunction
(2) will always have jaundice, since bilirubin will accumulate
(3) may not break down succinylcholine normally
(4) will not be able to break down lidocaine as a result of a lack of cholinesterase

86. The liver disease that results from alcohol ingestion

(1) can be prevented by a nutritious diet
(2) is usually present without hematologic involvement
(3) does not involve any gastrointestinal disorders
(4) is usually accompanied by vitamin deficiency

87. The effect of anesthesia on hepatic function is

(1) primarily due to toxic effects of the agents
(2) due to the effect of blood flow to the liver
(3) unaffected by the site of surgery
(4) independent of type used, ie, general or spinal

88. The glomerular capillaries

(1) originate from a small afferent and drain into a larger efferent arteriole
(2) are an extension of Bowman's capsule
(3) are many layers thick
(4) are the only capillaries in the body that drain into arterioles

89. Vasopressin

(1) is an antidiuretic hormone
(2) increases the permeability of the collecting duct to water
(3) is secreted by the posterior pituitary
(4) acts throughout the nephron system

90. Osmotic diuresis

(1) is produced only with agents administered intravenously
(2) is produced by agents that are filtered but not absorbed
(3) is caused by increased glomerular filtration rate (GFR)
(4) may follow if a substance is present in an amount exceeding the reabsorption capacity of the tubule

91. The secretion of ammonia by the kidney

(1) takes place in the proximal tubules, the distal tubules, and the collecting ducts
(2) involves combination with hydrogen ion to form ammonium ion
(3) depends on the pH of the tubular fluid
(4) increases in states of acidosis

92. Sweating may occur as a

(1) thermal-regulating mechanism
(2) response to anoxia
(3) response to emotional stimuli
(4) general reaction to sympathetic stimuli

$$pH = \log_{10} \frac{1}{H}$$

SUMMARY OF DIRECTIONS				
A	B	C	D	E
1, 2, 3 only	1, 3 only	2, 4 only	4 only	All are correct

93. Body temperature in the anesthetized patient

(1) is closely regulated by the hypothalamus
(2) is known to be elevated if the patient is sweating
(3) is best assessed by skin temperature
(4) will tend to drift to reach ambient temperature

94. Body temperature regulation involves

(1) heat production by the muscle
(2) heat production by the liver
(3) heat dissipation by the skin
(4) heat dissipation by the lungs

95. The set point of body temperature

(1) is the point at which the temperature usually is maintained
(2) never changes
(3) is elevated at the onset of fear
(4) is not altered by salicylate

96. The mechanism for active transfer of sodium out of the cell and potassium into the cell

(1) is referred to as the sodium–potassium pump
(2) requires no energy, being a passive movement
(3) is located in the cell membrane
(4) functions independently of the sodium concentration

97. Maintenance of a stable pH is essential for life. The pH

(1) of a solution is the logarithm to the base 10 of the reciprocal of the hydrogen ion concentration
(2) of a solution is the negative logarithm of the hydrogen ion concentration
(3) of water in which hydrogen ion and hydroxyl ion are in equal concentration is 7.0
(4) will decrease one unit for each ten-fold decrease in hydrogen ion concentration

98. Buffers are important to the maintenance of stable pH. A buffer

(1) is a substance that is present only in the red cell
(2) such as carbonic acid can only respond to the addition of hydrogen ion
(3) usually involves hydrochloric or phosphoric acid
(4) involves a weak acid and its salt

99. When evaluating renal function, one must consider that

(1) proteinuria is always abnormal
(2) a specific gravity of 1.023 or greater demonstrates good concentrating function
(3) BUN elevation is always abnormal
(4) creatinine is produced more in muscular persons

100. Extracellular fluid losses may occur with

(1) small bowel obstruction
(2) rapidly developing ascites
(3) burns
(4) fever and hyperventilation

Answers and Explanations

1. **(E)** Oxygen concentration does not affect body temperature in ranges useful in anesthesia. Exposure to room temperature may cause hypothermia if the room temperature is kept low. This is especially true in the very small patient. Intravenous fluids and humidification both may affect body temperature and can be used as a means of maintaining the temperature. Muscle relaxants prevent shivering, one of the body's methods of keeping temperature normal. (*1:458; 75:583*)

2. **(E)** Heat production in the body is decreased by anorexia. Shivering, hunger, and activity lead to an increase in temperature. Epinephrine increases temperature by leading to vasoconstriction, which conserves heat. (*15:617; 129:209*)

3. **(D)** The temperature setting mechanism is in the hypothalamus. This structure controls the set point for temperature. (*129:210*)

4. **(C)** The stimulus for the temperature-regulating center is the temperature of the blood perfusing the center. Several other activities are important in the regulation of temperature. Constriction or dilatation of blood vessels helps conserve or dissipate heat. Serotonin and norepinephrine may play a role in regulating temperature. Epinephrine is not a primary stimulus. (*129:210*)

5. **(E)** The total body water in the adult constitutes 60% of the body weight. (*1:569; 15:577; 75:738*)

6. **(A)** The difference between an osmolar and an osmolal solution lies in the method in which it is mixed. If 1 g molecular weight of a nonionized substance is dissolved in 1 L of solution, the concentration is 1 osmolar. If it is dissolved in 1 kg of solvent, it is osmolal. (*15:581; 75:738; 129:4*)

7. **(B)** The principal intracellular ion is potassium. The second most important is magnesium. Sodium is the most important extracellular ion. (*1:1319; 75:741*)

8. **(A)** Magnesium concentration is related to the irritability of nervous tissue. It has a high intracellular concentration. It is excreted in the urine even in the face of a low concentration in the blood. It is present in the bile and the gastric juice. (*132:80–81*)

9. **(E)** Ringer's lactate contains sodium, potassium, chloride, and calcium. It does not contain bicarbonate ions. (*1:1314; 2:584; 132:67*)

10. **(A)** The renal circulation is autoregulated over a wide range. There are many neural factors that control the vessel diameter and the renal blood flow, including the renin–angiotensin mechanism. Innervation comes from T4 to T12, the vagus, and the splanchnic. Epinephrine has an influence. Prostaglandin E_2 causes dilatation. (*1:1226; 75:1079; 129:598*)

11. **(B)** The glomerulus is a tuft of capillaries. The veins, Bowman's capsule, and the tubules are important structures but are not part of the glomerulus. (*2:969; 129:595*)

12. **(D)** The countercurrent mechanism involves the loops of Henle and the vasa recta. By this mechanism, the kidney is able to maintain concentration gradients. All of the renal structures, the nephron, the glomerulus, and the tubules, are involved in the process of excretion, but the parallel loops and the vasa recta are components of the countercurrent mechanism. (*15:769; 75:1080; 129:607*)

13. **(A)** Hydrogen ion is secreted by the proximal and distal tubules. It is actively transported and exchanged for sodium. The ion movement is interrelated, the hydrogen ion coming from the carbonic acid breakdown into hydrogen and bicarbonate. (*129:610*)

14. **(B)** Biotransformation of drugs in the liver includes all of the mechanisms listed except auto-oxidation. (*1:60,61; 75:146,147*)

15. **(C)** Glucuronyl transferase is produced in the endoplasmic reticulum. It has no function in the renal clearance of nitrogen. The conversion to bilirubin glucuronide produces a water-soluble compound. The enzyme is increased after barbiturate administration. It is important in other conversions in addition to bilirubin. *(129:426)*

16. **(B)** The enterohepatic circulation is the mechanism whereby some substances are reabsorbed from the gut into the portal blood and then from the liver back into the gut. The mechanism is most important for bile salts. It is of importance in the use of drugs that undergo this mechanism. The mechanism can function whether or not the substance is conjugated. *(75:148; 130:48–49)*

17. **(B)** Jaundice can result from all of the options except increased uptake of bilirubin into hepatic cells. The uptake is necessary to prevent jaundice. *(75:1137; 129:426)*

18. **(C)** The liver receives blood from the hepatic artery and the portal vein. The hepatic artery comes off the aorta. The vessels, except for the central vein, run in the interlobular spaces. *(15:780; 75:1134; 129:424)*

19. **(C)** Meralgia paresthetica is a condition marked by paresthesias on the anterior and lateral surfaces of the thigh. This condition is of importance to an anesthesiologist because it may develop after herniorrhaphy. It may also follow positioning in the lithotomy position if the legs are pushed back over the body, trapping the lateral femoral cutaneous nerve. *(75:812; 128:58)*

20. **(E)** The total volume of CSF is 120 to 150 ml. There is a constant turnover. CSF is produced at a rate of 0.35 to 0.40 ml/minute. *(15:588)*

21. **(A)** The formation of CSF involves passive filtration that accounts for about one third of the production. The other two thirds is due to active transport processes at the choroid plexus. The pons, the cerebellum, and cortex are not involved. None of the CSF is produced in the lumbar area. *(15:588; 112:1)*

22. **(A)** The third lumbar root is not involved in the makeup of the sciatic nerve. The lumbosacral trunk of L4 and L5 joins the sacral fibers to form the large trunk of the sciatic nerve. *(75:811)*

23. **(C)** The usual CSF pressure is 110 mm H_2O (about 15 mm Hg). *(2:765; 15:589; 112:1)*

24. **(B)** The absorption of CSF takes place through the arachnoid villi. The ependymal cells and the pia mater are not involved. The CSF flows through the foramina of Monro and Magendie. *(2:765; 15:589· 129:515)*

25. **(E)** CSF flows through the ventricles and the subarachnoid space after being formed in the choroid plexus. There is no CSF in the epidural space. *(2:765; 15:589; 129:515)*

26. **(C)** The specific gravity of CSF is 1.003 to 1.009. *(15:588)*

27. **(B)** The A-beta fibers are large fibers that are involved with deep touch and temperature. *(1:990; 15:598; 75:374)*

28. **(D)** A small fiber that is a preganglionic autonomic fiber is the B fiber. *(1:990; 15:598; 75:374)*

29. **(E)** A very small postganglionic fiber with slow conduction is the C fiber. *(1:990; 15:598; 75:374)*

30. **(C)** A medium-sized nerve that serves as an efferent to the muscle spindle is the A-gamma fiber. *(1:990; 15:598; 75:374)*

31. **(A)** The largest fiber, associated with motor and fast conduction is the A-alpha fiber. *(1:990; 15:598; 75:374)*

32. **(C)** Hepatic blood flow is decreased with sympathetic stimulation. The blood flow is difficult to regulate under anesthesia, and retraction and packing can grossly interfere with blood flow. Hypoxemia leads to increased resistance. Dopamine does not regulate liver blood flow. The blood flow responds quickly to body needs. *(1:1201; 75:1135)*

33. **(D)** Insulin production does not occur in the liver. Glycogen storage, gluconeogenesis, glycogenolysis, and the conversion of glycerol to glucose all take place in the liver and are important to glucose metabolism. *(1:1201; 75:1135)*

34. **(B)** The rate-limiting step in fat metabolism is the presence of acetyl-CoA. Fat is carried in the blood in chylomicrons. Cholesterol level and glucagon level are not rate limiting. Glucose availability is involved in fat metabolism, since excess glucose calories are stored as fat. *(1:1211; 75:1137)*

35. **(D)** Unconjugated bilirubin is conjugated with glucuronic acid to form a water-soluble compound that can be excreted. Unconjugated bilirubin is toxic in high concentrations and can lead to kernicterus. It is not secreted into the intestinal tract. Bilirubin results from the breakdown of red cells, not white cells. Biliverdin results from the breakdown of hemoglobin. Biliverdin is then converted to bilirubin. *(1:1211; 75:1137)*

36. (D) Ascites may be associated with severe cardiorespiratory symptoms. Ascites follows chronic increased portal vein pressure. It is usually accompanied by hyponatremia. Ascitic fluid should be removed slowly to avoid hypotension. *(1:1211; 75:1137)*

37. (D) Broca's area is an area in the nondominant hemisphere associated with speech. It is in the frontal area. *(54:9–157; 129:228)*

38. (E) The structure connecting the two hemispheres is the corpus callosum. The massa intermedius is a band of gray matter deep in the brain. The posterior commissure is a band of white matter that lies at the rostral end of the aqueduct of Sylvius. The anterior commissure connects the two olfactory bulbs. The cingulate gyrus lies immediately above the corpus callosum. *(54:9–128; 129:213)*

39. (C) The superior temporal lobe is the primary auditory center. The occipital lobe is the site of visual cortex. The precentral gyrus is involved with motor functions. The postcentral gyrus is involved with sensory function. *(8:333; 129:141)*

40. (B) Intention tremors may follow injury to the cerebellum. *(54:9–95)*

41. (D) Parkinsonism is due to pathology in the basal ganglia of the brain. A nonintention tremor may be a symptom. *(54:9–100; 129:179)*

42. (A) The cerebellum is primarily concerned with coordination of muscle activity. *(8:335; 129:181)*

43. (C) The dermatome serving the lateral aspect of the heel is S1. *(8:306; 75:760)*

44. (B) The foramen of Monro connects the lateral ventricle to the 3rd ventricle. The 3rd and 4th ventricles are connected by the sylvian aqueduct. From the 4th ventricle, the fluid passes into the cisterna and from the cisterna into the subarachnoid space of the spinal cord through foramina of Magendie and Luschka. *(8:339)*

45. (A) Alpha activity has a frequency range of 8 to 10 cycles/second. Beta activity has a frequency of 18 to 30 cycles/second. Theta rhythm has an activity of 4 to 7 cycles/second. Delta rhythm has an activity of 4 cycles/second. *(1:2262; 15:590)*

46. (B) The CSA presents data from the EEG in a format of amplitude, time, and frequency. This format is not more accurate but is more convenient. The CSA is not as accurate for sudden events. In spite of its convenience, a certain amount of training and familiarity is needed to interpret the tracing accu-

rately. CSA is not necessary for every anesthetic. *(1:2262; 15:590)*

47. (E) SSEPs are little affected by nitrous oxide. They are not disrupted by small doses of thiopental. Deep levels of halothane will disrupt the tracings. The tracings evaluate the latency and the amplitude. *(15:592; 75:833)*

48. (A) MRI gives superior anatomic resolution in comparison with CT. The procedure takes longer but does not require anesthesia in most cases. It cannot be used if metal implants are present because of the magnetic forces that are the basis of the technique. For this reason, it is not possible to have ferrous-containing anesthesia equipment or monitors nearby. *(1:1610; 75:838)*

49. (E) The lateral spinal column is made of both ascending and descending tracts. This is white matter. It is both motor and sensory. The anterior horn cells are in the gray matter. *(8:302–303)*

50. (A) The substantia gelatinosa has the highest concentration of opioids in the cord. This area is in the dorsal root of the spinal cord. *(15:596; 75:257)*

51. (E) The precentral gyrus is primarily involved with motor functions. Sensation involves the dorsal root ganglion cell, the lateral spinothalamic tract, the thalamic nuclei, and the postcentral gyrus. *(8:304, 334; 129:109)*

52. (E) All of the options are true. The liver has a diverse function in producing proteins. *(1:1209; 75:1147)*

53. (E) All of the options are true. Albumin production is higher in the neonate than in the adult. Oncotic pressure is largely determined by the presence of albumin, which is the main serum protein. Since albumin has a long half-life, it is not a good test for acute changes in liver function. If the albumin is low, the disease has been present for some time. *(1:1209)*

54. (E) All of the options are true. Albumin is a good test, but it has a long half-life, and recent changes may not be reflected. Coagulation factors, on the other hand, have a shorter half-life and will reflect recent changes. Dye-removal tests are not specific. Changes may reflect changes in blood flow, uptake, binding, and excretion. *(1:1216; 75:1146)*

55. (E) A decreased hematocrit in the patient with cirrhosis may reflect many factors: coagulation defect leading to bleeding, increased plasma volume leading to dilution of the red cells, megaloblastic anemia, and increased hemolysis. Many of these factors are interrelated. *(75:1141)*

56. **(E)** The major inhibitory transmitter in the central nervous system is GABA, but other transmitters may have inhibitory effects as well. All of the options have an inhibitory effect. *(8:335)*

57. **(C)** The reticular activating system (RAS) has both inhibitory and excitatory functions. The RAS is located in the brainstem. It has sensory and motor inputs. *(8:335)*

58. **(E)** Sodium conservation is important to homeostasis. Sodium is reabsorbed throughout the tubule system so that only about 1% of the filtered sodium is excreted by the kidney. *(75:1080; 129:613)*

59. **(A)** ADH release is in response to osmoreceptors in the hypothalamus to regulate fluid volume. It also responds to the stretch receptors in the atrium. ADH is secreted from the posterior pituitary. The principal effect is on the collecting tubules. *(8:359, 442; 75:1081)*

60. **(A)** Decreased urinary output in the patient being ventilated with PEEP is due to decreased cardiac output, increased sympathetic output, and release of renin. Most believe that ADH is not involved, but there are those who think that ADH secretion is important. *(75:739,1082)*

61. **(E)** Liver drug transformation involves all of the options cited. *(47:28)*

62. **(E)** All of the systems are responsible for buffering in the body. Bicarbonate and proteins are the most important. *(1:1295; 129:567)*

63. **(B)** Dextrose-containing fluid should be omitted in the patient for TUR and for intracranial procedures. The patient for TUR may absorb hypotonic fluids, and the intravenous administration will only make the symptoms worse. In the patient for brain surgery, cerebral edema may be aggravated by the administration of dextrose solutions. There is no problem in the use of these solutions for appendectomy or fracture repairs. *(1:1315)*

64. **(D)** Extracellular fluid status may be reflected in the heart rate. Tachycardia may accompany low volume status. The volume status is important to the conduct of anesthesia, since low volume status may lead to hypotension, and high volume may lead to heart failure. Blood pressure and laboratory studies may not reflect the volume status of patients. *(1:1317)*

65. **(A)** Hyperkalemia may be treated by the administration of glucose–insulin solutions, eliminating ex-

ogenous sources (one of the major causes), and correcting causes of endogenous sources. Treatment entails alkalinizing the blood, not acidifying it. *(1:1320; 8:421)*

66. **(A)** Blood volume of an adult is about 5 L. It is comprised 60% of plasma and averages 70 ml/kg in an adult. Blood volume does include the red cells. *(15:579)*

67. **(A)** The osmolarity of plasma is 280 mOsm/L, which is higher than that of interstitial or intracellular fluid. The higher osmotic pressure keeps a higher pressure in the capillaries. Sodium and chloride are important in maintaining the osmolarity. *(8:75,410; 15:581)*

68. **(B)** An isotonic solution exerts the same osmotic pressure as plasma. One need not use isotonic fluids for therapy. Saline, 0.9%, is isotonic. Glucose in a solution may be metabolized, changing the tonicity of the solution. *(15:581; 75:738)*

69. **(C)** Vasopressin causes a concentrated urine and antidiuresis. In addition, the urine has a high osmolality. Vasoconstriction also occurs. *(75:739; 129:200)*

70. **(E)** Inappropriate secretion of ADH is seen often after surgery. It includes hyponatremia and low serum osmolality. The kidneys excrete an excessive amount of sodium under the influence of ADH. The renal function is normal. *(75:740; 129:203)*

71. **(E)** Magnesium is an important intracellular ion. It may be mobilized from large stores in bone when needed for enzyme and protein synthesis. It is bound to plasma proteins. *(75:742; 132:81)*

72. **(E)** Parenteral nutrition is very important in the pre- and postoperative care of patients. There are problems associated with its use. It can be administered through a peripheral vein, and the problem with phlebitis is less if the glucose concentration is limited. Both lipids and proteins are used as sources of calories. *(8:425; 75:729)*

73. **(C)** The liver has a dual blood supply. Only 25% of the blood is supplied by the hepatic artery. The oxygen supply is evenly divided by the two vessels, even though the portal vein blood is more unsaturated. Most of the nutrients come from the portal vein. *(8:101; 75:1134)*

74. **(C)** The vitamin K-dependent factors are II, VII, IX, and X. *(15:533; 75:1141)*

75. **(B)** Autoregulation of the hepatic blood flow is predominantly in the hepatic artery and via the sympathetic nervous system. The portal vein is not primarily involved in the autoregulation nor is the

parasympathetic nervous system. *(8:103; 15:782; 75:1135)*

76. **(C)** During hemorrhage, the liver is an important source of blood. The sympathetic stimulation may squeeze blood from the liver into the general circulation. The vessels do not dilate under these circumstances. Anesthetic agents may interfere with this compensatory process. *(15:712; 75:1132)*

77. **(B)** The typical nerve cell has numerous dendrites that branch out and a dendritic zone that is a receptor membrane. The nerve cell has only one axon. The myelin sheath covers the axon only. *(15:598; 129:38)*

78. **(B)** CSF is formed by filtration and by active transport, the latter being responsible for about two thirds of the total amount. The active transport requires energy. The amount formed is 0.35 to 0.40 ml/minute. *(112:1; 129:515)*

79. **(B)** CSF values are pH of 7.32, P_{CO_2} of 50 torr, and bicarbonate of 25 mEq/L. Since the blood–brain barrier is more permeable to CO_2 than to bicarbonate, the CSF pH will change quickly with alterations of P_{CO_2} in the blood. *(15:588; 129:515)*

80. **(E)** All of the options are present in the reflex arc. Many problems in patients under anesthesia are attributed to a reflex. It is very difficult to describe the pathways in these reflexes. One should try to determine the cause before assuming all problems are related to some ill-defined reflex. *(129:100)*

81. **(C)** The EEG is not sufficient for the diagnosis of brain death. One must get a careful history, and the patient must be assessed carefully. Patients who are cold or under barbiturates may display a flat line. Cortical activity will increase with hypercapnia. Hysterical fits are not seen on the EEG. *(2:758; 15:591; 75:1471)*

82. **(D)** The RAS is a nonspecific area in the brainstem that is responsible for maintaining the conscious, alert state. It receives input from above and below. *(15:593; 129:158)*

83. **(E)** All of the substances listed are transmitters in the central nervous system. Their effects are not confined to the central nervous system but may be far-reaching. *(129:77)*

84. **(C)** The act of vomiting requires the activation of the vomiting center, which is located in the reticular formation of the medulla. It requires the opening of the esophageal and gastric cardiac sphincters. *(129:191)*

85. **(B)** A cirrhotic patient does not have normal hepatocytes and cannot produce protein normally. Succinylcholine may not be handled normally due to decreases in plasma pseudocholinesterase. Jaundice may not be present. Lidocaine is not broken down by pseudocholinesterase. *(75:1138; 165:1)*

86. **(D)** Alcohol ingestion in large amounts will lead to liver disease in spite of good nutrition. Hematologic disorders are due to clotting deficiencies and to the alcohol itself. Gastrointestinal problems, including pancreatitis, are common. *(1:1670; 75:411)*

87. **(C)** Anesthesia affects hepatic function by affecting hepatic blood flow. This may occur with general or regional anesthesia. The site of surgery, retractors, and preexisting hepatic disease also are important. *(1:1669; 75:1153)*

88. **(D)** The glomerular capillaries originate from a small afferent vessel and drain into a slightly smaller efferent vessel. This is the mechanism that effects filtration. Bowman's capsule is the tubular part of the nephron in which the glomerulus lies. The capillaries are very thin to achieve easy filtration. *(75:1079; 129:595)*

89. **(A)** Vasopressin increases the permeability of the collecting ducts to water. The hormone is an antidiuretic hormone, secreted by the posterior pituitary. It acts only on the collecting tubules. *(75:1208; 129:200)*

90. **(C)** Osmotic diuresis may follow ingestion of substances that are filtered by the kidney but not absorbed or if the substance is in an amount exceeding the capacity of the kidney to reabsorb it. Increased GFR is not involved. *(1:1238; 75:1085; 129:609)*

91. **(E)** Ammonia production takes place in the proximal and distal tubules and in the collecting ducts. Acidosis encourages ammonia production. Ammonia and hydrogen combine to form ammonium ion. *(129:610)*

92. **(E)** Sweating is an important temperature-regulating mechanism. It may also occur with hypoxia and in response to emotional stimuli. Sweating occurs with most sympathetic stimuli. *(6:759)*

93. **(D)** In the anesthetized patient, the temperature will tend to drift to equilibrate with the ambient temperature. It is important, especially in the patient with open cavities, to take steps to prevent heat loss and to actively treat hypothermia. *(6:759)*

94. **(E)** Body temperature regulation is a complex mechanism involving the muscles, the liver, the

skin, and the lungs. All of these are involved in the conduct of an anesthetic. *(129:209; 131:29)*

95. **(B)** The set point is the point at which body temperature usually is maintained. It is changed by fear, illness, and salicylates. The specific reasons for the changes in the set point are unknown. *(2:759; 131:30–31)*

96. **(B)** Sodium transport via the sodium–potassium pump is a process that involves energy. The pump is in the cell membrane. The process is related to the sodium concentration, since sodium is the rate-limiting step. *(129:24)*

97. **(A)** The pH will increase one unit for each 10-fold decrease in hydrogen ion concentration. *(129:4)*

98. **(D)** Buffers, such as bicarbonate, can respond to the addition of base as well as acid. Buffers are located in all body fluids and in the cells. Hydrochloric acid and phosphoric acid are strong acids, and most buffer pairs are weak acids and their salts. *(129:4)*

99. **(C)** Proteinuria may be normal with exercise or stress, and BUN elevation may occur with a high-protein diet. BUN may also be elevated by blood in the gastrointestinal tract. *(1:1644,2242)*

100. **(E)** Extracellular fluid may be lost by all of the mechanisms listed. The loss may not be apparent on examination and may require a careful history and examination to determine. For example, it the case of ascites, it is important to determine how fast the accumulation has occurred. In many cases, the accumulation is slow, and there is little cardiovascular instability. If the accumulation is fast, there may be great instability. *(132:34)*

Hyper-K+
Acidosis
HTN
Anemia
Pit dys.
Sepsis
↑ C.O.

CHAPTER 4

Pharmacology
Review

The practice of anesthesiology is essentially applied pharmacology. We use drugs extensively for producing anesthesia or pain control. Our knowledge must encompass the effects of the drugs themselves as well as interactions with other drugs. Our knowledge cannot be limited to anesthesia-related drugs, since our patients may be taking a variety of medications when they need surgical procedures.

The study of pharmacology is constantly changing. Drugs that were commonly used in the past are seldom used today. One must stay abreast of changes in the development of new drugs.

It is beyond the scope of this short review to present all drug groups. General concepts are reviewed, but the various drugs are not. In addition to the anesthetic agents, both local and general, you should be familiar with neuromuscular blocking agents, autonomic drugs, cardiac drugs, diuretics, and the various drugs that affect the central nervous system.

The *pharmacokinetics* of a drug deals with its absorption, distribution, metabolism, and excretion, in other words, what the body does to the drug.

The *pharmacodynamics* of a drug deals with the action and effects of a drug on the body.

The avenue of drug administration will affect the time taken to reach a blood level. If the administration is by mouth, the drug must be absorbed through the mucosa of the gastrointestinal tract. Some of the drug may be bound to the intestinal contents and become unabsorbable. Some of the absorbed drug may be eliminated as it passes through the liver, the first-pass effect. The total administered dose, therefore, is not available to the body.

A drug that is administered by the intramuscular route must be absorbed. The vehicle may retard its absorption into the bloodstream. In some cases, this is a desirable feature, and the drug is formulated to allow the slow release of the active ingredient. Various "depot" formulations are examples.

Intravenous administration leads to the fastest blood levels of drugs, but even this avenue may be affected by factors such as pH and protein binding.

The drug that is in the bloodstream must gain access to the tissues in most cases to be effective. The ability to cross cell membranes is dependent on the pH and the pKa.

The pKa is the pH at which the drug is 50% ionized and 50% nonionized. Membranes are more permeable to the nonionized form of the drug.

Drugs administered in one dose or concentration become available to the body at that dose or something less because of the factors already discussed. *Bioavailability* is defined as the amount of the drug that gets into the body. For intravenous drugs, bioavailability is 100%. For oral and intramuscular administration, it may be markedly less.

Once absorbed, the drugs must be distributed throughout the body. The term *half-life* describes the time required for the drug concentration to change by a factor of 2. This is affected by both the volume of distribution and the clearance. The *volume of distribution* is the total amount of tissue capacity for a drug. *Clearance* is the portion of the drug distribution from which the drug is removed in a given time.

In the case of inhalation agents, uptake of the gases is by way of the lungs. Factors that affect the uptake are solubility of the agent, ventilation, and cardiac output. Potency of anesthetic agents is defined by the minimum alveolar concentration (MAC), which is that concentration of an anesthetic measured in end-tidal gas that prevents a response to a standard painful stimulus in 50% of the subjects. Factors affecting the uptake of an agent are important in planning an anesthetic regimen: the circulatory status, known ventilation/perfusion abnormalities, and the characteristics of the particular agent must be considered.

Other definitions of importance are:

Tolerance: The need for increasing doses of a drug to achieve the same therapeutic effect. Many anesthetic drugs, eg, thiopental, may be subject to the development of tolerance. The extreme degree of tolerance is characterized by addiction to morphine in which very large doses are needed.

Tachyphylaxis: a rapidly developing tolerance.

Cumulative effect: the increase in amount of drug in the body due to administration in amount and/or frequency in excess of the body's ability to eliminate it.

One-compartment model: the model for drug distribution in which the drug behaves as though uniformly distributed in one large compartment, and a constant proportion is eliminated in a given time period.

Two-compartment model: the model in which the drugs behave as though they were distributed through two compartments, the first a central compartment and the second a larger peripheral compartment. There is a rapid fall in concentration followed by a less rapid decay of activity.

Recent drug advances and their use in the conduct of anesthesia are presented at the Annual Refresher Course Lectures of the American Society of Anesthesiologists and the International Anesthesia Research Society.

Questions

DIRECTIONS (Questions 1 through 219): Each of the numbered items or incomplete statements in this section is followed by answers or by completions of the statement. Select the ONE lettered answer or completion that is BEST in each case.

1. The most important site of drug transformation is usually the

   (A) liver
   (B) spleen
   (C) kidney
   (D) lungs
   (E) bloodstream

2. The first-pass effect refers to

   (A) the biotransformation of a drug in its vehicle of administration
   (B) the change of a drug by enzymes in muscle
   (C) biotransformation of a drug as it passes through the intestinal mucosa and liver
   (D) the drug lost by urinary excretion
   (E) the drug lost by being passed with feces

3. Systemic availability of a drug refers to the amount of drug

   (A) that is administered intramuscularly
   (B) that is administered orally
   (C) reaching the liver
   (D) that is excreted by the kidney
   (E) that reaches the general circulation

4. Renal clearance of a drug

   (A) is usually of little importance
   (B) has no relationship to creatinine clearance
   (C) is constant for a given drug
   (D) varies with pH, urine flow rate, and renal blood flow
   (E) may exceed renal blood flow

5. Halogenation of a hydrocarbon

   (A) usually increases its flammability
   (B) increases its narcotic activity
   (C) has no effect

   (D) makes it more of a cardiac irritant
   (E) makes it explosive

6. Halothane structurally is

   (A) an ether
   (B) a methane compound
   (C) an ethane compound
   (D) an ethane compound substituted with fluorine, chlorine, and iodine
   (E) an ethane compound substituted with fluorine, bromine, and iodine

7. The boiling point of halothane is

   (A) 30°C
   (B) 40.2°F
   (C) 40.2°C
   (D) 50.2°F
   (E) 50.2°C

8. Halothane is stored

   (A) in clear bottles with a preservative
   (B) in tinted bottles with the preservative butylated hydroxyl toluene
   (C) without a preservative
   (D) with provision to prevent photochemical decomposition
   (E) in plastic bottles

9. Halothane is

   (A) insoluble in rubber
   (B) soluble in rubber, and this may be a factor in induction with high flow rates
   (C) soluble in rubber but eliminated very rapidly
   (D) soluble in rubber, and the retained halothane may affect a second patient exposed to the same apparatus
   (E) soluble in rubber, and the rubber reacts with halothane to change its composition

10. Isoflurane

    (A) is a poor muscle relaxant compared with halo-
        thane
    (B) has a vapor pressure of 283 torr at 20°C
    (C) stimulates ventilation
    (D) has a MAC of 0.56% in 70% nitrogen (at age 26)
    (E) should be delivered by spontaneous ventilation

11. The most potent of the inhalation anesthetics is

    (A) halothane
    (B) cyclopropane
    (C) nitrous oxide
    (D) enflurane
    (E) methoxyflurane

12. The renal lesion associated with methoxyflurane

    (A) involves the glomerulus
    (B) is not dose related
    (C) causes decreased urine volume
    (D) is caused by the fluoride ion
    (E) will cause a decreased blood urea nitrogen

13. The cardiovascular effects of isoflurane are charac-
    terized by

    (A) stable cardiac rhythm
    (B) sensitization of the heart to epinephrine
    (C) a slowing of the heart rate
    (D) increased stroke volume
    (E) decreased cardiac output

    C.O. = HR + SV

14. The physical properties of isoflurane include

    (A) flammability in oxygen
    (B) red color
    (C) pungent odor
    (D) no breakdown when exposed to sunlight
    (E) addition of thymol as a preservative

15. Each of the following is an ether EXCEPT

    (A) halothane
    (B) fluroxene
    (C) enflurane
    (D) isoflurane
    (E) methoxyflurane

16. Sevoflurane

    (A) is an ether compound
    (B) has a blood-gas coefficient of 1.7
    (C) has a vapor pressure of 214
    (D) is irritating to the airway
    (E) contains no fluoride molecules

17. Enflurane is

    (A) a halogenated hydrocarbon with one double
        bond
    (B) a halogenated methyl compound

    (C) a hydrocarbon with a vapor pressure of 243 torr
    (D) a substituted hydrocarbon with two bromine
        sites
    (E) an ether

18. Enflurane

    (A) contains thymol as a preservative
    (B) is flammable at a concentration of 4%
    (C) gives poor muscle relaxation
    (D) causes central nervous system irritability
    (E) causes myocardial irritability

19. Sevoflurane

    (A) is highly lipid soluble
    (B) has a MAC of 2.6%
    (C) is highly water soluble
    (D) is a cardiovascular depressant
    (E) has a structure that contains all halogens

20. The action of thiopental after injection is termi-
    nated by

    (A) its elimination unchanged by the kidneys
    (B) its biotransformation by the liver
    (C) its being bound to proteins
    (D) its redistribution
    (E) being taken up in fatty tissues

21. The pH of a 2.5% solution of thiopental is

    (A) 2
    (B) 4
    (C) 6
    (D) 8
    (E) 10

22. Thiopental administration in humans is followed by

    (A) increased cardiac output, decreased stroke
        volume
    (B) decreased cardiac output, increased stroke
        volume
    (C) decreased cardiac output, decreased blood
        pressure
    (D) decreased cardiac output, increased blood
        pressure
    (E) decreased stroke volume, increased blood pres-
        sure

23. Thiopental is contraindicated in

    (A) porphyria congenita
    (B) porphyria cutanea tarda
    (C) acute intermittent porphyria
    (D) myotonia
    (E) chorea

24. In a patient with severe pain, administration of thiopental 80 mg will

(A) produce sleep
(B) will have an antianalgesic action
(C) will have no effect
(D) will sedate the patient but not induce sleep
(E) is more effective if given alone

25. Thiopental administration in hypnotic doses will

(A) increase cerebral blood flow
(B) have a depressant effect on uterine contractions
(C) decrease cerebral flow if P_{CO_2} is increased
(D) increase EEG activity
(E) decrease cerebral oxygen consumption

26. Injection of thiopental will lead to a dose-dependent

(A) decrease in arterial blood pressure
(B) increase in stroke volume
(C) increase in cardiac output
(D) bradycardia
(E) decreased coronary blood flow

27. After injection of thiopental, 4 mg/kg, there would be

(A) decreased heart rate
(B) arrhythmias
(C) baroreceptor-mediated decrease in sympathetic activity
(D) more pronounced changes in patients with heart disease
(E) no change in cardiovascular parameters

28. After the inadvertent injection of 15 ml 2% thiopental into the epidural space, you would expect

(A) immediate complaint of severe pain
(B) onset of drowsiness
(C) complete paralysis
(D) arachnoiditis
(E) cauda equina syndrome

29. After the administration of thiopental, the position of the oxyhemoglobin dissociation curve would

(A) be unchanged
(B) be shifted to the left
(C) be shifted to the right
(D) shift to the right but transiently
(E) shift to the left and remain so for 3 hours

30. A patient has been given an injection of ketamine in a dose calculated to be sufficient for anesthesia. His eyes remain open, and there is slight nystagmus and occasional purposeless movements. This is an indication that

(A) the dose is inadequate
(B) more ketamine should be given to stop the movements
(C) the dose is excessive
(D) the dose is adequate for anesthesia
(E) the patient is having a seizure

31. Expected changes in cardiovascular status after ketamine administration include

(A) elevated diastolic pressure, normal systolic pressure
(B) elevated diastolic and systolic pressure
(C) decreased diastolic and systolic pressure
(D) decreased diastolic pressure, increased systolic pressure
(E) no change in blood pressure

32. Administration of ketamine causes

(A) decreased heart rate
(B) increased heart rate
(C) decreased cardiac output
(D) no change in cardiac output
(E) no change in heart rate

33. Droperidol is

(A) a narcotic of intermediate potency
(B) a component of ketamine
(C) a butyrophenone derivative
(D) a short-acting (1 to 2 hours) tranquilizer
(E) eliminated totally by the kidney

34. The rigidity occasionally seen with Innovar injection is

(A) more likely to occur after intramuscular injection
(B) noted chiefly in the leg muscles
(C) due to droperidol
(D) due to fentanyl
(E) seen only after large doses

35. A local anesthetic that is an ester derivative is

(A) bupivacaine
(B) etidocaine
(C) mepivacaine
(D) lidocaine
(E) procaine

36. Local anesthetics have their effect at the

(A) nerve core
(B) axon hillock
(C) dendrite
(D) membrane
(E) synapse

37. Local anesthetics in the injectable form are

    (A) salts
    (B) acids
    (C) bases
    (D) proteins
    (E) lipids

38. Dibucaine is

    (A) a benzoic acid ester
    (B) eliminated by the kidneys
    (C) an alcohol
    (D) rapidly eliminated
    (E) a quinoline derivative

39. The addition of hyaluronidase to local anesthesia

    (A) increases the time to onset of action
    (B) decreases the success rate of blocks
    (C) increases the duration of the block
    (D) increases the incidence of toxic reactions
    (E) has no effect

40. A 9-year-old boy sustained a 40% burn to the anterior portion of his body. On the twentieth day after the burn, he is brought to the operating room for a skin graft. Anesthesia is induced with thiopental, and succinylcoline is injected for relaxation. The ECG shows a bizarre tracing followed by ventricular fibrillation. The most likely cause of the arrhythmia is

    (A) an overdose of thiopental
    (B) hypoxia
    (C) hyperkalemia
    (D) electrocution
    (E) administration of the wrong drug

41. Antibiotics that possess neuromuscular blocking properties include all of the following EXCEPT

    (A) neomycin
    (B) kanamycin
    (C) penicillin
    (D) gentamicin
    (E) streptomycin

42. The muscle relaxant metocurine

    (A) causes more histamine release than D-tubocurarine
    (B) causes more ganglionic blockade than D-tubocurarine
    (C) causes more blood pressure depression than D-tubocurarine
    (D) is structurally related to D-tubocurarine
    (E) always causes tachycardia

43. Echothiophate iodide eyedrops, chronically administered, will have an effect similar to

    (A) D-tubocurarine
    (B) intravenous narcotics
    (C) atropine
    (D) organophosphate insecticides
    (E) thiopental

44. A muscle relaxant with a steroid structure is

    (A) D-tubocurarine
    (B) metocurine
    (C) succinylcholine
    (D) pancuronium
    (E) gallamine

45. The most common arrhythmia seen on injection of a second dose of succinylcholine is

    (A) sinus arrest
    (B) sinus tachycardia
    (C) nodal rhythm
    (D) atrial fibrillation
    (E) bigeminy

46. A small dose of a nondepolarizing muscle relaxant given 3 minutes before an intubating dose of succinylcholine

    (A) will not alter the effectiveness of the succinylcholine
    (B) will not prevent the muscle pain
    (C) is useful in preventing arrhythmias
    (D) is especially helpful in patients who will be ambulatory after surgery
    (E) makes intubation easier

47. If your patient has a need for a high cardiac output and high systemic blood pressure, the relaxant of choice would be

    (A) D-tubocurarine
    (B) atracurium
    (C) pancuronium
    (D) decamethonium
    (E) succinylcholine

48. When succinylcholine is administered in a dose of 1 mg/kg, one may expect all of the following EXCEPT

    (A) an intraocular pressure increase
    (B) an increase in intragastric pressure in all cases
    (C) a low incidence of intragastric pressure increase in infants and children
    (D) an incidence of muscle pain in 0.2 to 89% of patients
    (E) no muscle pain if the depolarizing relaxant is preceded by a small dose of a nondepolarizer

49. A 58-year-old woman with a diagnosis of myasthenia gravis underwent a laparotomy. Her anesthesia consisted of thiopental, nitrous oxide, and oxygen, with pancuronium as a muscle relaxant in a total dose of 1 mg. At the end of the procedure,

thiotepa was instilled into the abdomen, and the patient received an intravenous dose of gentamicin. The patient remained apneic at the end of the procedure. The cause of the apnea could be ascribed to all of the following EXCEPT

(A) thiopental
(B) myasthenia gravis
(C) pancuronium
(D) thiotepa
(E) gentamicin

50. Muscle contraction

(A) in an individual fiber is an all-or-none phenomenon
(B) will vary in each fiber
(C) is uniform throughout an isolated muscle
(D) is independent of the number of fibers contracting
(E) is independent of membrane effects

51. Vecuronium

(A) has an activity of about 2 minutes
(B) is a depolarizing relaxant
(C) is difficult to reverse
(D) has very little cumulative effect
(E) depends on the kidney for elimination

52. The fasciculations seen with depolarizing agents are

(A) increased if the induction dose of thiopental is large
(B) increased if the relaxant is given by slow drip
(C) seldom seen with decamethonium
(D) not related to muscle pain
(E) increased with prior treatment with depolarizing agents

53. The administration of anticholinesterase drugs will

(A) prolong all neuromuscular blockade
(B) always reverse nondepolarizing agents
(C) shorten the block of a depolarizing agent
(D) reverse nondepolarizing agents if the plasma concentration of the drug is low enough
(E) reverse the action of a depolarizing agent if only partial paralysis is present

54. Myoglobin is a low molecular weight hemeprotein

(A) found only in cardiac muscle
(B) always found in the serum of children
(C) always found in serum after administration of succinylcholine
(D) related to fasciculation
(E) more commonly found in the blood of children than adults after administration of succinylcholine

55. A patient is admitted for emergency orthopedic surgery. Preliminary data show a BUN value of 85 and a serum potassium of 6.0 mEq/L. The drug of choice for intubation would be

(A) gallamine
(B) succinylcholine
(C) atracurium
(D) decamethonium
(E) D-tubocurarine followed by succinylcholine

56. Propofol

(A) is a halogenated liquid delivered by a vaporizer
(B) is very soluble in aqueous solutions
(C) is an intravenous anesthetic agent with a slow onset
(D) has little analgesic property
(E) has a longer sleep time than thiopental

57. Atracurium is a muscle relaxant that

(A) is a depolarizing drug
(B) is eliminated entirely by hydrolysis
(C) has few cardiovascular side effects
(D) has a half-life of 60 minutes
(E) is difficult to reverse

58. The test with the greatest sensitivity in detecting residual neuromuscular block is

(A) head lift
(B) hand grip
(C) inspiratory force
(D) normal tidal volume
(E) T4:T1 > 60%

59. All of the following are capable of antagonizing neuromuscular block EXCEPT

(A) edrophonium
(B) neostigmine
(C) pyridostigmine
(D) 4-aminopyridine
(E) atropine

Questions 60 and 61

A patient in the recovery room is apneic. His anesthesia consisted of thiopental, N_2O/O_2, a nondepolarizing relaxant, and fentanyl. Measurement of blood gases showed pH 7.20, P_{CO_2} 54, and P_{O_2} 85. Body temperature is 32°C. Neostigmine is administered to reverse the neuromuscular blockade.

60. Factors that will affect the amount of neostigmine needed include all of the following EXCEPT

(A) pH
(B) dose of relaxant
(C) time of last relaxant dose
(D) body temperature
(E) specific relaxant

61. The patient was given neostigmine until return of twitch was obtained. Over the next 40 minutes, his body temperature increased to 37°C. You would expect

(A) continued improvement in neuromuscular strength
(B) return to apnea
(C) no effect
(D) marked loss of twitch height but continued breathing
(E) sudden onset of muscarinic effects

62. Depolarization block is characterized by all of the following EXCEPT

(A) muscle fasciculation
(B) initial absence of fade
(C) posttetanic facilitation
(D) antagonism of block by D-tubocurarine
(E) potentiation of block by anticholinesterase

Questions 63 through 65

Please refer to the following figure:

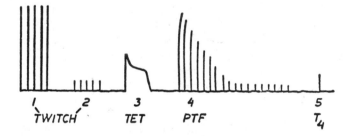

63. The graph shows the evoked twitch response following an unknown drug. The segment (1) is the baseline before drug administration, and (2) is the response in 3 minutes. From these two segments, you can say that the drug

(A) is not a muscle relaxant
(B) is a depolarizing muscle relaxant
(C) is a nondepolarizing muscle relaxant
(D) causes complete paralysis
(E) caused 90% depression

64. At the time interval (3), a tetanic stimulation was applied with the depicted result. Following this, one could state that

(A) the drug is not a muscle relaxant
(B) the drug is a depolarizing muscle relaxant
(C) the drug is a nondepolarizing muscle relaxant
(D) either the drug is a nondepolarizing muscle relaxant, or a dual block is present
(E) the tracing shown is due to artifact

65. The inability to sustain contraction (fade) during tetanic contraction is due to

(A) inability to transmit rapid electrical impulses
(B) cellular loss of potassium
(C) depletion of cellular DNA
(D) inability of recording apparatus to show all contractions
(E) the inability of the endplate to release sufficient acetylcholine

Questions 66 and 67

Please refer to the following figure:

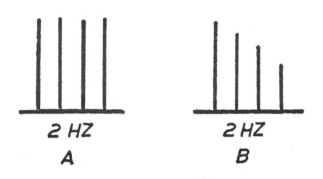

66. The train-of-four stimulus is depicted in the graph. Stimulation is at 2 Hz. The response in **A** is normal. By looking at **B** you know that

(A) a depolarizing block is present
(B) the patient is partially curarized
(C) the patient is partially curarized, but one would need a baseline recording to know how much
(D) the train-of-four ratio is 75%
(E) the patient could sustain a head lift

67. The train-of-four ratio for a depolarizing block is

(A) variable
(B) 50%
(C) 60%
(D) 75%
(E) 100%

68. The minimum alveolar concentration for isoflurane is

(A) 0.5
(B) 1.15
(C) 2.46
(D) 3.8
(E) 8.2

69. After administration of D-tubocurarine to a patient anesthetized with halothane, you would expect the maximum hypotensive effect at

(A) 1 minute
(B) 2 minutes
(C) 3 minutes
(D) 6 minutes
(E) 10 minutes

70. A patient who had been given D-tubocurarine received neostigmine, 3 mg, at the termination of the surgical procedure. Six minutes later, a large amount of white, frothy secretions was noted in the endotracheal tube. Vigorous suctioning was required to remove these secretions in order to ventilate the patient. The treatment of choice for such secretions is

(A) atropine
(B) digitalis
(C) more neostigmine
(D) recurarization
(E) use of a ventilator

71. The cardiovascular changes seen after administration of D-tubocurarine in the anesthetized patient may be due to all of the following EXCEPT

(A) the preservative in D-tubocurarine
(B) ganglionic blockade
(C) histamine release
(D) blood volume
(E) the dose of D-tubocurarine

72. Factors that affect the pharmacokinetics when using muscle relaxants include all of the following EXCEPT

(A) initial dose
(B) renal disease
(C) protein binding
(D) sex of patient
(E) advanced age

73. The patient with myasthenia gravis

(A) has normal reactions to muscle relaxants
(B) reacts abnormally to relaxants only when the condition is not controlled
(C) has a low sensitivity to nondepolarizing relaxants
(D) has an increased sensitivity to nondepolarizing relaxants
(E) has an increased sensitivity to depolarizing relaxants

74. A patient undergoes anesthesia for removal of a bronchial carcinoma. His anesthesia consists of thiopental, halothane, and N_2O/O_2, after intubation facilitated with 80 mg of succinylcholine. He was given D-tubocurarine, 6 mg, immediately after intu-

bation. At the end of the procedure, he is apneic. This may be due to all of the following EXCEPT

(A) D-tubocurarine
(B) succinylcholine
(C) bronchial carcinoma
(D) hyperventilation
(E) thiopental

75. If succinylcholine is given to facilitate intubation, and the patient is allowed to recover fully from the depolarizing block, and then is given pancuronium, one would expect

(A) a lower than normal amount of pancuronium is needed to reestablish neuromuscular blockade
(B) the pancuronium to have a shorter duration of action as a result of the succinylcholine
(C) no change in the duration of action of pancuronium
(D) no change in the duration of action of pancuronium but less intensity of relaxation
(E) the development of a phase II block

76. If a patient is to undergo an upper abdominal procedure that may require visceral traction, one should expect

(A) fewer side effects if the patient has not received relaxants
(B) fewer cardiovascular effects if D-tubocurarine is used rather than pancuronium
(C) fewer cardiovascular effects if pancuronium is used rather than D-tubocurarine
(D) the same cardiovascular response with or without relaxants
(E) increased systolic blood pressure with visceral traction

77. The formation of acetylcholine involves all of the following EXCEPT

(A) nerve terminal
(B) choline
(C) acetylCoA
(D) choline acetylase
(E) cholinesterase

78. Botulinus toxin interferes with neuromuscular transmission by

(A) preventing synthesis of acetylcholine
(B) increasing breakdown of acetylcholine
(C) preventing storage of acetylcholine
(D) preventing release of acetylcholine
(E) blocking receptors for acetylcholine

79. The administration of atropine may be followed by all of the following EXCEPT

    (A) unpredictable results in patients with Mobitz II block
    (B) unpredictable results in older patients
    (C) angina pectoris
    (D) decreased AV conduction time
    (E) decreased oxygen use

80. Propranolol hydrochloride

    (A) is an alpha blocker
    (B) is a beta agonist
    (C) causes increased heart rate
    (D) causes decreased cardiac output
    (E) causes increased cardiac contractility

81. Propranolol is useful in the treatment of

    (A) sinus bradycardia
    (B) chronic bronchitis
    (C) congestive heart failure
    (D) AV block
    (E) atrial flutter

82. You see a patient preoperatively and note that she is on propranolol 40 mg daily for hypertension. This drug

    (A) should be stopped immediately, and the procedure can be done the next day
    (B) should be stopped and surgery postponed for 2 weeks
    (C) should be continued during surgery and then stopped
    (D) will not affect the anesthetic regimen in any way
    (E) should always be discontinued gradually to avoid a sympathetic stimulation response

83. The drug that has only alpha agonist effects is

    (A) epinephrine
    (B) norepinephrine
    (C) methoxamine
    (D) isoproterenol
    (E) ephedrine

84. Quinidine is

    (A) useful only when given intravenously
    (B) 85% bound to plasma protein
    (C) useful only for atrial arrhythmias
    (D) known to counteract neuromuscular blockers
    (E) not useful in patients with renal disease

85. Procainamide

    (A) is eliminated chiefly through the liver
    (B) slows conduction of cardiac impulses

    (C) may not be administered orally
    (D) is easily hydrolyzed by plasma cholinesterase
    (E) increases ventricular automaticity

86. Lidocaine

    (A) is eliminated chiefly by the liver
    (B) is effective orally
    (C) is toxic at levels over 1 μg/ml
    (D) toxicity is noted by the appearance of hematuria
    (E) is useful in supraventricular tachycardia

87. Phenytoin

    (A) is the drug of choice for complete heart block
    (B) is broken down chiefly by cholinesterase
    (C) is useful in treatment of arrhythmias associated with digitalis
    (D) increases diastolic depolarization
    (E) increases automaticity

88. The calcium channel blocking drugs

    (A) are all antiarrhythmics
    (B) all have a peak effect in about 3 minutes
    (C) are poorly bound to proteins
    (D) interfere with the flow of calcium ion through cellular membranes
    (E) are all about equally effective

89. The drug pentazocine is

    (A) a nonaddicting narcotic
    (B) a pure narcotic agonist
    (C) a mixed agonist–antagonist
    (D) a pure narcotic antagonist
    (E) useful only orally

90. Lorazepam is a premedicant that

    (A) is a butyrophenone
    (B) has good antianxiety properties
    (C) has no sedative effect
    (D) is a respiratory depressant
    (E) is a cardiovascular depressant

91. A patient who is taking lithium for treatment of manic-depressive attacks is about to have an anesthetic. The lithium

    (A) need not be considered in the anesthetic regimen
    (B) may affect both depolarizing and nondepolarizing drugs
    (C) shortens the activity of muscle relaxants
    (D) should be stopped 2 weeks before surgery
    (E) may increase anesthetic requirements

92. If a patient is taking monamine oxidase (MAO) inhibitors, which of the following should be avoided?

    (A) local anesthetics
    (B) halothane
    (C) vecuronium
    (D) meperidine
    (E) aspirin

93. All of the following are adverse effects of furosemide EXCEPT

    (A) renin release
    (B) ototoxicity
    (C) hypokalemia
    (D) acidosis
    (E) hyperglycemia

94. The most common electrolyte alteration caused by the thiazide diuretics is

    (A) hypokalemia
    (B) hypoglycemia
    (C) hyperchloremia
    (D) hypernatremia
    (E) hyperuricemia

95. A diuretic that exerts its effect on the ascending loop of Henle is

    (A) hydrochlorothiazide
    (B) ethacrynic acid
    (C) chlorthalidone
    (D) triamterene
    (E) benzthiazide

96. Nifedipine is a calcium channel blocker that

    (A) is quite effective in supraventricular tachycardia
    (B) is used for the treatment of ischemic heart disease
    (C) has a half-life of 30 minutes
    (D) is a peripheral vasoconstrictor
    (E) is an effective drug for ventricular tachycardia

Questions 97 and 98

A 25-year-old man is admitted after abdominal trauma. After induction of anesthesia, a Foley catheter is inserted. There is little urine output. Blood pressure is 90/60. The urine/plasma osmolality ratio is found to be 2.5.

97. The treatment of choice is

    (A) ethacrynic acid
    (B) mannitol
    (C) furosemide
    (D) rapid infusion of 500 ml of balanced salt solution
    (E) fluid restriction

98. Later, the patient's central venous pressure (CVP) is found to be 22 cm H_2O. The treatment of choice should be

    (A) a loop diuretic
    (B) mannitol
    (C) 50% glucose
    (D) rapid infusion of balanced salt solution
    (E) 500 ml plasmanate

99. Certain drugs, such as phenylbutazone, aspirin, and radiographic contrast media, can prolong the action of thiopental by

    (A) competition for binding sites
    (B) leading to increased protein binding of thiopental
    (C) forming a more potent compound
    (D) causing a slower excretion
    (E) leading to enhanced distribution

100. The interaction of D-tubocurarine and acetylcholine at the myoneural junction is one of

    (A) synergism
    (B) competition for binding sites
    (C) chemical combination
    (D) alteration of metabolism
    (E) altered protein binding

101. The interaction of protamine and heparin to terminate anticoagulation is of

    (A) competition for binding sites
    (B) a chemical interaction leading to an inactive compound
    (C) pH change
    (D) a conformational change
    (E) platelet stimulation

102. Echothiophate causes prolongation of succinylcholine by

    (A) chemical interaction
    (B) interaction at site of absorption
    (C) altered protein binding
    (D) competition for binding sites
    (E) altered metabolism

103. Epinephrine causes a prolongation of activity for local anesthetics by

    (A) chemical interaction
    (B) interaction at site of absorption
    (C) altered protein binding
    (D) competition for binding sites
    (E) altered metabolism

104. The interaction of phenobarbital and phenytoin can be described as one of

    (A) chemical interaction
    (B) interaction at site of absorption
    (C) altered protein binding
    (D) competition for binding sites
    (E) altered metabolism

105. The interaction of a mixture of thiopental and meperidine is one of

    (A) synergism
    (B) interaction at site of absorption
    (C) altered protein binding
    (D) precipitation
    (E) altered metabolism

106. The combination of nitrous oxide at 0.5 MAC plus isoflurane 0.5 MAC is one of

    (A) antagonism
    (B) potentiation
    (C) additive effect
    (D) synergism
    (E) no effect

107. Isoflurane is to be used in a patient who has a history of chronic alcohol abuse. The interaction of alcohol and isoflurane is one of

    (A) antagonism
    (B) potentiation
    (C) additive effect
    (D) synergism
    (E) no effect

108. In the patient in Question 107, the MAC of isoflurane would be

    (A) increased
    (B) decreased
    (C) unchanged
    (D) at least doubled
    (E) dependent on liver function

109. The chemical formula for methoxyflurane is

    (A) $CFHCl\text{-}CF_2\text{-}O\text{-}CHF_2$
    (B) $CH_3\text{-}O\text{-}CF_2\text{-}CCl_2H$
    (C) $CF_3\text{-}CHCl\text{-}O\text{-}CHF_2$
    (D) $CHClBr\text{-}CF_3$
    (E) $C_2H_5\text{-}O\text{-}C_2H_5$

110. The chemical formula for halothane is

    (A) $CFHCl\text{-}CF_2\text{-}O\text{-}CHF_2$
    (B) $CH_3\text{-}O\text{-}CF_2\text{-}CCl_2H$
    (C) $CF_3\text{-}CHCl\text{-}O\text{-}CHF_2$
    (D) $CHClBr\text{-}CF_3$
    (E) $C_2H_5\text{-}O\text{-}C_2H_5$

111. The chemical formula for enflurane is

    (A) $CFHCl\text{-}CF_2\text{-}O\text{-}CHF_2$
    (B) $CH_3\text{-}O\text{-}CF_2\text{-}CCl_2H$
    (C) $CF_3\text{-}CHCl\text{-}O\text{-}CHF_2$
    (D) $CHClBr\text{-}CF_3$
    (E) $C_2H_5\text{-}O\text{-}C_2H_5$

112. The chemical formula for diethyl ether is

    (A) $CFHCl\text{-}CF_2\text{-}O\text{-}CHF_2$
    (B) $CH_3\text{-}O\text{-}CF_2\text{-}CCl_2H$
    (C) $CF_3\text{-}CHCl\text{-}O\text{-}CHF_2$
    (D) $CHClBr\text{-}CF_3$
    (E) $C_2H_5\text{-}O\text{-}C_2H_5$

113. The chemical formula for isoflurane is

    (A) $CFHCl\text{-}CF_2\text{-}O\text{-}CHF_2$
    (B) $CH_3\text{-}O\text{-}CF_2\text{-}CCl_2H$
    (C) $CF_3\text{-}CHCl\text{-}O\text{-}CHF_2$
    (D) $CHClBr\text{-}CF_3$
    (E) $C_2H_5\text{-}O\text{-}C_2H_5$

114. The minimal alveolar concentration (MAC) for methoxyflurane is

    (A) 0.77
    (B) 1.68
    (C) 1.15
    (D) 105
    (E) 0.16

115. The MAC for isoflurane is

    (A) 0.77
    (B) 1.68
    (C) 1.15
    (D) 105
    (E) 0.16

116. The MAC for enflurane is

    (A) 0.77
    (B) 1.68
    (C) 1.15
    (D) 105
    (E) 0.16

117. The MAC for nitrous oxide is

    (A) 0.77
    (B) 1.68
    (C) 1.15
    (D) 105
    (E) 0.16

118. The MAC for halothane is

    (A) 0.77
    (B) 1.68
    (C) 1.15
    (D) 105
    (E) 0.16

119. The drug thiopental is a(n)

    (A) isopropylphenol
    (B) butyrophenone
    (C) eugenol
    (D) barbiturate
    (E) benzodiazepine

120. The drug propofol is a(n)

    (A) isopropylphenol
    (B) butyrophenone
    (C) eugenol
    (D) barbiturate
    (E) benzodiazepine

121. The drug propanidid is a(n)

    (A) isopropylphenol
    (B) butyrophenone
    (C) eugenol
    (D) barbiturate
    (E) benzodiazepine

122. The drug droperiodol is a(n)

    (A) isopropylphenol
    (B) butyrophenone
    (C) eugenol
    (D) barbiturate
    (E) benzodiazepine

123. The drug diazepam is a(n)

    (A) isopropylphenol
    (B) butyrophenone
    (C) eugenol
    (D) barbiturate
    (E) benzodiazepine

124. The drug methohexital is a

    (A) phencyclidine derivative
    (B) butyrophenone
    (C) benzodiazepine derivative
    (D) drug whose action is terminated by rapid redistribution
    (E) drug that may cause skeletal muscle rigidity

125. The drug ketamine is a

    (A) phencyclidine derivative
    (B) butyrophenone
    (C) benzodiazepine derivative
    (D) drug whose action is terminated by rapid redistribution
    (E) drug that may cause skeletal muscle rigidity

126. The drug fentanyl is a

    (A) phencyclidine derivative
    (B) butyrophenone

    (C) benzodiazepine derivative
    (D) drug whose action is terminated by rapid redistribution
    (E) drug that may cause skeletal muscle rigidity

127. The drug lorazepam is a

    (A) phencyclidine derivative
    (B) butyrophenone
    (C) benzodiazepine derivative
    (D) drug whose action is terminated by rapid redistribution
    (E) drug that may cause skeletal muscle rigidity

128. The drug althesin is a

    (A) phencyclidine derivative
    (B) butyrophenone
    (C) benzodiazepine derivative
    (D) drug whose action is terminated by rapid redistribution
    (E) drug that may cause skeletal muscle rigidity

129. A drug that is a mixed agonist–antagonist is

    (A) butorphanol
    (B) naloxone
    (C) bleomycin
    (D) methohexital
    (E) midazolam

130. A drug that is a pure narcotic antagonist is

    (A) butorphanol
    (B) levallorphan
    (C) naloxone
    (D) neostigmine
    (E) edrophonium

131. A drug that is associated with pulmonary toxicity is

    (A) adriamycin
    (B) bleomycin
    (C) vincristine
    (D) methotrexate
    (E) L-asparaginase

132. Methohexital

    (A) is metabolized to a greater extent than thiopental
    (B) is broken down to active metabolites
    (C) has a longer elimination half-life than thiopental
    (D) causes histamine release from mast cells
    (E) is contraindicated in asthma

133. Midazolam

(A) is contraindicated in the child
(B) is shorter-acting than thiopental
(C) is associated with less frequent venous irritation than diazepam
(D) suppresses adrenal cortical function
(E) has a high incidence of histamine release

134. Lidocaine in a 1% solution

(A) is highly protein bound
(B) has a duration of 60 to 120 minutes
(C) is not effective topically
(D) is frequently associated with allergic reactions
(E) frequently causes tachycardia

135. The addition of epinephrine to a local anesthetic

(A) prolongs the duration of the drug's activity
(B) causes a higher peak level of the drug
(C) decreases intensity of the block
(D) increases surgical bleeding
(E) causes increased toxicity

136. Prilocaine

(A) is an ester derivative
(B) may be associated with methemoglobinemia
(C) is a fast-onset local anesthetic with long duration
(D) is associated with little liver metabolism
(E) is the drug of choice for the obstetric patient

137. Procaine and other ester local anesthetics are

(A) metabolized to a great extent in the lung
(B) metabolized in the cerebrospinal fluid (CSF)
(C) excreted unchanged in the urine
(D) broken down into active metabolites
(E) more slowly metabolized in patients with liver disease

138. Bupivacaine

(A) is an ester local anesthetic with short duration
(B) should be used in a concentration of 0.75% for epidurals
(C) is associated with cardiac toxicity due to its effect on sodium
(D) is not a problem unless injected directly intravenously
(E) cardiotoxicity is noted by the onset of tachycardia

139. Flecainide is

(A) an antidysrhythmic drug
(B) a lidocaine analog
(C) a muscle relaxant
(D) the drug of choice for local anesthesia reactions
(E) administered only orally

140. Alfentanil

(A) has a larger volume of distribution when compared to fentanyl
(B) is one-third more potent than fentanyl
(C) is longer acting than fentanyl
(D) has its effect terminated by being redistributed
(E) does not affect the MAC of enflurane

141. Sufentanil

(A) is less potent than fentanyl
(B) decreases intracranial pressure more than fentanyl
(C) is redistributed to terminate its effect
(D) has a more prolonged effect in the elderly
(E) has a longer duration of action than fentanyl

142. Prostaglandin E_1

(A) is a potent vasoconstrictor
(B) should be given by bolus
(C) should always be stopped before inducing anesthesia
(D) is useful in closing a patent ductus arteriosus
(E) may cause hypotension

143. Physostigmine

(A) may cause central anticholinergic syndrome
(B) does not cross the blood–brain barrier
(C) is less effective than neostigmine in treating emergence delirium
(D) may reverse the sedative effect of opioids
(E) is a long-acting drug

144. The patient on tricyclic antidepressants

(A) may have an increased number of arrhythmias
(B) should have halothane and pancuronium as drugs of choice
(C) should be cautioned to stop the medications before surgery
(D) may become hypotensive with ketamine
(E) may have short emergence with thiopental

145. A patient is to have a herniated disc injected with chymopapain. When you see the patient preoperatively, you should

(A) explain that general anesthesia will decrease the chance of allergic reactions
(B) check the history for any previous allergic reactions
(C) avoid all antihistamines in the perioperative period
(D) avoid use of cortisone, since it may increase the chance of an allergic reaction
(E) be aware that the chance of reaction is greater in men

146. A patient is brought to the operating room with an infusion of vancomycin running. You should

(A) stop the drug
(B) run the infusion as fast as possible to get the drug in before induction
(C) disconnect the intravenous line and place in a piggyback to give more control
(D) disregard the fact that vancomycin is present
(E) use atracurium as your choice of relaxant

147. Terbutaline

(A) is an alpha agonist
(B) is a selective beta$_2$ agonist
(C) causes more tachycardia than isoproterenol
(D) should be avoided in patients with heart disease
(E) cause hyperkalemia .

148. The patient who has abused cocaine

(A) will be calm and sedated
(B) may be treated with propranolol
(C) exhibits signs of sympathetic blockade
(D) will have bradycardia
(E) will have hypotension

149. Meperidine

(A) is a naturally occurring opioid
(B) is more potent than morphine
(C) is excreted unchanged in the urine
(D) is primarily metabolized in the liver
(E) is not useful orally

150. An asthmatic patient comes to the operating room with an infusion of aminophylline. The anesthetic of choice is

(A) high-dose fentanyl
(B) halothane
(C) morphine
(D) isoflurane
(E) a thiopental infusion

151. Ranitidine

(A) is a histamine (H$_2$) receptor antagonist that decreases gastric volume
(B) will decrease the pH of gastric fluid
(C) has a very short half-life
(D) must be given parenterally
(E) has a low incidence of CNS depression

152. Cromolyn sodium is used in the treatment of asthma because it

(A) has a direct effect on bronchioles
(B) stimulates cyclic AMP
(C) releases catecholamines
(D) prevents histamine release from mast cells
(E) decreases bronchiole reactivity

153. Verapamil is a calcium entry blocker that

(A) is very useful in the treatment of supraventricular tachycardia
(B) is contraindicated in patients with asthma
(C) is especially useful when combined with propranolol
(D) is a potent vasoconstrictor
(E) has no effect on the pacemaker cells

154. Chemical substances released at the time of an anaphylactic reaction include all of the following EXCEPT

(A) histamine
(B) slow-reacting substance A (SRS-A)
(C) eosinophilic chemotactic factor A (ECF-A)
(D) epinephrine
(E) prostaglandin

155. Glycopyrrolate

(A) is a quaternary amine
(B) crosses the blood–brain barrier with ease
(C) is associated with the central cholinergic syndrome
(D) is a cholinergic drug
(E) is a naturally occurring belladonna alkaloid

156. Amrinone

(A) is a catecholamine used for treatment of congestive failure
(B) is an antidysrhythmic drug
(C) causes peripheral vasoconstriction
(D) is effective orally or parenterally
(E) is associated with rapid onset of tachyphylaxis

157. The xanthine group of drugs

(A) includes caffeine
(B) has a strong beta$_1$ mimetic effect
(C) stimulates production of phosphodiesterase
(D) has a direct effect on bronchioles
(E) leads to a decrease in cyclic AMP

158. Hydralazine is an antihypertensive that

(A) is a vasodilator due to its catecholamine inhibitor properties
(B) may cause bradycardia
(C) may lead to a lupuslike syndrome
(D) leads to diuresis and sodium loss
(E) has beneficial effects in patients with angina

159. You are using trimethaphan for deliberate hypotension. This drug

(A) is a ganglionic blocker
(B) is associated with bradycardia
(C) causes pupillary constriction
(D) can be used at the same dose for long time periods
(E) may cause increases in catecholamines

160. A major side effect of valproic acid is

(A) renal failure
(B) hepatic failure
(C) muscle relaxation
(D) cardiac toxicity
(E) anemia

161. Sublingual drug administration

(A) leads to lower drug levels
(B) is effective for ionized drugs
(C) eliminates the first-pass effect
(D) leads to rapid liver breakdown of the drug
(E) requires a much larger dose for effectiveness

162. If a patient is to receive a calcium infusion for hypocalcemia, the calcium

(A) should be mixed with sodium bicarbonate
(B) can be given as the chloride or the gluconate
(C) may lead to tachycardia
(D) should be given via a peripheral vein to avoid cardiac effects
(E) gluconate salt is preferred

163. Your patient is a 45-year-old male with a history of hypertension. The hypertension has been controlled with diuretics alone. He is scheduled for a hernia repair. He is completely asymptomatic, but his potassium is 3.0 mEq/L. You should

(A) cancel the procedure
(B) start a potassium infusion and proceed
(C) do the procedure but not infuse potassium
(D) give 40 mEq of potassium before starting
(E) do the procedure only if it can be done under regional anesthesia

164. Metoclopramide

(A) is a dopamine stimulating drug
(B) decreases gastric acid secretion
(C) stimulates motility of the upper gastrointestinal tract
(D) may lead to vomiting
(E) leads to an ileus and increased small intestinal transit time

165. Bretylium

(A) inhibits release of norepinephrine
(B) is useful in the treatment of supraventricular tachycardia
(C) may lead to persistent hypertension
(D) has its effect on the renal–angiotensin system
(E) leads to tachycardia

166. Sodium nitroprusside is to be used for treatment of intraoperative hypertension. This drug

(A) causes venous dilatation only
(B) will be needed in increased doses if the patient receives propranolol
(C) may cause cyanide toxicity in high doses, evidenced by alkalosis and increasing drug dosage needed to achieve the same result
(D) may cause acidosis as a sign of toxicity
(E) may cause a toxicity that is evidenced by an acidosis that is responsive to sodium bicarbonate

167. Diazoxide is an antihypertensive that

(A) is little affected by protein binding
(B) has its primary effect on the capacitance vessels
(C) is administered by an infusion and titrated to effect
(D) is administered by bolus infusion
(E) causes decreased cardiac output

168. The drug dobutamine

(A) is primarily an alpha agonist
(B) is primarily a beta$_1$ agonist
(C) causes decreased renal blood flow
(D) is associated with severe increases in heart rate
(E) is a naturally occurring catecholamine

169. Edrophonium, in a dose of 1 mg/kg

(A) has a slower onset time than neostigmine
(B) has a much shorter duration than neostigmine
(C) has greater muscarinic side effects than neostigmine
(D) has a faster onset and decreased duration than neostigmine
(E) should be preceded by atropine

170. A patient with hypertension is being treated with clonidine. This drug

(A) has its primary effect in the brainstem
(B) should be quickly tapered before surgery
(C) should be given by infusion during surgery
(D) is a central analgesic that is reversed by naloxone
(E) increases the MAC of halothane

171. Your patient, who has a known history of heart disease and asthma, is seen in the recovery room with hypertension. You start an infusion of labetalol. The following statements about this drug are true EXCEPT

(A) it will not precipitate wheezing in this patient
(B) it is a beta blocker
(C) it is an alpha blocker
(D) it is conjugated in the liver
(E) the intravenous and oral doses are the same

172. A diabetic patient on NPH insulin is given protamine to neutralize heparin. There is a drop in blood pressure and wheezing is heard. All of the following are true EXCEPT

(A) patients on protamine-containing insulin are at risk for reactions to intravenous protamine
(B) protamine is a synthetic salt
(C) protamine can cause anaphylactic reactions
(D) patients suspected of being susceptible to a reaction should be given a small dose at first
(E) protamine given into a peripheral vein is less likely to cause histamine release

173. Esmolol

(A) is a beta$_1$ agonist
(B) has a half-life of 4 hours
(C) is contraindicated in the patient with AV block
(D) is more likely than propranolol to cause bronchospasm
(E) is broken down in the liver

174. A 45-year-old male is to have a gallbladder procedure. He has had heart disease and is on amiodarone. This drug

(A) should be stopped before surgery
(B) has a half-life of 4 hours
(C) is used for ventricular arrhythmias
(D) is eliminated by the kidneys
(E) should be stopped and any arrhythmias treated with diltiazem

175. Major side effects of amiodarone include all of the following EXCEPT

(A) hepatitis
(B) exacerbation of arrhythmias
(C) congestive heart failure
(D) pneumonitis
(E) renal failure

176. You are about to induce anesthesia in a patient who is a Jehovah's Witness. She adamantly refuses to receive blood. The procedure may require volume replacement. A product that may be used is

(A) packed red cells
(B) washed red cells
(C) autologous blood
(D) hetastarch
(E) platelets to decrease bleeding, thus making transfusion unnecessary

177. Hetastarch

(A) is a crystalloid solution
(B) is a synthetic colloid
(C) is free of allergenic potential
(D) does not interfere with coagulation
(E) is eliminated chiefly through the lungs

178. A local anesthetic that inhibits the reuptake of norepinephrine is

(A) procaine
(B) cocaine
(C) bupivacaine
(D) etidocaine
(E) lidocaine with epinephrine

179. The narcotic heroin

(A) is a naturally occurring substance
(B) has less brain penetration than morphine
(C) is less soluble than morphine
(D) causes more nausea than morphine
(E) is more addicting than morphine

180. The drug hydroxyzine

(A) is an antihistamine
(B) is a phenothiazine derivative
(C) is a potent analgesic
(D) produces amnesia
(E) is useful when given intravenously

181. Postoperative pain control with methadone

(A) is limited by its short half-life
(B) is more effective with oral administration
(C) is used on an every 2 hour regimen
(D) may take 48 hours to obtain a stable effect
(E) does not depress respiration

182. Therapeutic agents can affect hypoxic pulmonary vasoconstriction (HPV). A drug that potentiates HPV is

(A) isoflurane
(B) ibuprofen
(C) nitroglycerin
(D) halothane
(E) nitroprusside

183. Dopamine

(A) is a transmitter confined to the central nervous system
(B) stimulates dopaminergic receptors when the dose exceeds 10 µg/kg/minute
(C) decreases renal blood flow
(D) increases cardiac output by stimulating beta$_1$ receptors
(E) decreases pulmonary artery pressure

184. A patient is undergoing a procedure under non-depolarizing neuromuscular blockade. Near the end of the procedure, succinylcholine is given to facilitate closing the incision. This combination

    (A) will always lead to good closing conditions
    (B) will produce a block that will last about 10 minutes
    (C) may produce a long block
    (D) may then be antagonized by edrophonium
    (E) will lead to the same results regardless of the amount of succinylcholine given

185. Vecuronium

    (A) may be associated with bradycardia in patients on beta-blocking drugs
    (B) has an onset time independent of dose
    (C) is totally eliminated by the kidneys
    (D) activity is not prolonged by hepatic disease
    (E) must be used in reduced dose in patients with renal disease

186. Cimetidine may impede the metabolism of all of the following EXCEPT

    (A) lidocaine
    (B) propranolol
    (C) diazepam
    (D) atracurium
    (E) theophylline

187. The instillation of phenylephrine eyedrops used before eye muscle surgery may

    (A) be beneficial because of its mydriatic effect
    (B) lead to hypertension
    (C) be ineffective if used in 2.5% solution
    (D) lead to increased conjunctival bleeding
    (E) be used in the same concentration regardless of age

188. A patient is scheduled for glaucoma surgery. Timolol eyedrops have been in use for 2 months. This drug

    (A) is a beta agonist
    (B) may be beneficial in the patient with asthma
    (C) may lead to tachycardia under anesthesia
    (D) is not absorbed systemically
    (E) does not affect the size of the pupil

189. Drug elimination may be via all of the following EXCEPT

    (A) the liver
    (B) the kidneys
    (C) the lungs
    (D) sweat
    (E) muscles

190. Scopolamine is an anticholinergic drug that

    (A) increases heart rate better than atropine
    (B) is a better antisialogogue than atropine
    (C) has poorer amnestic properties than glycopyrrolate
    (D) has poorer sedative properties than glycopyrrolate
    (E) is better for decreasing gastric acid than glycopyrrolate

191. Nitrous oxide

    (A) always leads to increased blood pressure due to release of catecholamines
    (B) will lead to decreased cardiac output when combined with halothane
    (C) causes sympathetic inhibition
    (D) administered with an opioid will maintain cardiac output and peripheral vascular resistance
    (E) causes cardiovascular changes only when administered as the sole agent

192. Dantrolene is available to treat episodes of malignant hyperthermia (MH). This drug

    (A) has a half-life of 36 hours
    (B) reduces levels of intracellular calcium
    (C) causes marked cardiac depression
    (D) should be administered daily for 3 days after an MH episode
    (E) causes hepatotoxicity

193. Glucagon is a hormone with all of the following effects EXCEPT

    (A) decreased insulin secretion
    (B) inotropic cardiac effects
    (C) chronotropic cardiac effects
    (D) increased hepatic gluconeogenesis
    (E) anorexia

194. Atracurium is an intermediate duration neuromuscular blocker that

    (A) has only postjunctional effects
    (B) liberates histamine at all dose levels
    (C) liberates histamine if administered over 75 seconds
    (D) breaks down into laudanosine, which has caused seizures in humans
    (E) causes increased blood pressure

195. Drugs to be avoided in the patient with deficiency of glucose 6-phosphate dehydrogenase include all of the following EXCEPT

    (A) aspirin
    (B) methylene blue
    (C) primaquine
    (D) penicillin
    (E) isoflurane

196. Certain drugs may affect or are affected by cytochrome P-450. Which of the following is true?

(A) after treatment with phenobarbital, cytochrome P-450 is decreased
(B) diltiazem binds to cytochrome P-450, inhibiting drug metabolism
(C) cimetidine stimulates production of cytochrome P-450
(D) ranitidine causes increased biotransformation
(E) once the enzyme is induced, the level stays elevated for 10 days

197. The patient is a 72-year-old male with Parkinson's disease. He is on levodopa. Your anesthetic plan should include

(A) stopping levodopa for 24 hours before induction
(B) avoidance of droperidol
(C) use of phenothiazine to decrease the concentration of halothane
(D) use of ketamine as the drug of choice
(E) use of succinylcholine

198. A patient who has had surgical ablation of the pituitary gland is scheduled for surgery. She is on desmopressin twice daily. The drug

(A) should be given intravenously during the procedure
(B) may lead to an increase in blood pressure
(C) has a half-life of 3 hours
(D) is equally effective in nephrogenic diabetes insipidus
(E) may increase blood loss at the time of surgery

199. Dextran is a volume expander that

(A) may lead to fatal allergic reactions
(B) may lead to clot formation by accelerating coagulation
(C) interferes with crossmatching of blood due to the hemolysis it causes
(D) stays in the intravascular space for 3 hours
(E) blocks release of histamine

200. Reversal drugs are used at the end of many cases. All of the following are true EXCEPT

(A) reversal agents should be used if pancuronium was the relaxant
(B) reversal agents need not be used if atracurium was the relaxant
(C) reversal agents need not be used if vecuronium was the relaxant
(D) reversal agents need not be used if pipecuronium was the relaxant
(E) reversal agents are needed if BWA938U was the relaxant

201. The muscle relaxant BW1090U (mivacurium)

(A) is a steroidal compound
(B) is eliminated unchanged by the kidneys
(C) has a faster onset than succinylcholine
(D) has a longer duration than vecuronium
(E) is suitable for use by infusion

202. Edrophonium

(A) inhibits acetylcholinesterase by the same mechanism as neostigmine
(B) inhibits acetylcholinesterase by the same mechanism as pyridostigmine
(C) has a longer duration than neostigmine
(D) forms a chemical bond with the subsites on acetylcholinesterase
(E) has a shorter time of inhibition than neostigmine or pyridostigmine

203. A patient with hemiplegia is scheduled for open reduction of an ankle fracture. Pancuronium is administered. The patient may respond with

(A) hyperkalemia
(B) neuromuscular block on the normal side with decreased block on the affected side
(C) neuromuscular block on the affected side with decreased block on the normal side
(D) an exaggerated response
(E) a normal response on both sides

204. Age-related differences in dose responses include

(A) MAC increases with age
(B) slower induction in children
(C) lower induction dose of thiopental in the elderly
(D) shorter recovery time for ventilation in the elderly who have received fentanyl
(E) higher dose of fentanyl needed to achieve burst suppression in the elderly

205. Preanesthetic medication

(A) should be given in a standard dose to achieve standard effects
(B) need not take into consideration the patient's physical status
(C) need not take into consideration the patient's elective status
(D) should always include an antisialogogue
(E) may be given by mouth

206. Some patients may take their preanesthetic medication with a small amount of water. Patients who should be kept NPO even for the premedication include all of the following EXCEPT

(A) the obese
(B) those with hiatus hernias
(C) diabetics
(D) obstetric patients
(E) a 4-year-old-child

207. Nonparticulate antacid preanesthetic medication

(A) should be given 3 hours before surgery
(B) is shown to decrease gastric volume
(C) may lead to pulmonary distress if aspiration occurs
(D) has a lag time of 1 hour for effectiveness
(E) is aimed at raising the pH to >2.5

208. H$_2$ antagonists administered preoperatively

(A) facilitate gastric emptying
(B) should be used in all patients
(C) increase the pH of fluid in the stomach as well as fluid secreted after administration
(D) protect one against aspiration of gastric juice
(E) do not change the need for a cuffed tube

209. The drugs listed all decrease gastric acid EXCEPT

(A) cimetidine
(B) glycopyrrolate
(C) metoclopramide
(D) ranitidine
(E) scopolamine

210. All of the following statements are true of the use of diazepam used in preanesthetic medication EXCEPT

(A) will decrease anxiety
(B) will decrease recall
(C) will decrease the likelihood of local anesthetic toxicity
(D) should be given intramuscularly
(E) is a better amnestic if scopolamine is given with it

211. An induction agent that contains ethylene glycol in its formulation is

(A) thiopental
(B) methohexital
(C) lorazepam
(D) midazolam
(E) thiamylal

212. An induction agent that causes increases in intracranial pressure is

(A) thiopental
(B) methohexital
(C) ketamine
(D) thiamylal
(E) midazolam

213. The induction agent etomidate

(A) has no anticonvulsant activity
(B) releases histamine
(C) has analgesic properties
(D) does not decrease hepatic perfusion
(E) increases intraocular pressure

214. An induction agent causing postoperative adrenal suppression is

(A) thiopental
(B) midazolam
(C) ketamine
(D) etomidate
(E) propofol

215. A drug that can potentiate a depolarizing neuromuscular block and antagonize a nondepolarizing block is

(A) cytoxan
(B) azathioprine
(C) cyclosporin
(D) cimetidine
(E) cocaine

216. Patients with alcohol abuse

(A) will have increased anesthetic requirements in the acute state of intoxication
(B) will have reduced anesthetic requirement in the chronic abuse state
(C) will develop tolerance to the CNS effects with chronic usage
(D) will develop tolerance to the respiratory effects with chronic usage
(E) will develop tolerance to the cardiovascular effects with chronic usage

217. Which of the following is a beta antagonist?

(A) isoproterenol
(B) dobutamine
(C) nadolol
(D) albuterol
(E) ritodrine

218. A drug that is a tricyclic antidepressant is

(A) pargyline
(B) phenelzine
(C) isocarboxazid
(D) isosorbide
(E) doxepin

219. A patient who has abused cocaine is to be anesthetized for emergency surgery. All of the following are recommended EXCEPT

(A) avoid vasopressors
(B) avoid halothane
(C) avoid pancuronium
(D) avoid sympathomimetics
(E) avoid isoflurane

DIRECTIONS (Questions 220 through 390): For each of the items in this section, ONE or MORE of the numbered options is correct. Choose the answer

A if only 1, 2, and 3 are correct,
B if only 1 and 3 are correct,
C if only 2 and 4 are correct,
D if only 4 is correct,
E if all are correct.

220. (An) agent(s) known to increase cerebral blood flow is (are)

(1) halothane
(2) enflurane
(3) sevoflurane
(4) thiopental

221. If a patient has increased intracranial pressure and a volatile agent is to be used, methods that can be used to mitigate problems include

(1) use of an agent with the least potential to elevate cerebral blood flow
(2) use of hyperventilation before use of the volatile agent
(3) use of intravenous drugs to reduce intracranial pressure
(4) use of as low a dose as possible of the volatile agent

222. Elevation of the intracranial pressure seen with succinylcholine is

(1) due to increase of P_{CO_2} from fasciculation
(2) due to CNS activation from proprioceptors
(3) not seen in patients who are hyperventilated and given thiopental
(4) due to tightness of the neck muscles

223. Nifedipine

(1) is not available intravenously because of its photosensitivity
(2) may cause tachycardia as a compensatory effect
(3) is not suited for treatment of arrhythmias
(4) is a coronary vasoconstrictor

224. Calcium channel blockers

(1) should be continued through the perioperative period
(2) may be potentiated by amrinone
(3) will be additive with anesthetics
(4) may antagonize the effect of muscle relaxants

225. In the distribution phase of an intravenous drug

(1) blood is distributed to the vessel-rich group
(2) there is an equilibrium between blood and tissues

(3) a high perfusion causes slow equilibration
(4) diffusion factors may determine the time to equilibration

226. Drug clearance

(1) may be due to metabolism to an inactive product
(2) may be due to metabolism to less active products
(3) may be due to elimination of an unchanged drug
(4) is independent of drug concentration

227. The loading dose of a drug

(1) helps reach a tissue concentration in a shorter time
(2) causes a higher level than needed for a short time
(3) decreases the time to a steady-state plasma concentration
(4) may lead to undesirable effects

228. Noncatecholamine sympathomimetics include

(1) ephedrine
(2) dopamine
(3) methoxamine
(4) isoproterenol

229. Methoxamine

(1) is a pure alpha receptor stimulator
(2) is associated with reflex tachycardia
(3) increases afterload
(4) is used to treat bradycardia

230. Endogenous catecholamines include

(1) epinephrine
(2) norepinephrine
(3) dopamine
(4) dobutamine

231. Epinephrine

(1) stimulates alpha and beta receptors
(2) causes decreased systemic vascular resistance
(3) may lead to cardiac arrhythmias
(4) has strong chronotropic effects

232. Ephedrine

(1) is a catecholamine
(2) is a direct-acting pure alpha stimulator
(3) can be used for long periods without tachyphylaxis
(4) does not decrease uterine blood flow

SUMMARY OF DIRECTIONS				
A	B	C	D	E
1, 2, 3 only	1, 3 only	2, 4 only	4 only	All are correct

233. Amrinone

(1) is useful orally
(2) causes vasoconstriction
(3) has little effect on heart rate
(4) stimulates phosphodiesterase

B

234. Isoproterenol is useful

(1) in treating heart failure with pulmonary hypertension
(2) as a temporary pacemaker
(3) as a bronchodilator
(4) to treat overzealous beta blockade

235. Droperidol, used for preanesthetic medication

(1) may produce dysphoria
(2) increases intraoperative rhythm disturbance
(3) may produce extrapyramidal symptoms
(4) increases postoperative nausea and vomiting

236 Preanesthetic anticholinergics

(1) have a predictable effect on gastric pH
(2) have a predictable effect on gastric volume
(3) are all good amnestic drugs
(4) produce an antisialogogue effect

237. Conduction blockade by local anesthetics is by blockade of flow of

(1) calcium ions
(2) potassium ions
(3) magnesium ions
(4) sodium ions

238. Systemic signs of local anesthetic toxicity include

(1) numbness of lips and tongue
(2) tinnitus
(3) difficulty in focusing
(4) drowsiness

E

239. Toxic effects of local anesthetics

(1) are more prone to affect the cardiovascular system than the nervous system
(2) occur at about the same dose for all agents
(3) may be manifest as a shortened P-R interval
(4) may involve depression of the SA node

240. The cardiac effects of local anesthetics

(1) occur by interference with sodium conductance
(2) may be associated with ventricular fibrillation

(3) are worse with bupivacaine because the effect is longer
(4) are easily treated with diazepam

241. The use of the priming principle to shorten the onset time for neuromuscular blocking agents

(1) uses divided doses of the drug
(2) is a consistent method for obtaining blockade in an emergency
(3) may lead to the patient having difficulty in swallowing and protecting the airway in the interval period
(4) requires an interval period of 120 seconds

242. Drug elimination from the body

(1) is faster than distribution
(2) may occur by metabolism
(3) is usually complete after 2 half-lives
(4) may occur by excretion

243. Vecuronium administered to infants

(1) has the same ED_{50} as in adults
(2) has a longer duration
(3) has an altered effect, since infants are more sensitive
(4) has a greater volume of distribution

E

244. When using an infusion of a muscle relaxant

(1) monitoring is not necessary once the steady state is reached
(2) the first twitch should be maintained
(3) volatile agents will not affect relaxant requirements
(4) atracurium should not be mixed in Ringer's lactate solution

245. Administration of phenylephrine

(1) is useful in treating cyanotic episodes in tetralogy of Fallot
(2) always leads to an increased cardiac output
(3) causes increases in pulmonary artery occlusion pressure
(4) is given in doses of 10 to 25 mg/70 kg

246. Aminophylline is

(1) a catecholamine
(2) a beta agonist
(3) an adrenergic drug
(4) a phosphodiesterase inhibitor

247. Halothane sensitizes the heart to catecholamines. This sensitization

(1) is accentuated by hypoxemia
(2) is accentuated by hypercarbia
(3) can be abolished by beta blockers
(4) can be abolished by calcium channel blockers

248. Epinephrine regimen(s) that is (are) relatively safe when halothane is employed include(s)

(1) concentration no greater than 1:100,000
(2) adult dose not greater than 10 ml of 1:100,000 within 10 minutes
(3) adult dose not greater than 20 ml of 1:200,000 within 10 minutes
(4) adult total dose not to exceed 30 ml of 1:100,000 within 1 hour

249. The decrease in cerebral metabolic rate by inhaled anesthetics is

(1) most profound with isoflurane
(2) independent of dose
(3) linked with cerebral electrical activity
(4) not affected by seizure activity with enflurane

250. Cardiovascular changes seen with halogenated hydrocarbons are

(1) blood pressure decrease due to depression of cardiac output with halothane
(2) blood pressure decrease due to vasodilatation and depression of contractility with enflurane
(3) blood pressure decrease due to decreased peripheral vascular resistance with isoflurane
(4) more pronounced heart rate changes with halothane than with isoflurane

251. Nitrous oxide

(1) decreases pulmonary vascular resistance
(2) increases cardiac output when given with opioids
(3) decreases blood pressure when administered with isoflurane
(4) increases blood pressure when given with halothane

252. Hepatic blood flow is decreased by

(1) halothane
(2) enflurane
(3) isoflurane
(4) nitrous oxide

253. Drug(s) considered safe for the patient with a history of malignant hyperthermia is (are)

(1) barbiturates
(2) local anesthetics
(3) droperidol
(4) atracurium

254. Increasing the dose of pancuronium from its ED$_{95}$ to twice the ED$_{95}$

(1) shortens the onset of block to 1.8 minutes
(2) increases the intensity of the block
(3) lengthens the time of recovery
(4) has no effect on heart rate

255. The metabolic breakdown of halothane results in

(1) trifluoroacetic acid
(2) chloride ion
(3) fluoride ion
(4) bromine ion

256. Physostigmine has been shown to reverse the CNS effects of

(1) Benadryl
(2) Sominex
(3) diazepam
(4) meperidine

257. Intravenous benzodiazepines

(1) are equally effective amnestic agents
(2) produce little cardiovascular depression
(3) are not associated with respiratory depression
(4) are metabolized by the liver

258. Digoxin

(1) increases contractile force
(2) slows heart rate
(3) causes an effect in sodium-potassium ATPase
(4) is potentiated by calcium

259. Digitalis toxicity may be manifest in

(1) prolonged P-R interval
(2) nausea and vomiting
(3) multifocal PVCs
(4) tachycardia

260. The histamine release seen with administration of muscle relaxants may cause

(1) bradycardia
(2) erythema
(3) increases of peripheral vascular resistance
(4) hypotension

261. Doxorubicin (Adriamycin) produces a toxic cardiomyopathy that

(1) is present only during therapy
(2) is dose dependent
(3) is not affected by radiation therapy
(4) can be evaluated with echocardiography

262. Esmolol

(1) is an ester
(2) has a longer half-life if succinylcholine is used
(3) can blunt response to intubation
(4) has a prolonged effect

SUMMARY OF DIRECTIONS				
A	**B**	**C**	**D**	**E**
1, 2, 3 only	1, 3 only	2, 4 only	4 only	All are correct

263. Doxapram

    (1) is a centrally acting analeptic
    (2) requires an intact carotid body
    (3) is not useful in drug-induced coma
    (4) should not be used for postoperative hypoventilation

264. A child is brought to the emergency room for evaluation of his disoriented state. This was first noticed after he ate some berries. He is also noted to be very warm, to be flushed, and to have dilated pupils. Your suggested treatment should be

    (1) CT scan
    (2) aspirin
    (3) sponge baths for the fever
    (4) physostigmine

265. A patient has been on steroid therapy for a dermatologic problem for 2 years. She is to undergo a cholecystectomy. Your approach to steroid coverage should include

    (1) use of a mineralocorticoid
    (2) use of a parenteral dose with induction
    (3) use of glucocorticoid the night before surgery
    (4) use of an infusion for 24 hours

266. A patient who has been on steroids within a year preceding surgery

    (1) may not have any problem
    (2) has little risk with low-dose supplementation
    (3) is at risk of having a stress reaction without coverage
    (4) should be covered with supplemental steroids

267. You have begun to administer intravenous methicillin when there is a sudden increase in airway pressure, wheezing, tachycardia, and a decreased blood pressure. Your treatment should include

    (1) stop the methicillin infusion
    (2) administer 100% oxygen
    (3) give volume expanders
    (4) given a bolus of epinephrine of 5 μg

268. Tachyphylaxis is seen when using

    (1) thiopental
    (2) trimethaphan
    (3) isoproterenol
    (4) epinephrine

269. Mannitol

    (1) is filtered at the glomerulus
    (2) is an osmotic diuretic
    (3) causes an immediate increase in intravascular volume
    (4) is of value in congestive failure

270. Relative contraindications to the use of osmotic diuretics include

    (1) congestive heart failure
    (2) renal failure with oliguria
    (3) cerebral AV malformations
    (4) cerebral aneurysms

271. Alpha receptors in the adrenergic nervous system

    (1) are stimulated by norepinephrine
    (2) are blocked by labetalol
    (3) cause vasoconstriction
    (4) cause bronchial dilatation

272. Beta$_2$ receptors in the adrenergic nervous system

    (1) are stimulated by isoproterenol
    (2) are antagonized by esmolol
    (3) cause glycogenolysis
    (4) cause vasoconstriction

273. Magnesium deficiency may

    (1) be seen in the chronic alcoholic
    (2) occur as cardiac arrhythmias
    (3) be associated with skeletal muscle spasm
    (4) be associated with CNS irritability

274. The opioids produce

    (1) dilated pupils
    (2) nausea and vomiting mediated through the gastrointestinal tract
    (3) good amnesia
    (4) unconsciousness at high doses

275. A patient scheduled for an emergency procedure gives a history of drug abuse. Problems that must be anticipated include

    (1) full stomach
    (2) exposure to AIDS
    (3) exposure to hepatitis
    (4) decreased need for anesthetics

276. Drugs that are helpful in the treatment of the opioid addict include

    (1) clonidine
    (2) butorphanol
    (3) propranolol
    (4) nalbuphine

277. Cyanide toxicity from administration of sodium nitroprusside

   (1) occurs at blood levels >100 μg/100 ml
   (2) is aggravated by the previous treatment with captopril
   (3) is seen more often in patients who are nutritionally deprived
   (4) will not occur if the dose is kept under 2 mg/kg/hour

278. Drugs that depend on renal elimination and, therefore, must be avoided or used in reduced dosage in the patient with renal failure include

   (1) penicillin
   (2) gallamine
   (3) digoxin
   (4) vecuronium

279. Drugs suitable for the patient with hyperthyroidism include

   (1) ketamine
   (2) succinylcholine
   (3) pancuronium
   (4) thiopental

280. The mechanism of the coronary steal seen with isoflurane involves

   (1) preferential dilatation of intramyocardial arterioles
   (2) increased flow through stenotic vessels
   (3) greater pressure drop across stenotic vessels
   (4) lesser flow through pressure-dependent collaterals

281. Corticosteroids given for the treatment of asthma

   (1) have an immediate onset of action
   (2) have no use in the anesthetized patient
   (3) are best given by the inhalation route to decrease onset time
   (4) should involve only those drugs with little mineralocorticoid effect

282. Drug therapy appropriate for ventricular arrhythmias includes

   (1) lidocaine
   (2) procainamide
   (3) bretylium
   (4) magnesium sulfate

283. Mechanism(s) that accurately describe the effect of the drugs used to produce deliberate hypotension is (are)

   (1) sodium nitroprusside dilates capacitance vessels

   (2) trimethaphan is a ganglionic blocker
   (3) nitroglycerin dilates resistance vessels
   (4) isoflurane dilates peripheral vasculature

284. Disadvantage(s) of the use of halogenated hydrocarbons for deliberate hypotension is (are)

   (1) seizure activity stimulated by halothane
   (2) increased perfusion pressure
   (3) increased myocardial blood flow due to coronary stimulation
   (4) loss of autoregulation

285. Anesthetic management of the patient in renal failure should include

   (1) increased dose of thiopental because of decreased protein binding
   (2) use of a combination of midazolam and an opioid
   (3) succinylcholine for intubation
   (4) maintenance of anesthesia with isoflurane

286. Anesthetic agents that are appropriate for the patient with asthma include

   (1) thiopental
   (2) enflurane
   (3) isoflurane
   (4) halothane

287. Drugs that increase the production of cerebrospinal fluid include

   (1) acetazolamide
   (2) reserpine
   (3) digoxin
   (4) theophylline

288. Ionization of a drug

   (1) is a function of pH of the fluid it is in
   (2) may render a drug inactive
   (3) is a function of the pKa
   (4) may affect the drug's ability to cross membranes

289. The action of thiopental in the obese patient is affected by the

   (1) fat/blood partition coefficient of 11
   (2) fact that the concentration of thiopental in the blood is greater than in fat
   (3) fact that adipose tissue is capable of great uptake of thiopental
   (4) pH of thiopental

SUMMARY OF DIRECTIONS				
A	B	C	D	E
1, 2, 3 only	1, 3 only	2, 4 only	4 only	All are correct

290. When providing anesthesia for an obese patient

(1) thiopental should be administered on a milligram per kilogram basis
(2) emergence may be prolonged due to volatile agents leaching out of fat stores
(3) thiopental equilibrium will not occur between blood and tissue
(4) isoflurane is a good drug because of its low metabolism

291. The usual, or normal, reaction to an intravenous anesthetic agent, such as thiopental, may be altered by

(1) hypovolemia
(2) compromised hepatic function
(3) obesity
(4) alkalosis

292. The principal disadvantage(s) of methohexital is (are)

(1) poor solubility
(2) pain on injection
(3) low pH
(4) involuntary muscle movements

293. A patient with intermittent porphyria

(1) voids dark urine
(2) voids urine containing uroporphyrins, which is pathognomonic of the disease
(3) will have urine negative for porphobilinogen
(4) will give a positive Watson-Schwartz test

294. The short duration of methohexital is due to

(1) its low pH
(2) its inactivation by metabolism
(3) low fat solubility
(4) its redistribution

295. After intravenous injection, the distribution of thiopental will show

(1) rapidly falling concentration in the central pool
(2) increasing concentration in the viscera
(3) a rising concentration in the lean tissues that follows the concentration in the viscera
(4) a slowly rising concentration in the fatty tissue

296. The rapidly perfused (vessel-rich) tissues include

(1) heart
(2) kidney
(3) central nervous system
(4) muscle

297. The graph depicts the relative effect of thiopental in three physiologic states. From this we can say that

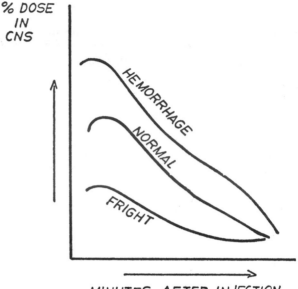

(1) in the normal patient, there is an initial high concentration followed by rapidly decreasing concentration
(2) a patient in shock will have decreased effect from thiopental
(3) the anxious patient will require a larger dose
(4) the bleeding patient has a faster loss of level as a result of the thiopental being lost with the blood

298. Tissue perfusion will affect the thiopental concentration. The shock patient is an example of this, since

(1) cerebral blood flow is poorly maintained in shock
(2) vasoconstriction occurs in skin and skeletal muscles in shock
(3) the dose of thiopental going to the brain is lower in shock
(4) cardiac output is reduced and cerebral blood flow is relatively higher in the shock patient

299. A comparison of a dissociative and a conventional anesthetic shows that

(1) the relaxed, nonresponding state is present in each

(2) the eyes remain open in dissociative anesthesia

(3) the presence of movement is a sign of insufficient dosage in each

(4) there is increased muscle tone in dissociative anesthesia

300. Cardiovascular changes noted after ketamine administration include

(1) decreased systolic blood pressure

(2) decreased diastolic blood pressure

(3) decreased heart rate

(4) increased cardiac output

301. Under ketamine anesthesia, the eye effects include

(1) open lids with an adequate level of anesthesia

(2) diplopia occurring in the postoperative period

(3) nystagmus

(4) lacrimation

302. The pharmacologic effects of ketamine include

(1) depression of the medial thalamic nuclei

(2) retention of visceral sensation

(3) maintenance of respiratory rate and tidal volume at near normal levels

(4) loss of gag reflex

303. Emergence sequelae with ketamine include delirium and dreaming, which

(1) is always of an unpleasant nature

(2) occurs equally in men and women

(3) is decreased by a vigorous stir-up regimen in the recovery room

(4) can be minimized by medication

304. Local anesthetic agents block nerve conduction by

(1) blocking conduction through the myelin sheath

(2) forming a salt in the nerve membrane

(3) depolarizing the membrane

(4) blocking the ionic movement through membrane pores

305. The blocking property of a local anesthetic

(1) is greatly affected by pH

(2) involves the penetration of the nerve membrane by the basic component of the agent

(3) is decreased if injected into inflamed tissue

(4) is enhanced by the addition of buffer

306. Comparison of duration of action of local anesthetics shows that the

(1) duration of lidocaine is approximately 60 minutes

(2) duration of procaine is approximately 30 minutes

(3) duration of mepivacaine is approximately 120 minutes

(4) addition of epinephrine increases the duration of lidocaine more than that of mepivacaine

307. Systemic toxicity to a local anesthetic is related to the

(1) dose of drug

(2) rapidity of injection

(3) vascularity of the site injected

(4) inherent toxicity of the drug injected

308. If a patient has an allergic reaction to lidocaine administered from a multidose vial, he or she

(1) will probably also react to mepivacaine

(2) will probably have no reaction to procaine

(3) may be exhibiting a reaction to methylparaben

(4) can be given an additional dose of lidocaine with impunity

Questions 309 through 311

A 46-year-old woman enters the hospital for correction of strabismus. She has been using echothiophate iodide drops for 2 years. She undergoes induction of anesthesia with thiopental, and succinylcholine is given to facilitate intubation. Anesthesia is maintained with N_2O/O_2 and a narcotic. At the end of the procedure, the patient is apneic.

309. The cause of the apnea in this patient may be

(1) low P_{CO_2} due to hyperventilation

(2) prolonged succinylcholine effect

(3) narcotic depression from premedication

(4) depression due to thiopental

310. Maneuvers that can be done to ascertain the cause of this depression include

(1) use of a nerve stimulator

(2) determination of arterial P_{CO_2}

(3) administration of a narcotic antagonist

(4) allowing the P_{CO_2} to build up by withholding ventilation for 3 minutes

311. Your tests show that your patient has no twitch or tetanic response to nerve stimulation. P_{CO_2} is 38 torr, and there is no response to narcotic antagonism. The proper treatment is

(1) administration of a CO_2 mixture

(2) administration of a stimulant, eg, doxapram

(3) administration of neostigmine

(4) artificial ventilation as long as necessary

SUMMARY OF DIRECTIONS

A	B	C	D	E
1, 2, 3 only	1, 3 only	2, 4 only	4 only	All are correct

Questions 312 and 313

A 49-year-old white male underwent induction of anesthesia for repair of an abdominal aneurysm. During induction, he received thiopental and succinylcholine followed by halothane 1% in N_2O/O_2 at 2 L each per minute. Within 5 minutes of intubation, massive swelling of the salivary glands was noted, accompanied by profuse sialorrhea.

312. Possible cause(s) of this condition is (are)

(1) succinylcholine
(2) endotracheal intubation
(3) overactive pharyngeal reflex
(4) thiopental

313. To treat this patient, one should

(1) stop the succinylcholine
(2) cancel the procedure
(3) observe the patient for at least 1 hour to determine if the swelling will subside
(4) perform an emergency tracheostomy at once

314. The resting membrane potential of a muscle cell is

(1) about −90 mV
(2) primarily dependent on the relative concentration of intracellular and extracellular potassium
(3) dependent on the selective permeability of the cell membrane
(4) changed rapidly with depolarization

315. Myoglobinemia

(1) may occur after a single dose of succinylcholine
(2) is a well-known but harmless side effect of succinylcholine administration in children
(3) is more common in children
(4) is known to result from smooth muscle breakdown

316. Succinylcholine is given to a 35-year-old primipara for an elective cesarean section in the 38th week of pregnancy. At the end of the procedure, the patient is apneic. Succinylcholine given to a pregnant patient

(1) may lead to prolonged block in a patient with a high dibucaine number
(2) may lead to a prolonged block as a result of low pseudocholinesterase level
(3) will lead to increased uterine motility
(4) may cross the placenta if given in large dose (over 300 mg)

317. Succinylcholine may cause prolonged apnea in patients

(1) exposed to organophosphate insecticides
(2) with severe liver disease
(3) receiving echothiophate eyedrops
(4) with heterozygous atypical pseudocholinesterase

318. The signs of nondepolarizing block include

(1) fade of response to twitch rate
(2) fade of response to tetanic rate
(3) posttetanic facilitation
(4) no change after administration of anticholinesterase drug

319. A patient has been receiving lithium for a psychiatric disorder. At the time of surgery, you could expect which of the following drugs to be potentiated?

(1) pancuronium
(2) succinylcholine
(3) gallamine
(4) D-tubocurarine

320. The release of acetylcholine at the motor nerve terminal is dependent on the

(1) ionic conditions
(2) intensity of the depolarization
(3) duration of the depolarization
(4) resting level of the presynaptic membrane

321. In an anesthetized patient, hemodynamic responses to neuromuscular blockers may be altered by

(1) anesthetic depth
(2) surgical stimulation
(3) blood volume
(4) sex of the patient

322. Injection of succinylcholine is normally followed by

(1) the presence of myoglobinemia
(2) profound bradycardia
(3) muscle pain noted mainly in the arms
(4) an increase in potassium value by 0.5 to 1.0 mEq/L

323. A change in heart rate may be noted after injection of succinylcholine. This usually is

(1) a tachycardia with the first dose in children
(2) a bradycardia if a repeat injection is used
(3) not related to the type of general anesthesia being used
(4) associated with an increase in blood pressure

324. Injection of succinylcholine may be followed by increased intragastric pressure, which

(1) will not lead to regurgitation unless the pressure exceeds 75 cm of water pressure

(2) may lead to regurgitation more readily if the patient has a hiatus hernia

(3) may be accentuated by prior injection of atropine, 0.6 mg, intravenously

(4) may be attenuated by pretreating the patient with 4 to 6 mg of D-tubocurarine

325. Atracurium is a muscle relaxant that

(1) has little renal clearance

(2) has minimal cardiovascular effects

(3) is easily antagonized

(4) is broken down by hydrolysis

326. The development of dual (phase II, desensitization) block

(1) only follows prolonged treatment with high doses of succinylcholine

(2) is both time and dose dependent

(3) cannot be detected clinically

(4) follows a stage of tachyphylaxis

327. The cholinergic receptor at the motor endplate

(1) is activated (depolarized) by acetylcholine

(2) may be activated by molecules, such as succinylcholine

(3) is refractory to further depolarization for a few milliseconds after activation

(4) is the only site of activity of acetylcholine

328. Muscle relaxant side effects caused by activation or inhibition of cholinergic receptor sites include

(1) muscle fasciculation

(2) increased intraocular pressure

(3) bradycardia

(4) histamine release

329. Histamine release is associated with

(1) erythema of the upper chest

(2) hypertension

(3) bronchospasm in susceptible patients

(4) bradycardia

330. The enzyme acetylcholinesterase is composed of two subsites, the anionic site and the esteratic site. Inhibitors of the enzyme block either one or both of these sites. The inhibitor(s) that block by forming a carbamyl ester at the esteratic site is (are)

(1) neostigmine

(2) pyridostigmine

(3) physostigmine

(4) edrophonium

331. Plasma cholinesterase

(1) has no known physiologic function

(2) is specific for succinylcholine

(3) is inhibited by hexafluorenium

(4) is activated by echothiophate

332. Succinylcholine is contraindicated in

(1) amyotrophic lateral sclerosis

(2) massive tissue trauma

(3) paraplegia

(4) burns

333. Studies of the hemodynamic effect of nondepolarizing drugs show that

(1) the hypotensive effect of D-tubocurarine is not dose related

(2) the tachycardia of pancuronium is not dose related

(3) the tachycardia of gallamine is only present at above relaxant doses

(4) metocurine has much less cardiovascular effect than D-tubocurarine

334. The dosage of relaxant drugs

(1) varies widely from patient to patient

(2) should be individualized

(3) should be sufficient to abolish 90 to 95% of twitch

(4) should be given on a fixed time scale

335. When reversing nondepolarizing neuromuscular blockers

(1) the peak effect of atropine occurs in 10 to 15 mintues

(2) the peak effect of neostigmine occurs in 10 to 15 minutes

(3) the twitch height is the best indicator of reversal

(4) adequate reversal is more important in patients with renal failure

336. The relaxation achieved with succinylcholine

(1) varies little from patient to patient for a specific dose

(2) is more prolonged when administered by infusion than by single doses

(3) is always prolonged with onset of desensitization block

(4) cannot be readily antagonized

337. Factors that may affect the dosage of D-tubocurarine include

(1) premedication

(2) acid-base status

(3) anesthetic concentration

(4) anesthetic used

SUMMARY OF DIRECTIONS				
A	**B**	**C**	**D**	**E**
1, 2, 3 only	1, 3 only	2, 4 only	4 only	All are correct

338. The action of pancuronium may be modified by

(1) previous injection of succinylcholine, which decreases the action of pancuronium
(2) deep halothane anesthesia, which will potentiate pancuronium
(3) the site of administration
(4) the use of atropine in premedication

339. Pyridostigmine, when compared with neostigmine, has

(1) a longer duration of action
(2) greater dependence on the kidneys for elimination
(3) fewer side effects
(4) a more rapid onset of action

340. The myasthenia gravis patient

(1) has weakness of muscle groups commonly involving cranial muscles, eg, ocular and oropharyngeal
(2) has neurologic defects
(3) is very sensitive to nondepolarizing agents
(4) has a constant degree of paralysis

341. Dual block

(1) develops immediately after injection of a large dose of succinylcholine
(2) follows a stage of tachyphylaxis
(3) only occurs after doses of succinylcholine in excess of 5 mg/kg
(4) will respond to anticholinesterase

342. The myasthenic syndrome (Eaton-Lambert syndrome) is a condition in which

(1) patients show sensitivity to depolarizing muscle relaxants
(2) the neuromuscular block is readily reversed by neostigmine
(3) sensitivity to nondepolarizing relaxants is increased
(4) resection of the tumor does not effect a cure

343. Local anesthetics

(1) increase the effectiveness of succinylcholine
(2) antagonize acetylcholine
(3) potentiate nondepolarizing drugs
(4) depolarize the neuromuscular junction

344. In a patient with myotonia, you would expect

(1) muscle spasm that occurs after succinylcholine
(2) muscle spasm that does not relax with D-tubocurarine
(3) increased muscle tone that is alleviated by quinine
(4) increased muscle tone aggravated by procainamide

345. The activity of muscle relaxants is affected by many conditions. You would expect

(1) a limb with high blood flow to have a prolonged block
(2) curare to be potentiated by respiratory acidosis
(3) gallamine reversal to be faster in a state of acidosis
(4) a patient with renal disease to have a prolonged block from curare

346. Gallamine

(1) cannot be mixed with thiopental
(2) increases the heart rate independently of the autonomic nervous system
(3) is broken down in the liver
(4) has a shorter duration than curare

347. The effects of acetylcholine that are accentuated by the use of neostigmine include

(1) bradycardia
(2) sweating
(3) skeletal muscle stimulation
(4) urinary retention

348. Tetanus is a disease characterized by muscle stiffness and paroxysmal spasms. In the treatment

(1) sedation with diazepam may also relieve the spasm
(2) D-tubocurarine is helpful to relieve the spasm
(3) labetalol may relieve the sympathetic overactivity
(4) pancuronium may increase heart rate and cause hypertension

349. In a patient paralyzed by neuromuscular blocking drugs, depth of anesthesia can be assessed by

(1) blood pressure
(2) eye movement
(3) pulse rate
(4) muscle tone

Questions 350 through 352

Two or more drugs administered to the same patient may interact in many ways, or their effects can be entirely independent.

350. Drug antagonism may occur when two drugs

(1) actually combine in the body
(2) both affect a physiologic system in a similar way
(3) compete for the same receptor site
(4) displace the dose–response curve in the same direction

351. Two drugs are said to have an additive effect when

(1) one drug will accelerate the speed of onset of the other
(2) one drug will prolong the action of the other
(3) both drugs are of the same chemical family
(4) the combined effect of the two drugs is the algebraic sum of the individual actions

352. Two drugs, A and B, may also interact by which of the following complex reactions?

(1) Drug A may interfere with the gastrointestinal absorption of drug B
(2) drug A may interfere with the protein binding of drug B
(3) drug A may interfere with the renal excretion of drug B
(4) drug A may alter electrolyte patterns, which, in turn, affect drug B

Questions 353 and 354

Please refer to the following figure:

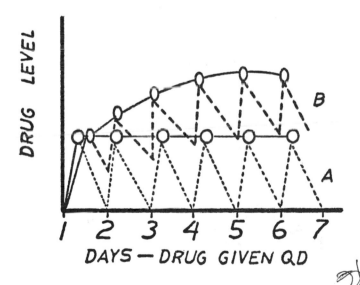

353. The graph shows the results of cumulative drug effect. From the graph, you can say that

(1) drug A does not maintain therapeutic levels when administered every 24 hours
(2) drug A exhibits cumulative properties

(3) drug B is cumulative when administered every 24 hours
(4) drug B is completely destroyed in less than 24 hours

354. The graph shows that

(1) drug A has a long half-life in the body
(2) a large initial dose of both drugs was given
(3) different doses are given for initial doses and maintenance doses
(4) in the case of drug B, the body does not remove one dose before another is administered

Questions 355 and 356

Please refer to the following figure:

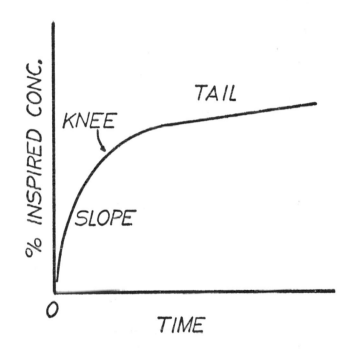

355. In the graph, the factor(s) affecting the initial slope is (are)

(1) cardiac output
(2) temperature
(3) alveolar ventilation
(4) age of patient

356. The knee of the initial slope

(1) will vary with the type of vaporizer used
(2) is independent of blood gas solubility
(3) will vary with the temperature
(4) is dependent on the concentration of the inspired anesthetic

SUMMARY OF DIRECTIONS				
A	B	C	D	E
1, 2, 3 only	1, 3 only	2, 4 only	4 only	All are correct

357. The factor(s) that determine the rate at which a certain partial pressure is reached include(s)

(1) concentration in the inspired gas
(2) uptake by blood
(3) alveolar concentration
(4) tissue uptake

358. The alveolar concentration of a gas

(1) is independent of the lung volume
(2) will vary with alveolar ventilation
(3) will vary with the type of soda lime used
(4) is dependent on uptake of the blood

359. Uptake of an agent by blood is determined by

(1) passage across the alveolar membrane
(2) the Ostwald coefficient
(3) the cardiac output
(4) the types of system being used

360. The administration of halothane

(1) may cause a decrease in respiratory resistance
(2) decreases respiratory resistance by direct effect
(3) decreases respiratory resistance through its anesthetic effect
(4) is always useful in bronchospastic conditions

361. The sympathetic stimulating properties of nitrous oxide are

(1) intensified in patients on gangliolytics
(2) decreased in the elderly
(3) lowest in young, healthy patients
(4) decreased in debilitated patients

362. The addition of nitrous oxide to a halothane anesthetic

(1) will have the greatest effect early in the course of the anesthesia
(2) will have its greatest effect at deeper levels of anesthesia
(3) may cause antagonism of halothane
(4) will cause intense vasodilatation

363. The circulatory effects of halothane include

(1) increased contractile force of the ventricle
(2) ganglionic blockade
(3) increased cardiac output
(4) reduced total peripheral resistance

364. The circulatory effects of halothane are

(1) insignificant at 0.5%
(2) due to a single mechanism
(3) essentially the same at 1% and 2%
(4) all due to its central action

365. Enflurane is a volatile anesthetic agent that causes

(1) generalized electroencephalographic hyperexcitability
(2) seizure patterns similar to minor motor seizures
(3) more seizure activity in the hypocapnic state
(4) an electroencephalographic pattern similar to that caused by ketamine

366. MAC-BAR

(1) is the anesthetic concentration at which adrenergic response to surgical stimulus is blocked
(2) is the desired concentration for most surgical procedures
(3) is higher than MAC
(4) will not block response to tracheal intubation

367. The addition of nitrous oxide to an enflurane–oxygen anesthetic with controlled ventilation causes

(1) decreased cardiac output more than with enflurane alone
(2) decreased stroke volume more than with enflurane alone
(3) decreased blood pressure more than with enflurane alone
(4) sympathetic stimulation

368. A patient is breathing a nitrous oxide–oxygen mixture and has an endotracheal tube cuff filled with a gas. You would expect an increase in

(1) volume of the cuff if it is filled with air
(2) volume of the cuff if it is filled with a nitrous oxide–oxygen mixture
(3) volume and pressure of a large volume cuff
(4) pressure but not volume of a small volume cuff

369. Nitrous oxide administered in a 40% concentration to patients with coronary artery disease

(1) decreases mean arterial blood pressure
(2) decreases left ventricular end-diastolic pressure (LVEDP)
(3) decreases left ventricular contractile force
(4) increases cardiac output

370. The beta receptors prepare the body for flight or fright by

(1) increasing the cardiac output
(2) bronchoconstriction
(3) increasing the circulating glucose
(4) decreasing insulin release

371. Beta blockers have therapeutic usefulness in

(1) coronary artery disease
(2) cardiac arrhythmias
(3) pheochromocytoma
(4) obstructive cardiomyopathy

372. An imbalance of the sympathetic nervous system may be precipitated by treatment with beta blockers. Examples of this effect may be seen in

(1) thyrotoxicosis
(2) congestive heart failure
(3) peripheral vascular disease
(4) diabetes mellitus

373. Metoprolol

(1) is a selective beta$_1$ adrenergic blocker
(2) inhibits the vasodilator effect of isoproterenol
(3) inhibits the chronotropic effect of isoproterenol
(4) is synergistic with the inotropic effect of isoproterenol

374. A diabetic patient is to undergo anesthesia for a vein stripping. On the morning of surgery, he receives one-half dose of his insulin requirement and his usual morning dose of 40 mg of propranolol. Anesthesia is maintained with isoflurane. In the recovery room 4 hours later, his blood sugar is 52 mg/dl. The cause of this could be

(1) stress of surgery
(2) propranolol
(3) isoflurane
(4) insulin

375. Digitalis intoxication may be manifest by

(1) gynecomastia
(2) hunger
(3) dizziness
(4) alopecia

376. The purpose of digitalis therapy is to

(1) increase depressed myocardial contractility
(2) achieve higher stroke volume at lower filling pressure
(3) move the patient onto a better Frank-Starling cardiac function curve
(4) control severe tachyarrhythmias

377. The use of digitalis in the treatment of pulmonary heart disease

(1) is the treatment of choice
(2) is prone to produce arrhythmias
(3) is the most effective way to treat congestive symptoms
(4) should follow the treatment of pulmonary disease

378. The administration of digitalis

(1) causes increased contractility
(2) increases oxygen consumption
(3) increases the P-R interval
(4) increases heart rate

379. The effectiveness of digitalis in a given individual may be affected by

(1) thyroid status
(2) acid-base balance
(3) serum electrolytes
(4) concomitant drugs

380. The drug propanidid is

(1) a barbiturate
(2) a premedicant administered intramuscularly
(3) hepatotoxic
(4) short acting

381. Diazepam

(1) is a benzodiazepine
(2) is specific for the limbic system
(3) causes little analgesia
(4) causes retrograde amnesia in moderate doses

382. Intravenous ethanol is characterized by

(1) sedative effect
(2) marked cardiovascular instability
(3) diuretic effect
(4) hypoglycemia

383. The neuroleptic state is characterized by

(1) increased reflexes
(2) amnesia
(3) continued awareness of environment
(4) analgesia

384. Large doses of intravenous morphine for anesthetic use

(1) are always accompanied by loss of consciousness
(2) cause increased liberation of catecholamines
(3) cause cardiac instability
(4) cause decreased cardiac output if nitrous oxide is added

SUMMARY OF DIRECTIONS				
A	B	C	D	E
1, 2, 3 only	1, 3 only	2, 4 only	4 only	All are correct

385. The anesthetic state achieved with ketamine is characterized by

(1) analgesia to somatic pain
(2) inhibition of reflexes, eg, gag reflex
(3) cardiovascular stimulation
(4) marked respiratory depression

386. The patient who has been receiving large doses of central nervous system stimulants, eg, amphetamines

(1) has increased anesthetic requirements
(2) may have altered cardiovascular compensatory mechanisms
(3) may have aberrations of temperature
(4) may have angiitis

387. A patient with a history of narcotic addiction admitted for surgery may have complications related to

(1) pulmonary disease
(2) liver disease
(3) cardiovascular disease
(4) renal disease

388. If a patient has been taking monamine oxidase (MAO) inhibitors

(1) elective surgery should be delayed until a 2-week drug-free interval has elapsed
(2) the premedication of choice is meperidine
(3) drug effects may be exaggerated
(4) the main complication to guard against is emotional instability

389. Hypotension associated with morphine administration results from

(1) vasodilatation due to direct effects on arteries and veins
(2) vasodilatation due to histamine release
(3) increased vagal stimulation
(4) myocardial depression

390. High doses of fentanyl may cause hypotension as a result of

(1) supraventricular tachycardia
(2) direct vasodilatation
(3) direct myocardial depression
(4) bradycardia

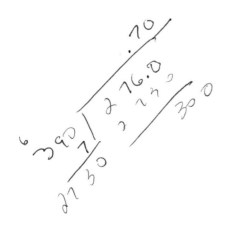

Answers and Explanations

1. **(A)** The liver is the most important site of drug transformation. The kidney is responsible for the removal of many drugs, many after they have been transformed in the liver to a water-soluble form. There are some drug reactions that occur in the lung. There are few that occur in the spleen. *(1:61; 15:11)*

2. **(C)** The first-pass effect is the biotransformation of a drug as it passes through the intestinal mucosa and liver. In some cases, much of the effective concentration is lost at this point, leaving little of the drug to have its desired effect. Some drugs are poorly soluble and never diffuse through the mucosa to be picked up in the bloodstream. There are other sites where drugs are altered, but this is important for the drugs that are administered orally. *(1:58; 15:5)*

3. **(E)** Systemic availability is the amount of drug that is free to circulate after it has passed through the intestine or the liver and is still active. Many drugs are bound to protein and are rendered inactive. *(1:59; 15:5)*

4. **(D)** Renal clearance of a drug in an individual with normal renal function may vary from patient to patient and from time to time, depending on the variables as stated in option D. The excretion is correlated with renal blood flow. Drug elimination is correlated with creatinine clearance, and one may use changes in creatinine clearance to gauge how doses must be altered. *(1:61; 15:11)*

5. **(B)** Halogenation decreases flammability and increases anesthetic potency. Cardiac irritation is not increased. *(15:37; 75:294)*

6. **(C)** Halothane is a halogenated hydrocarbon of the ethane series. The halogen substitutions are fluorine, chlorine, and bromine. *(1:730; 15:36)*

7. **(E)** The boiling point of halothane is 50.2° C. *(15:36; 75:294)*

8. **(D)** Halothane is stored in tinted bottles, and the preservative is thymol. The bottles are glass, not plastic. *(15:37)*

9. **(D)** Halothane is soluble in rubber and, if one uses rubber delivery hoses, the agent can be absorbed into the rubber. The halothane can then have an effect on subsequent patients. The rubber does not change the composition of halothane. If high flow rates are used, the halothane will be washed out of the system faster. *(75:295)*

10. **(D)** Isoflurane is a better relaxant when compared to halothane. The vapor pressure is 238 torr at 20° C. Isoflurane depresses ventilation and should be delivered by assisted or controlled ventilation. The data for MAC are correct. *(75:294)*

11. **(E)** The MAC for methoxyflurane is 0.16 at 1 atmosphere, making it the most potent of the inhalation anesthetics. In comparison, enflurane has a MAC value of 1.7. *(1:558; 15:30; 75:297)*

12. **(D)** The renal lesion associated with methoxyflurane is caused by the fluoride ion. The disease is dose dependent, and an attempt was made to establish a MAC hour limit. With the arrival of other agents that are better and the problem with methoxyflurane, hepatic as well as renal, the agent has fallen into disuse. *(1:722; 75:311,1464)*

13. **(A)** Isoflurane is characterized by a stable cardiac rhythm that is maintained in the face of epinephrine injection in conservative doses. A tachycardia is noted that leads to a decrease in stroke volume. Cardiac output is maintained. *(1:651; 15:41)*

14. **(C)** Isoflurane is a clear, colorless, stable, volatile liquid with a pungent odor. The blood-gas coefficient is 1.43 at 37° C. It contains no preservative and undergoes little biotransformation. *(15:37)*

15. **(A)** All of the options have an ether structure with the exception of halothane, which is a straight-chain hydrocarbon. *(1:730; 15:36)*

16. **(A)** Sevoflurane is a fluorinated ether. The blood-gas coefficient is 0.6, and the vapor pressure is 160. The vapor is not irritating. *(15:37; 75:294)*

17. **(E)** Enflurane is a substituted ether with no double bonds. The vapor pressure is 172. Halogenation is limited to 5 fluorine and 1 chlorine sites. *(15:36,37; 75:294)*

18. **(D)** Enflurane contains no preservative. It is not flammable. The agent produces good muscle relaxation, and there is little cardiac irritability. There is a tendency to cause CNS irritability, especially at low P_{CO_2} levels. *(15:37,39)*

19. **(B)** Sevoflurane has a MAC of 2.6%. The structure contains only fluorine as the halogen. The cardiac profile is similar to that of other inhalation agents. The agent has a very low solubility. Sevoflurane is not on the market, having been withdrawn because of its metabolism to fluoride ion. *(15:37; 75:294)*

20. **(D)** The action of thiopental is terminated by its redistribution. The drug is bound to protein, and the binding may be interfered with by various concomitant drugs. It is taken up in fatty tissues, but that is not the mechanism of terminating the effect. *(1:801; 15:104)*

21. **(E)** Thiopental is a very alkaline solution. When administered concomitantly with acid solutions, eg, narcotics or antibiotics, a precipitate will occur. *(1:801; 15:102)*

22. **(C)** When thiopental is administered, the cardiac output falls, and there is decreased blood pressure. The other options are incorrect. *(1:806; 15:111)*

23. **(C)** Thiopental is contraindicated in patients with acute intermittent porphyria. The other porphyrias listed as options are not associated with drug induction. Two others are variegate porphyria and hereditary coproporphyria. Thiopental should also be avoided in those. *(15:112; 75:476; 140:567)*

24. **(B)** Thiopental is known to have an antianalgesic effect. If given in small doses for sedation to one who is experiencing severe pain, the pain will be aggravated. The drug is a poor choice for sedation in this type of patient. *(1:806; 15:108)*

25. **(E)** Thiopental will decrease cerebral oxygen consumption. Cerebral blood flow and EEG activity will decrease. If P_{CO_2} is increased, the cerebral blood flow will stay elevated. Uterine contractions are not halted. *(1:805; 15:109)*

26. **(A)** Thiopental injection is followed by decreased blood pressure and increased heart rate. Coronary blood flow is increased. Stroke volume is decreased, as is cardiac output. *(1:806; 75:240)*

27. **(C)** Injection of a sleep dose of thiopental leads to an increased heart rate, probably brought about by baroreceptor-mediated changes in sympathetic activity. There are other changes, cited in previous questions. These changes are more pronounced in the patient with moderately severe heart disease. Some of the change is dependent on the rate of injection. *(1:804; 75:240)*

28. **(B)** After the inadvertent injection of thiopental into the epidural space, the patient would become drowsy but would have no complaints of severe pain, nor would paralysis, arachnoiditis, or cauda equina syndrome follow. The fact that the patient becomes drowsy suggests that significant absorption occurs through the epidural vessels. This reference also points up the fact that we must always identify what we are injecting. *(142:406)*

29. **(A)** Administration of thiopental does not shift the oxyhemoglobin dissociation curve. *(143:817)*

30. **(D)** Traditional signs of the anesthetic state are not seen with ketamine administration. Purposeless movements are seen, and these do not indicate the need for more anesthesia. *(15:134; 144:1127)*

31. **(B)** Ketamine administration is associated with increases in both systolic and diastolic blood pressure. The mechanism for the increases are direct central nervous system stimulation as well as the liberation of catecholamines. *(15:138; 75:237; 144:1129)*

32. **(B)** Ketamine administration is associated with changes in cardiovascular parameters similar to those seen with sympathetic stimulation. Therefore, the heart rate is increased, and there is an increase in cardiac output. *(15:138; 75:237; 144:1129)*

33. **(C)** Droperidol is a butyrophenone derivative. It is a component of Innovar. It is a tranquilizer with a long half-life. It is eliminated from the body by hepatic mechanisms. *(15:351; 75:490)*

34. **(D)** The chest wall rigidity seen with Innovar injection is due to the fentanyl component. The rigidity can be seen with fentanyl alone, and although usually seen with large doses, it may be seen with small doses. The rigidity is usually seen in the muscles of the chest wall and may make ventilation difficult. *(15:86; 75:261)*

35. **(E)** Procaine is the only choice that is an ester. All of the other options are amide derivatives. *(1:986; 15:148; 75:382)*

36. (D) Local anesthetics have their action at the membrane. The local anesthetics block sodium channels so that the membrane cannot conduct nerve impulses. All of this takes place in the peripheral area of the nerve, not at the nerve core. *(1:995; 15:156; 75:377)*

37. (A) Local anesthetics in the free base form are poorly soluble and are prepared as hydrochloride salts in water or saline. The acid solution helps solutions that contain epinephrine, since basic solutions promote the breakdown of catecholamines. *(1:993; 15:148; 75:372)*

38. (E) Dibucaine is a quinoline derivative with an amide bond. It is the most slowly eliminated of the amide local anesthetics. It is metabolized in the liver. *(15:154)*

39. (D) Hyaluronidase increases the incidence of toxic reactions by allowing more widespread distribution of the drug, thereby increasing the uptake of the drug. This spread also increases the success rate of the block and decreases the duration of the block. The time of onset of the block is decreased. *(1:1912; 75:395)*

40. (C) Succinylcholine in the susceptible patient causes the release of potassium from the cell membrane. The efflux of potassium, which is normal at the motor end plate, is seen over a much wider area of the membrane. This may result in a massive outpouring of potassium and cardiac arrest. *(1:919; 15:195; 75:352)*

41. (C) Penicillin does not have neuromuscular blocking properties. The aminoglycoside-type antibiotics are associated with decreased muscle function or potentiation of muscle relaxants in a dose-related fashion. This is probably due to a prejunctional inhibition of acetylcholine release. *(1:930; 15:461; 75:363)*

42. (D) Metocurine is related structurally to D-tubocurarine but causes less histamine release. It also has a less pronounced effect on the autonomic nervous system, with less ganglionic blockade and blood pressure depression. *(1:909; 15:189; 75:348)*

43. (D) Echothiophate eyedrops, chronically administered, may cause a problem in patients who are then given succinylcholine. In most cases, this presents no problem, but it must be borne in mind when succinylcholine is being administered for short cases. It is also important in these patients to allow the respirations to return before any other relaxant is administered. The organophosphate insecticides act by causing an inhibition of

cholinesterase. After the patient has been on the drops for a few weeks, the level of cholinesterase will drop to about 20% of normal. *(1:1846; 15:218; 75:1056)*

44. (D) Of the drugs listed, only pancuronium is a steroid. Metocurine and D-tubocurarine are cogeners of ring compounds. Succinylcholine is a straight-chain compound consisting of two acetylcholine molecules joined together. Gallamine has a substituted ring structure. *(1:895; 15:171; 75:351)*

45. (C) There are many types of arrhythmia seen on the second dose of succinylcholine, but the most frequent is nodal rhythm. The most threatening arrhythmia is sinus arrest, which, fortunately, is not common. *(1:918; 15:178; 41:498)*

46. (D) The small blocking dose of a nondepolarizing muscle relaxant given before an intubating dose of succinylcholine decreases the effectiveness of succinylcholine and may make intubation more difficult. However, Churchill-Davidson makes the point that in patients who are to be up and about soon after surgery, the prevention of muscle pain is beneficial. There is no guarantee that the small dose will be effective. *(1:922; 15:178; 41:498; 75:345)*

47. (C) Churchill-Davidson makes the point that we should choose a relaxant that is consistent with our needs in regard to hemodynamics and relaxation. D-tubocurarine is associated with decreased pressure due to histamine release; succinylcholine may cause heart rate drops that may affect pressure. Atracurium also may be associated with histamine release. *(1:913; 41:500; 75:348)*

48. (B) Succinylcholine causes an increase in intraocular pressure and an increase in intragastric pressure in some, but not all, patients. It is not seen in young children. There is a definite incidence of postoperative pain that is not always successfully blocked by pretreatment. *(1:919; 15:177)*

49. (A) In the case cited, any of the options except thiopental may be involved in the apnea. Thiopental, in usual doses, should not cause apnea after a procedure as long as a laparotomy. Any of the options or a combination of the options can be the cause. *(1:930; 75:354; 149:220)*

50. (A) Muscle contraction is an all-or-none phenomenon. The action potential is a membrane event. The strength of contraction is dependent on the number of fibers contracting, but in the individual fibers, it is all-or-none. *(75:342; 148:16)*

51. **(D)** Vecuronium has little cumulative effect. It is a nondepolarizing relaxant with an activity of about 30 minutes. It is not difficult to reverse. Vecuronium is eliminated chiefly in the bile. *(15:202; 75:351)*

52. **(C)** Fasciculation is decreased with a large dose of thiopental and decreased if the drug is given by a slow drip. Fasciculations are not always seen with decamethonium but may be. The fasciculations are associated with muscle pain. Pretreatment may attenuate the pain in some cases. *(1:852; 15:174; 148:33)*

53. **(D)** Administration of anticholinesterase drugs will reverse the block of a nondepolarizing agent only if the drug is in low enough concentration. They may prolong the block produced by depolarizers. If there is free succinylcholine in the circulation, administration of an anticholinesterase will prolong the block. *(1:924; 15:225)*

54. **(E)** Myoglobin is more commonly found in the serum of children than adults after the administration of succinylcholine. The reason is not definitely known. It is found in skeletal muscle, and its appearance in the serum is due to loss of integrity of the muscle cell. *(15:179,728; 26:824)*

55. **(C)** In this patient, it would be wise to avoid the use of a depolarizing relaxant. The usual potassium increase seen with succinylcholine is 0.5 to 1.0 mEq. Gallamine is eliminated by the kidney and, therefore, should be avoided. Pretreatment with curare does not guarantee that potassium will not increase. *(1:898; 15:183; 75:350)*

56. **(D)** Propofol is an intravenous agent with a fast onset and short time to awakening. It is essentially insoluble in water. There is very little analgesic effect. When compared to thiopental, the sleep time is shorter. *(1:824; 15:143; 75:229)*

57. **(C)** Atracurium is a nondepolarizing relaxant that has few cardiovascular side effects. It is broken down by two mechanisms: Hoffman degeneration and ester hydrolysis. It is not difficult to reverse. The half-life is about 25 minutes. *(1:894; 15:199; 75:350)*

58. **(E)** If the patient has an objective measurement of recovery from neuromuscular block, it is better than a clinical assessment. All of the options are indicators of recovery, but only the T4 ratio is specific. At 60% ratio, the patient has a sustained head lift for 3 seconds; at 75% recovery, the correlation is for head lift for 5 seconds. Normal tidal volume is not sufficient to protect the airway. There must be enough force to generate a cough, and about 15 ml/kg is needed. Hand grip is a clinical assessment and must be sustained to correlate with recovery. Inspiratory force is a good measurement. It should be at least 25 cm H_2O negative pressure. The advantage of inspiratory force is that it can be assessed in the patient who is still asleep and unable to respond. *(1:881; 75:357)*

59. **(E)** Atropine is part of the regimen to reverse a neuromuscular blockade but in itself has no ability to reverse a block. Edrophonium, neostigmine, and pyridostigmine are all cholinesterase inhibitors. 4-Aminopyridine does not inhibit cholinesterase but has its effect by facilitating calcium entry into the nerve ending. *(15:226; 75:361)*

60. **(D)** Reversal by neostigmine is not affected by body temperature per se. With hypothermia there is decreased elimination of the relaxant due to decreased hepatic and renal blood flow. If more relaxant is given than is needed, it may be difficult to antagonize the block, but that is due to relaxant overdose. Respiratory acidosis makes it very difficult to reverse a block. The total dose and the time of the last dose are factors in reversibility. The specific relaxant is important, since some relaxants resist reversal. Gallamine reportedly is harder to reverse than other nondepolarizers. *(1:924; 75:360; 156:324)*

61. **(A)** Assuming that the dose of neostigmine is adequate and the dose of relaxant is not excessive, the patient should have no problem when his body temperature increases. If the decreased body temperature led to an overdose of relaxant, it would be difficult to reverse and would probably lead to a problem in getting a return of the twitch. *(1:904; 75:360; 156:325)*

62. **(C)** A depolarization block does not have any post-tetanic facilitation. The block is characterized by fasciculation and is antagonized by nondepolarizers and potentiated by anticholinesterase compounds. There is no fade initially, but fade may appear with the onset of a phase II block. *(1:923; 15:175; 75:361)*

63. **(E)** From the data presented in the two segments, the only statement that can be made is that there is a 90% block. The block could represent either type of blockade. There is not complete relaxation. *(1:877; 75:358)*

64. **(D)** The drug is a muscle relaxant, since tetanic stimulation produces fade. The drug may be either a depolarizing or nondepolarizing relaxant. If the dose of a depolarizer is sufficient to cause a phase II block, fade may be demonstrated. *(1:877; 15:175; 75:358)*

65. (E) When a nondepolarizing muscle relaxant is present, acetylcholine cannot be mobilized in sufficient quantities to sustain contraction. It is not a result of recording inabilities or potassium. Cellular DNA is not the factor. *(1:877; 75:581)*

66. (B) The patient is partially curarized. The block that is present is not a depolarizing block. The train-of-four ratio is 50% and, therefore, could not sustain a head lift. The advantage of the train-of-four is that it is not necessary to have a control tracing, since it serves as its own control. *(1:877, 882; 75:581; 158:224)*

67. (E) The train-of-four ratio for a depolarizing block is 100%, since there is no fade. The fourth twitch will be as high as the first. *(159:110)*

68. (B) The minimum alveolar concentration for isoflurane is 1.15. *(1:558; 15:30; 75:297)*

69. (C) Studies done by Stoelting show the maximal effect at about 3 minutes. It is important to wait for the maximal effect before giving more drugs. Values tend to return toward baseline over the subsequent 10 minutes. *(1:912; 15:188; 75:349)*

70. (A) Anticholinesterase drugs have potent muscarinic stimulating effects. These may be exhibited in the heart, bronchioles, or gut. It is important to consider each of these areas in the particular patient whose relaxants are being reversed. Atropine or glycopyrrolate should be used with the reversal drug. Although the muscarinic manifestations are not common, their occurrence may be quite troublesome. *(75:359)*

71. (A) Ganglionic blockade may lead to cardiovascular changes. Drugs administered to a patient with a low blood volume may also lead to marked changes in cardiovascular values. The dose of D-tubocurarine is important from the standpoint of the amount of drug effect and the release of histamine. There were some studies that implicated the preservative in the drug, but work by Stoelting did not confirm these studies. *(1:912; 15:188)*

72. (D) Factors that affect the pharmacokinetics of muscle relaxants include the initial dose. If a large dose is given initially, Feldman believes that less relaxant is needed for the procedure. Other workers have not confirmed Feldman's theory. Renal disease prolongs the effect of many relaxants. Protein binding may have positive and negative effects, but the overall clinical effect is variable with the individual patient. The sex of the patient has no effect. Advanced age has an effect in that the older patient

has less requirement for relaxants that are cleared by the kidney. *(1:898; 75:355)*

73. (D) The patient with myasthenia gravis has an altered sensitivity to relaxants. These patients are more sensitive to nondepolarizing agents. This sensitivity is present with or without control of the disease. *(1:933; 75:35)*

74. (E) Thiopental should not be a factor in the apnea after a time period needed to complete a thoracotomy. The muscle relaxants may be involved because of altered metabolism. Hyperventilation may lead to apnea due to lack of carbon dioxide drive to ventilation. The patient may also be exhibiting the Eaton-Lambert syndrome with muscle weakness due to the carcinoma. This alone, or in combination with the relaxants, may lead to apnea. *(1:933; 75:351)*

75. (A) After a patient has had and recovered from a dose of succinylcholine, it takes a smaller amount of drug than normal to establish a neuromuscular block. This may be due to continued desensitization of the endplate. A longer duration of the nondepolarization block also occurred. *(1:923; 75:361)*

76. (D) When traction is applied during a laparotomy, the cardiovascular effects will be the same whether or not a relaxant is being used. The vagolytic effects of the relaxants are limited to the receptors in the sinus node. The muscarinic sites in the bowel are not affected. *(1:911; 166:388)*

77. (E) Cholinesterase is involved in the breakdown rather than the formation of acetylcholine. In the nerve terminal, choline is acetylated under the control of the enzyme choline acetylase. The acetyl molecule is derived from acetylCoA. *(1:841; 15:173; 75:341)*

78. (D) Botulinus toxin leads to muscular weakness by preventing the release of acetylcholine at the nerve endings. The release of acetylcholine is necessary for muscle function. Calcium and cyclic AMP also are involved in the release of acetylcholine at the nerve ending. *(15:624; 75:342)*

79. (E) Atropine is not always predictable, especially in those with heart block and in the elderly. Its administration will lead to increased heart rate, increased oxygen use, and possibly angina pectoris. It causes decreased conduction time. *(1:2132; 75:1404; 168:15)*

80. (D) Propranolol, a beta blocker, causes decreased cardiac output. It will decrease heart rate. The contractility is decreased. *(1:970; 15:283)*

81. **(E)** Propranolol is useful in the treatment of atrial flutter. Since it causes bradycardia, it is not useful in treatment of that disorder. It may aggravate both congestive heart failure and bronchitis. *(1:970; 15:283; 75:211)*

82. **(E)** Propranolol should not be terminated suddenly, since a withdrawal syndrome has been reported with sudden termination. In general, most antihypertensive agents should be continued and the induction planned around them. This makes heart rate and blood pressure easier to control. *(1:978; 15:282; 75:216)*

83. **(C)** Methoxamine is the drug with pure alpha effects. Epinephrine, norepinephrine, and ephedrine have mixed effects. Isoproterenol has all beta effects. *(1:964; 15:252; 75:195)*

84. **(B)** Quinidine is highly bound to protein. It is useful orally. It is effective against ventricular arrhythmias. Quinidine is known to potentiate neuromuscular blockers. It is the drug of choice for people with renal disease. *(15:324; 75:596–597)*

85. **(B)** Procainamide is eliminated mostly by the kidneys. Some is metabolized in the liver, but the metabolite is excreted by the kidneys. It is useful orally. It decreases ventricular automaticity. It is resistant to hydrolysis by cholinesterase. *(15:326; 75:596–597)*

86. **(A)** Lidocaine is eliminated chiefly by the liver. It is not effective orally. The toxic level is at 5 μg/ml. The symptoms of toxicity are usually CNS stimulation. Lidocaine is useful in ventricular arrhythmias. *(15:327; 75:596–597)*

87. **(C)** Phenytoin is useful in treatment of arrhythmias associated with digitalis overdose. It is eliminated through the kidneys after being conjugated with glucuronic acid. It decreases diastolic depolarization and automaticity. *(15:323,328; 75:516)*

88. **(D)** The calcium channel blockers have an effect by interfering with the flow of calcium through membranes. All are highly bound to protein. The peak effect is about 20 minutes. Some are good for treatment of arrhythmias; others are poor. *(1:853; 15:335; 75:596)*

89. **(C)** Pentazocine is a mixed narcotic agonist–antagonist that is useful both orally and parenterally. Although originally thought to have no addiction potential, it has been found to cause dependence in some people. *(1:776; 15:91; 75:274)*

90. **(B)** Lorazepam is a benzodiazepine derivative with good antianxiety properties. It does not cause respiratory depression and maintains good cardiovascular function. It is a good sedative. *(1:811; 15:129; 75:489)*

91. **(B)** Lithium may prolong the effect of both depolarizing and nondepolarizing relaxants. It is not necessary to stop the drug before induction, but it is necessary to consider the drug when planning the anesthesia. In addition to the effect on relaxants, the drug may lead to a reduction of anesthetic requirements. *(1:332; 15:355; 75:364)*

92. **(D)** Drugs that release histamine, eg, meperidine and morphine, should be avoided. Local anesthetics, halothane, vecuronium, and aspirin should not cause problems. *(1:331; 15:362; 75:209)*

93. **(D)** Use of furosemide leads to alkalosis. Renin release follows decreased volume. Hypokalemia is one of the most common problems in the patient on diuretics. Hyperglycemia is not as common as with thiazides. Ototoxicity usually is seen with chronic treatment with high doses. It is probably related to changes in the endolymph. *(1:1237; 15:428; 75:428)*

94. **(A)** Hypokalemic, hypochloremic alkalosis is one of the most common problems in the patient being treated with thiazides. Hyperuricemia may occur, but it is not as common as decreased potassium. Hyponatremia and hyperglycemia also may occur. *(1:1319; 15:424)*

95. **(B)** Ethacrynic acid has its effect on the ascending portion of the loop of Henle. The thiazides, eg, hydrochlorthiazide, chlorthalidone, and benzthiazide, have their effect between the ascending loop and the distal tubule. Triamterene is a potassium-sparing diuretic that has its effect in the distal convoluted tubule. *(1:1237; 15:426; 75:1086)*

96. **(B)** Nifedipine is a drug effective for coronary vasospasm. It has no antiarrhythmia effect. It is a vasodilator. The half-life is about 4 hours. *(1:330; 15:336; 75:214)*

97. **(D)** In this patient with oliguria, the first thing to establish is that the volume is replaced. A fluid challenge is appropriate. *(1:1317; 22:115; 75:1095; 181:1439)*

98. **(A)** This type of patient is seen frequently by an anesthesiologist. The question is whether the oliguric patient has renal disease, needs fluids, or should receive a diuretic. By determining the urine/plasma osmolar ratio, some help can be obtained. Oliguria resulting from fluid depletion with normal kidneys is invariably associated with a ratio of >2. This patient then has a rapid infusion of 500 ml of

balanced salt solution, and the urine output is determined again. If this same patient should later develop a high CVP, the treatment of choice would be a loop diuretic. If mannitol or an osmotic-type diuretic is administered in this situation, a further increase in CVP would be expected initially. *(1:1317; 22:115; 75:1095)*

99. **(A)** The drugs that are mentioned prolong the action of thiopental by competing with it for binding sites. When this occurs, a higher amount of the thiopental is available. The more pronounced effect is not due to a more potent compound being formed or an altered elimination or distribution. *(1:803; 15:104)*

100. **(B)** The interaction of D-tubocurarine and acetylcholine at the myoneural junction is one of competition for binding sites. As the relaxant occupies the receptors, the action of acetylcholine cannot have an effect. *(1:846; 15:174; 75:346)*

101. **(B)** The combination of protamine and heparin results in a compound with no anticoagulation effect. There is no other mechanism involved. *(15:448)*

102. **(E)** Echothiophate treatment leads to a prolongation of succinylcholine effect by altering the metabolism. This occurs because echothiophate is a cholinesterase inhibitor with a prolonged effect. Since pseudocholinesterase is needed for the breakdown of succinylcholine, problems may arise in patients who are taking these eyedrops. *(1:1846; 15:219; 75:192)*

103. **(A)** Epinephrine causes vasoconstriction, which leads to decreased absorption of the local anesthetic, thus prolonging its effect. This also leads to altered time to metabolism but more directly by change of absorption. Protein binding, chemical interaction, and binding site competition are not involved. *(1:1000; 15:155; 75:393)*

104. **(E)** The interaction of phenytoin and phenobarbital is one of altered metabolism due to enzyme induction. If a patient has a stable drug level, this can be changed by starting another drug that may induce the enzyme system that metabolizes the drug. *(75:148)*

105. **(D)** When meperidine, an acid compound, and thiopental, a basic compound, are mixed in the same syringe or the same intravenous tubing, a precipitate is formed. This may completely plug an intravenous line. When using multiple drugs, such as antibiotics and anesthetic agents, the compatibility must be known. *(1:801; 15:102; 75:228)*

106. **(C)** The combination of nitrous oxide in 0.5 MAC concentration and isoflurane in 0.5 MAC concentra-

tion will lead to an anesthetic combination of 1 MAC potency. For all practical purposes, nitrous oxide and a halogenated agent are the only agents that are administered together, but if two halogenated agents could be used together, their effect would be additive. *(1:565; 15:30; 75:297)*

107. **(A)** Alcohol abuse leads to an increased MAC for anesthetic agents. The increase is about 40%. In the patient with acute alcohol abuse, the MAC value is decreased. *(1:572; 15:31; 75:297)*

108. **(A)** The MAC would be increased. *(1:572; 15:31)*

109. **(B)** Methoxyflurane is an ether with fluorine substitutions on the second carbon atom. *(1:730; 15:30; 75:294)*

110. **(D)** Halothane is an ethane compound with bromine, chlorine, and fluorine substitutions. *(1:730; 15:30; 75:294)*

111. **(A)** Enflurane is an ether with fluorine substitutions on the second carbon atom. *(1:730; 15:30; 75:294)*

112. **(E)** *(1:730; 15:30; 75:294)*

113. **(C)** Isoflurane is an ether compound with three fluorine substitutions on the first carbon atom. *(1:730; 15:30; 75:294)*

114. **(E)** The MAC for methoxyflurane is 0.16, making it the most potent of the inhalation agents. *(1:558; 15:30; 75:297)*

115. **(C)** The MAC for isoflurane is 1.15. *(1:558; 15:30; 75:297)*

116. **(B)** The MAC for enflurane is 1.68. *(1:558; 15:30; 75:297)*

117. **(D)** The MAC for nitrous oxide is 105, which makes it a very weak anesthetic agent. *(1:558; 15:30; 75:297)*

118. **(A)** The MAC for halothane is 0.77. *(1:558; 15:30; 75:297)*

119. **(D)** Thiopental is a barbituric acid derivative. *(1:801; 15:103; 75:229)*

120. **(A)** Propofol is an isopropylphenol derivative. This is a newer induction agent. *(1:823; 15:143; 75:229)*

121. **(C)** Propanidid is a eugenol derivative. This drug has been withdrawn from the market because of the high incidence of anaphylactoid reactions. *(1:821; 15:144; 75:228)*

122. (B) Droperidol is a butyrophenone derivative. *(1:385; 15:350; 75:490)*

123. (E) Diazepam is a benzodiazepine derivative. *(1:809; 15:119; 75:150)*

124. (D) Methohexital is an oxybarbiturate whose activity is terminated by redistribution. It is not associated with muscle rigidity. *(1:801; 15:103; 75:229)*

125. (A) Ketamine is a phencyclidine derivative. Metabolism is by the liver, although redistribution plays a part in the termination of effect. Random involuntary movement is seen under ketamine anesthesia, but rigidity is not a part of the normal anesthetic course. *(1:813; 15:134; 75:229)*

126. (E) Fentanyl is a narcotic associated with muscle rigidity. The rigidity usually occurs with high dosage but may occur with low dosage. The exact cause of the rigidity is not known. Fentanyl is broken down in the liver. *(1:764; 15:86; 75:261)*

127. (C) Lorazepam is a benzodiazepine derivative. It is metabolized in the liver. *(1:808; 15:118; 75:150)*

128. (D) The effect of althesin is terminated by redistribution. This drug is now off the market because of its propensity for causing hypersensitivity reactions. *(1:819; 15:144; 75:228)*

129. (A) Butorphanol is a mixed agonist–antagonist. This drug has an addictive potential. The drug has more analgesia than morphine but is not as useful as morphine in the patient with cardiac disease, since it has the potential to increase pulmonary artery pressure. *(1:776; 15:31; 75:273)*

130. (C) Naloxone is a pure narcotic antagonist, meaning that the drug has no narcotic effect of its own. Butorphanol and levallorphan are both mixed agonist–antagonists. Neostigmine and edrophonium are cholinesterase inhibitors. *(1:774; 15:70; 75:275)*

131. (B) Bleomycin is associated with pulmonary toxicity. This is manifest as pulmonary fibrosis, sometime long after the drug has been stopped. Adriamycin has cardiac toxicity. Vincristine is associated with myelosuppression. Methotrexate toxicity is manifest as immunosuppression. L-Asparaginase is associated with hepatic toxicity. *(1:324; 15:492)*

132. (A) Methohexital is metabolized to a greater extent than thiopental. The drug is metabolized to hydroxymethohexital, which is inactive. The elimination half-life is shorter than that of thiopental. Meth-

ohexital does not release histamine from mast cells and is not contraindicated in asthma. *(1:804; 15:106; 75:248)*

133. (C) Midazolam is associated with fewer cases of venous irritation than diazepam. The drug is not contraindicated in children; in fact, it is very useful in children. The duration is longer than thiopental. There is no adrenal cortical depression and no histamine release. *(1:810; 15:224; 75:245)*

134. (B) Lidocaine, 1%, has a duration of action of about 60 to 120 minutes. It is about 70% protein bound compared to bupivacaine, which is 95% bound to protein. Lidocaine is effective topically. There are few allergic reactions. The drug is not associated with tachycardia. *(1:999; 15:151; 75:382)*

135. (A) Addition of epinephrine prolongs the action of a local anesthetic by decreasing the absorption. This leads to decreased peak effect and decreased toxicity. The vasoconstrictor leads to decreased surgical bleeding. It does not decrease the intensity of the block. *(1:1008; 15:155)*

136. (B) Prilocaine is associated with methemoglobinemia. It is an amide derivative. The drug has a fast onset but a short duration. Prilocaine is broken down in the liver. It is not the drug of choice for obstetrics, since the occurrence of methemoglobinemia interferes with newborn assessment, and newborns lack the enzyme systems to reduce methemoglobin. *(1:1010; 15:154; 75:391)*

137. (E) The ester compounds are more slowly metabolized in patients with liver disease, since the metabolism is via cholinesterase. The metabolism takes place in the plasma and the liver. No metabolism occurs in the CSF, since there is no cholinesterase in the CSF. The drugs are broken down to inactive metabolites and excreted by the kidneys. *(1:1010; 15:154; 75:386)*

138. (C) The toxicity associated with bupivacaine is due to interference with sodium channels. The drug is an amide of long duration. It should not be used in concentrations above 0.5% for epidurals. Toxicity may occur after injection other than intravenously. *(1:1004; 15:160; 75:390)*

139. (A) Flecainide is an antidysrhythmic drug that is a procaine analog. The drug is not a muscle relaxant. It can be administered orally or parenterally. It is not the drug of choice for local anesthetic reactions. *(15:327; 75:596)*

140. (D) Alfentanil effect is terminated by redistribution. The volume of distribution is smaller than that of fentanyl. The drug has about one-fifth the

potency of fentanyl. It is shorter acting. There is an effect to reduce the MAC of enflurane. *(1:781; 15:327; 75:596)*

141. **(D)** Sufentanil has a more prolonged effect in the elderly. The drug is more potent than fentanyl by a factor of about 10. Most of the breakdown takes place in the liver. Sufentanil has a shorter duration of action and has been reported to increase intracranial pressure more than fentanyl. *(1:781; 15:86; 75:596)*

142. **(E)** Prostaglandin E_1 may cause hypotension. The drug should not be stopped before induction, since it may be required to keep a ductus open. The drug is administered by infusion, since it has a short duration. *(1:2336; 15:368; 75:1004)*

143. **(D)** Physostigmine may be used to reverse the sedative effects of opioids. It is a short-acting drug and may have to be repeated if used to counteract the effects of longer-acting drugs. The drug does cross the blood–brain barrier, since it is a tertiary amine. It is used in the treatment of central anticholinergic syndrome. *(1:962; 15:226; 75:194)*

144. **(A)** Arrhythmias are common in the patient on tricyclic antidepressants. The combination of halothane, pancuronium, and tricyclics has been reported to have been associated with intraoperative problems. The drugs should not be stopped, but we must be aware of their effects on induction. Ketamine may cause hypertension in these patients. Patients on tricyclics may have prolonged sedation with thiopental. *(1:331; 15:358; 75:209)*

145. **(B)** Chymopapain is associated with allergic reactions, which are decreased with local anesthetics. The reactions are more common in women and in those with allergic histories. Cortisone and antihistamines are given in the intraoperative period to alleviate the reaction. *(1:299; 15:413; 75:1379)*

146. **(C)** Vancomycin is associated with histamine release when given with any speed. The drug should not be given in the primary intravenous line but should be piggybacked so that the infusion can be controlled. Other drugs that may release histamine, eg, atracurium, should be avoided. *(1:335; 15:468; 75:1386)*

147. **(B)** Terbutaline is a selective beta$_2$ agonist. It causes less tachycardia than isoproterenol. It is preferred in the patient with heart disease. *(1:329; 15:226; 75:909)*

148. **(B)** The patient showing signs of cocaine toxicity may be excited, anxious, and restless and have hypertension and tachycardia. *(1:1864)*

149. **(D)** Meperidine is primarily metabolized in the liver. About 5% is excreted unchanged. The drug is a synthetic opioid. It is used orally. The potency is about one-tenth that of morphine. *(1:779; 15:82; 75:265)*

150. **(D)** Halothane anesthesia in the patient with therapeutic levels of aminophylline may cause arrhythmias. It is better to use a drug that is a bronchodilator and not as prone to arrhythmias. Fentanyl anesthesia may be associated with chest stiffness and should be avoided as the primary anesthetic. Morphine releases histamine, which may aggravate the asthma. A thiopental infusion will not prevent pain, and the light anesthesia will be detrimental. *(1:333)*

151. **(E)** Ranitidine has lower CNS depression problems than has cimetidine. It is an H_2 blocker that increases pH but does not necessarily decrease volume of the gastric fluid. It has a half-life of about 9 hours. It is effective orally as well as parenterally. *(1:390; 15:381; 75:494)*

152. **(D)** Cromolyn prevents release of histamine from the mast cells. It has no direct effect on bronchioles. It does not stimulate cyclic AMP, nor does it release catecholamines. It does not decrease bronchiole reactivity. *(1:1379; 15:382; 75:909)*

153. **(A)** Verapamil is a calcium entry blocker that is useful in the treatment of supraventricular tachycardia. It is useful in the patient with asthma but should not be combined with propranolol, since it may cause profound bradycardia. The drug causes vasodilatation. Its effect is on the pacemaker cells. *(15:332; 75:214)*

154. **(D)** Epinephrine is not released at the time of anaphylaxis. Histamine is released from the mast cells. The other three options, SRS-A, ECF-A, and prostaglandins, all are mediators of the reaction. *(1:298; 15:813; 75:1384)*

155. **(A)** Glycopyrrolate is a quaternary amine that is an anticholinergic agent. It is synthetic, not a naturally occurring alkaloid, such as atropine and scopolamine. Since it is a quaternary amine, it does not cross the blood–brain barrier and is not associated with the central cholinergic syndrome. *(1:386; 15:232; 75:192)*

156. **(D)** Amrinone is a noncatecholamine inotropic drug. It has little antidysrhythmic effect. It is effective orally or parenterally. It causes mild vasodilatation. There is no tachyphylaxis. *(15:277; 75:206; 76:455)*

157. (A) The xanthine group of drugs includes caffeine. This group has strong beta$_2$ mimetic effects. The mechanism of action is by phosphodiesterase inhibition, which leads to an increase of cyclic AMP. *(1:333; 15:267; 75:205)*

158. (C) Hydralazine may be associated with a lupuslike syndrome. It is a direct vasodilator. It may cause a reflex tachycardia, which limits its usefulness in the patient with angina. There may be a retention of sodium and water that may require diuretics. *(1:1951; 15:299; 75:217)*

159. (A) Trimethaphan is a ganglionic blocker that may cause pupillary dilatation. This limits its usefulness in the neurosurgical patient, since patient assessment may be difficult. Tachyphylaxis is common. Tachycardia is common. Catecholamines are decreased, not increased. *(1:960, 1956; 15:316; 75:188)*

160. (B) Valproic acid has been associated with some minor problems, but the most serious is hepatic failure. It is important to be aware of this if the patient develops jaundice in the perioperative period. *(15:505; 75:445)*

161. (C) Sublingual administration avoids the first-pass effect and bypasses the liver. This route is not useful in all drugs, only in those that are un-ionized, eg, nitroglycerin. This route leads to higher blood levels if the drug can be absorbed. *(1:58; 15:6; 75:139)*

162. (B) Either formulation of calcium can be used. Calcium infusions should not be given into a peripheral vein because of the irritation it may cause. Infusions may lead to bradycardia. The gluconate formulation can be used, but there is no preference. The combination of calcium and sodium bicarbonate will form a precipitate. *(15:538)*

163. (C) There is a growing feeling that the concern over potassium is unfounded. Reference 77 speaks to this. If the cause of the hypokalemia is known and the patient is asymptomatic, there is no need to cancel the procedure in an otherwise healthy patient. Intraoperative infusions may cause hyperkalemia, and it is important that the potassium be infused slowly. It is not possible to replenish the intracellular potassium over a short period of time. *(1:315; 77:132)*

164. (C) Metoclopramide stimulates upper gastrointestinal motility. It has no effect on the acid secretion of the stomach. It is an antiemetic. The transit time should be shorter. There is no ileus, since motility is stimulated. *(1:1820; 15:437; 75:495)*

165. (A) Bretylium inhibits the release of norepinephrine. It is useful in the treatment of ventricular arrhythmias. The major side effect is hypotension, but there may be a transient hypertension. Bradycardia also may result. *(1:515; 15:330; 75:598)*

166. (D) Sodium nitroprusside may lead to cyanide toxicity, which is detected by an acidosis and a tolerance to the drug's effects. This drug has an effect on venous and arterial vessels. The acidosis that is seen is treated by stopping the drug. It should not be treated by sodium bicarbonate. *(1:1954; 15:309; 75:217)*

167. (D) Diazoxide is an antihypertensive that is administered by bolus infusion. This is necessary, since the drug is so highly protein bound that little effective drug is available if given by a slow infusion. The drug causes an increased cardiac output. *(1:1937; 15:317; 75:218)*

168. (B) Dobutamine is primarily a beta$_1$ agonist. At higher dosage levels, alpha agonist effects may be seen. It causes increased renal blood flow. The drug is a synthetic catecholamine. It is associated with little change in heart rate. *(1:975; 15:262; 75:202)*

169. (E) Edrophonium should be used with atropine. The drug has a fast onset but, in the dose cited, a duration as long as neostigmine. The muscarinic effects are fewer than neostigmine. *(1:929; 15:224; 75:1265)*

170. (A) Clonidine has its primary effect in the brainstem. The drug should not be tapered quickly because that can precipitate a withdrawal syndrome with hypertension. Clonidine is not available for intravenous use. The central analgesia is not reversed by naloxone. The MAC of halothane is decreased. *(1:329,569; 15:297; 75:217)*

171. (E) Labetalol is subject to the first-pass effect, and the oral dose must be higher to obtain a therapeutic level. The drug may precipitate wheezing. It is both an alpha and a beta blocker. Labetalol is conjugated in the liver. *(1:976; 15:302; 75:212)*

172. (B) Protamine is a naturally occurring protein salt. Patients who have been sensitized to protamine are more susceptible to reactions. In those patients, a small dose should be given first. The drug seems to cause fewer reactions if injected into a peripheral vein, probably due to less histamine release. *(1:1508; 15:449; 75:715)*

173. (C) Esmolol is contraindicated in the patient with AV block. The drug has a half-life of under 15 minutes. It is a beta$_1$ blocker. It is less likely than propranolol to cause bronchospasm, since it blocks beta$_1$ receptors, not beta$_2$ receptors. *(15:12; 75:212)*

174. (C) Amiodarone is useful for both atrial and ventricular arrhythmias, but it is usually reserved for arrhythmias that are refractory to other therapy, since there are many side effects with this drug. Amiodarone has a half-life of up to 100 days; therefore, stopping it before surgery would be to no avail. It is thought to be eliminated through the liver. The interaction with diltiazem has been associated with sinus arrest. *(15:331; 75:596; 76:455)*

175. (E) Renal failure has not been associated with amiodarone. All of the other options have been reported. The pneumonitis is seen in patients who have x-ray evidence of previous lung disease. *(15:331; 75:596; 76:459)*

176. (D) Hetastarch is a synthetic colloid. The other options all include administration of blood products. Some people of this belief will accept blood that is autologous; others will require that the blood be in circuit continuously, eg, in a cell saver. It is important to understand the particular patient's requirements before undertaking the procedure. *(15:553; 75:857)*

177. (B) Hetastarch is a synthetic colloid. The drug interferes with coagulation by diluting platelets and coagulation factors. The allergy potential is about the same as with Dextran. Hetastarch is eliminated through the kidneys. If large doses are used, elimination may be troublesome. *(15:553)*

178. (B) Cocaine is the only local anesthetic that blocks the reuptake of norepinephrine. The addition of epinephrine does not make a difference. *(1:568; 15:627; 75:391)*

179. (E) Heroin is more addicting than morphine. Heroin is a synthetic compound of morphine. It is more soluble than morphine and is able to enter the brain more easily. There is less nausea with heroin. *(15:90; 75:1434)*

180. (A) Hydroxyzine is an antihistamine and a tranquilizer. It has limited analgesic properties and is not an amnestic agent. It is not approved for intravenous use. *(1:386; 75:491)*

181. (D) Postoperative pain control with methadone requires some time to obtain stable levels. The drug has a long half-life and is usually given in twice daily dosage. It does depress respiration. The oral dose is only about 50% as effective as the same parenteral dose. *(1:1106; 15:89; 75:1433)*

182. (B) Ibuprofen potentiates HPV. All of the other options inhibit the effect. *(1:677; 15:674; 75:927)*

183. (D) Dopamine has different mechanisms depending on the dosage: at levels >10 μg/kg/minute, there is a stimulation of alpha receptors. At lower levels, dopaminergic receptors are stimulated. This leads to an increase in renal blood flow. Dopamine leads to an increase in pulmonary artery pressure, making it a poor choice in the patient with right heart failure. Dopamine is a transmitter in both the central and peripheral nervous system. *(1:693; 15:260; 75:202)*

184. (C) The sequence that is proposed may result in a long block. This is a common situation to be in—to be at the end of a procedure with a patient who is showing full return of muscle function, yet the surgeon needs more time to close the incision. A small dose of succinylcholine may give the relaxation that is needed, but a large dose may lead to a longer block. The dilemma then is whether to try to reverse that block. *(1:923; 75:361)*

185. (A) Vecuronium is associated with bradycardia when the patient is on beta blockers, since the drug has so little autonomic activity itself. The onset time will be faster if the dose is increased. About 10% is eliminated through the kidneys. The activity is prolonged by hepatic disease. Renal disease does not have a significant effect. *(1:899; 15:202; 75:351)*

186. (D) Cimetidine may affect the metabolism of all of the drugs except atracurium. The effect may be through the P-450 cytochrome system or protein binding. *(1:385; 15:380; 75:494)*

187. (B) Phenylephrine eyedrops may be absorbed and lead to hypertension. It is important to know the concentration being used. The effect that is needed by the surgeon is achieved by the 2.5% concentration. The 10% concentration can lead to elevations of blood pressure and evidence of ischemia. I have seen a resident squirt the solution into the eye with abandon. One must remember that it is a potent solution. The purpose of the solution for eye muscle surgery is to constrict the vessels and decrease bleeding. *(1:1846; 15:265; 75:1057)*

188. (E) Timolol does not affect the size of the pupil. It is absorbed systemically and may lead to a bradycardia, since it is a beta blocker. Asthma may be precipitated. *(1:1846; 15:286; 75:1057)*

189. (E) Drug elimination is principally by the liver, kidneys, and the lung. Other avenues are sweat, saliva, and breast milk, although these are not of significance in most cases. *(1:68; 75:140)*

190. (B) Scopolamine is a potent antisialogogue. It also has potent amnesic properties and is a good sedative. It is not as effective as atropine in increasing heart rate, nor is it as effective as glycopyrrolate in decreasing gastric secretion. *(1:387; 15:234; 75:193)*

191. **(B)** Nitrous oxide will decrease cardiac output when combined with halothane. It is important when reading of drug effects to know if the drug is being used alone or in combination. Narcotics offer stable hemodynamic conditions when used alone, but when combined with nitrous oxide, the stability may be lost. *(1:658; 15:49; 75:302)*

192. **(B)** Dantrolene decreases intracellular calcium. The half-life is about 12 hours. Cardiac muscle effect is not seen in the usual clinical doses. Hepatoxicity is not a factor in the treatment of MH but may be a factor in prolonged treatment. There is no need for daily treatment in most cases of MH. *(1:1984; 15:523; 75:460)*

193. **(A)** Glucagon increases insulin secretion. The drug is a cardiac stimulant causing both inotropic and chronotropic effects. Hepatic gluconeogenesis is stimulated. *(1:1211; 15:277; 75:206)*

194. **(C)** The histamine release of larger doses of atracurium is not seen if the drug is administered over a 75 second period. Atracurium has both pre- and postjunctional effects. Laudanosine is theoretically a problem in higher doses, but no problem has been reported in humans. Blood pressure will decrease due to the release of histamine. *(1:912; 15:200; 75:350)*

195. **(E)** None of the inhalation anesthetics have been implicated in the patient with glucose 6-phospate dehydrogenase deficiency. The other options are all implicated. *(1:321; 75:449)*

196. **(B)** Diltiazem does bind to cytochrome P-450, leading to inhibition of drug metabolism. Phenobarbital leads to an induction of the enzyme. Cimetidine blocks binding sites. Ranitidine leads to decreased biotransformation but has less effect than cimetidine. The enzyme levels remain elevated only about 24 hours after induction. *(1:1203; 15:14; 75:146)*

197. **(B)** Droperidol may induce antagonism of the drug effect at the basal ganglia, leading to muscle spasms. Phenothiazines should be avoided for the same reasons. Levodopa has a short duration and should be continued through the perioperative period. Ketamine may lead to increased blood pressure. Succinylcholine may lead to increased levels of potassium. *(1:1203; 15:14; 75:146)*

198. **(B)** Desmopressin may lead to increased blood pressure, although the effect is less than that seen with vasopressin. Desmopressin is available only for intranasal use for treatment of diabetes insipidus. Recent reports have noted the decreased bleeding in some procedures when intravenous infusions were

used. The half-life is over 8 hours. The drug has no effect on nephrogenic diabetes insipidus. *(1:278; 15:410; 75:1209)*

199. **(A)** Dextran has precipitated fatal allergic reactions. The coagulation picture is changed by a prolonged bleeding time. Crossmatching of blood is affected by rouleau formation, which interferes with the crossmatch. The solution stays in the intravascular space about 12 hours. Histamine is released. *(1:1361; 15:552; 75:1374)*

200. **(D)** Reversal agents should be used for all long-acting muscle relaxants. Many believe that it is not necessary to reverse the newer intermediate-duration relaxants, but others would opt to reverse all patients who have received relaxants. If the relaxants are not reversed, there should be documentation that full muscle tone has returned. The drug BWA938U is not as short acting as atracurium or vecuronium. *(1:925; 75:361; 84:3)*

201. **(E)** BW1090U (mivacurium) is short acting and may be administered by infusion. It is a benzylisoquinoline derivative. It is broken down by plasma cholinesterase. The drug has a slower onset than succinylcholine and a shorter duration than vecuronium. *(75:1351; 84:2)*

202. **(E)** Edrophonium does not form a chemical bond with the subsites on acetylcholinesterase. The inhibition is shorter than neostigmine or pyridostigmine. *(15:218; 83:1)*

203. **(B)** Patients with hemiplegia may have a normal block on the normal side but decreased block on the affected side. If one is monitoring the degree of block on the affected side, there may be a false interpretation of the results and more relaxant administered when none is needed. *(15:196; 88:1)*

204. **(C)** Elderly patients require less thiopental. MAC values decrease with age. Induction is faster in children. Elderly patients have a longer time to recover from the ventilatory effects of fentanyl, and they require a lower dose to burst suppression with fentanyl. *(89:1)*

205. **(E)** Preanesthetic medication may be given by mouth and may be administered with a small amount of water. There is no need for an anti-sialogogue in every patient. The premedication regimen should be individualized for each patient, taking into consideration the patient's psyche, procedure, and desires. *(90:1)*

206. **(E)** Some patients who will not empty the stomach will not benefit from oral medications and will be put at more risk with an added amount of water.

Most 4-year-old children can take oral premedication without problems. The other options are those who are at risk for emptying the stomach. *(90:1)*

207. **(E)** The aim of antacid administration is to raise the pH. It should be given 15 to 30 minutes before surgery. Antacids will not decrease gastric volume but may increase it. Nonparticulate antacids should not cause any problem if aspirated. There is no lag time. *(15:435; 90:5)*

208. **(E)** Pharmacologic preparation of the patient does not preclude good airway management. There is no protection against aspiration. H_2 antagonists do not facilitate gastric emptying nor do they have any effect on fluid that is already present. There is no need to use the H_2 blockers in all patients. *(15:374; 90:5)*

209. **(C)** Metoclopramide increases gastric emptying but has no effect on the secretion of gastric acid. All of the other options have an effect on gastric acid, some more efficiently than others. *(15:237; 90:4)*

210. **(D)** Diazepam used for premedication should be administered orally or intravenously. Intramuscular injections are erratically absorbed and painful. There are data in animals that local anesthetic toxicity may be thwarted, but that is not true in humans. Diazepam will decrease anxiety and prevent recall. The latter affect is better if scopolamine is given with it. *(15:124; 90:4)*

211. **(C)** Lorazepam is formulated with propylene glycol. All of the other agents are water soluble. Diazepam is another agent with propylene glycol in its formulation. *(15:119,129; 91:2)*

212. **(C)** Ketamine is known to cause increases in intracranial pressure. The other induction agents will decrease the pressure. *(1:1262; 91:4)*

213. **(D)** Etomidate does not decrease hepatic perfusion. There is no histamine release with injection. It has some anticonvulsant activity. It does not have any analgesic property. Intraocular pressure is decreased. *(1:818; 91:5)*

214. **(D)** Etomidate is the only induction agent known to decrease steroid production. *(1:819; 91:5)*

215. **(C)** Azathioprine is known to affect both depolarizers and nondepolarizers. The mechanism is not known. The other options do not have a neuromuscular effect. *(92:5)*

216. **(C)** Patients who abuse alcohol have a tolerance to the CNS effects but not to the respiratory and cardiovascular effects. The acutely intoxicated person takes less anesthesia, whereas the chronic alcoholic requires more. *(92:5)*

217. **(C)** Of the group listed, only nadolol is a beta blocker. Isoproterenol is a beta agonist. Dobutamine is a $beta_1$ and $beta_2$ agonist. Albuterol and ritodrine are $beta_2$ agonists. *(1:970; 92:3)*

218. **(E)** Doxepin is a tricyclic antidepressant. Pargyline, phenelzine, and isocarboxazid are monamine oxidase inhibitors. Isosorbide is a vasodilator. *(15:356; 92:4)*

219. **(E)** Isoflurane is not a problem in the patient with cocaine abuse. Since cocaine prevents the reuptake of norepinephrine, we must avoid anything that will cause an increased response of norepinephrine. Vasopressors and sympathomimetics may cause an increase in blood pressure that is excessive. Halothane may predispose to arrhythmias. Pancuronium may lead to a tachycardia. *(1:1864; 75:412; 92:5)*

220. **(A)** The halogenated hydrocarbons increase cerebral blood flow to various degrees, halothane having the most profound effect. Thiopental decreases cerebral blood flow. *(1:1265; 94:4)*

221. **(E)** If it is necessary to use a volatile agent for a procedure, steps should be taken to decrease the effect as much as possible. Intravenous drugs, such as thiopental, should be administered when practical, and hyperventilation and as low a dose as possible should be used. The choice of an agent with the least effect on cerebral blood flow is also helpful. *(94:4)*

222. **(A)** The elevation of intracranial pressure seen with succinylcholine is due to the transient increase in Pco_2 seen with fasciculation and to CNS proprioceptors. If the patient is hyperventilated and given thiopental, the effect is not seen. This concept is important in intubating the patient who has increased intracranial pressure. If the patient has a full stomach, one may not want to wait the time necessary for a nondepolarizer to act. If thiopental is given, the patient hyperventilated and then intubated, further damage should be mitigated. The fasciculation and tightness of neck muscles are not involved. *(1:1275; 94:5)*

223. **(A)** At the present time, nifedipine is not available for parenteral use, since it is very light sensitive. There may be a reflex tachycardia to compensate for the vasodilatation that is a therapeutic effect. This calcium channel blocker is not as useful as an antidysrhythmic. It is useful as a coronary vasodilator. *(1:330; 96:2)*

224. **(B)** Calcium channel blockers should be continued into the perioperative period, but care must be taken, since they may be additive with the anesthetics. They may be antagonized by amrinone. They will potentiate the effects of muscle relaxants. *(92:4; 96:4)*

225. **(D)** After injection of a drug, there is a rapid mixing of the drug in the blood and vessel-rich group. In the distribution phase, the drug equilibrates with the lesser perfused tissues. High perfusion increases the rate of equilibration. Diffusion factors may affect the speed of equilibration. *(1:59; 97:2)*

226. **(E)** Drug clearance may occur by metabolism to inactive or less active products or by elimination of the unchanged drug. Clearance is independent of drug concentration. *(1:68; 97:3)*

227. **(E)** The loading dose of a drug is the dose given to achieve a faster blood concentration. This decreases the time needed to achieve a steady state. In some drugs, the larger dose can have detrimental effects; eg, a larger dose of relaxants may lead to a longer time of paralysis or cardiovascular effects. *(75:160; 97:5)*

228. **(B)** All sympathomimetic drugs are not catecholamines. Ephedrine and methoxamine are examples. Both dopamine and isoproterenol are catecholamines. *(15:252; 98:2)*

229. **(B)** Methoxamine is a pure alpha receptor stimulator. It is associated with a reflex bradycardia. This effect can be used to treat tachycardias. Afterload is increased by the vasoconstriction. *(1:964; 75:195; 98:4)*

230. **(A)** Endogenous catecholamines are epinephrine, norepinephrine, and dopamine. Dobutamine is a synthetic drug. *(15:252; 98:2)*

231. **(E)** Epinephrine is the most widely used catecholamine. It has many uses because of its effects on alpha and beta receptors. Arrhythmias have been noted. There are strong chronotropic effects that may limit its use as an inotrope. *(15:275; 98:4)*

232. **(D)** Ephedrine is useful in obstetrics, since it does not decrease uterine blood flow. The drug has an indirect action, liberating norepinephrine. This causes tachyphylaxis. *(15:262; 98:5)*

233. **(B)** Amrinone is an orally effective inotrope that has little effect on heart rate. It causes some vasodilatation. Amrinone is a phosphodiesterase inhibitor, which causes an increase in cyclic AMP. *(15:277; 98:6)*

234. **(E)** Isoproterenol is useful in the treatment of heart failure with associated pulmonary hypertension. The drug can be used as a temporary pacer, since it has good chronotropic effects. The beta effects lead to bronchodilatation. The drug is a beta stimulator and, therefore, can be used for treatment of overzealous beta blockade. *(15:261; 98:6)*

235. **(B)** Droperidol is known to cause a dysphoria that limits its usefulness as a premedicant. Extrapyramidal symptoms may occur, and this must be considered in the patient with parkinsonism. Droperidol is useful for preventing catecholamine-related intraoperative dysrhythmias. It has been proposed in many studies to prevent postoperative nausea and vomiting, especially in the child having strabismus surgery. *(15:351; 90:3)*

236. **(D)** Antisialogogue effects are consistent, although of varying degree, among the anticholinergics. Amnestic effects and effects on gastric volume and pH are not consistent among this group of drugs. *(15:234; 90:4)*

237. **(D)** Conduction blockade by local anesthetics is primarily due to blockade of sodium conductance. This is a minimal block of potassium, but it is not significant. Calcium and magnesium are not involved. *(1:993; 99:1)*

238. **(E)** Systemic signs of local anesthetic toxicity involve all of the options. When a block is being administered, it is important to look for these signs. *(1:1002; 99:2)*

239. **(D)** The toxic effects of local anesthetics are seen at lower doses in the nervous system. There is a varying toxic level among the various drugs. One of the signs of toxicity is a longer P-R interval. Depression of the SA node does occur. *(1:1004; 99:3)*

240. **(A)** The cardiac effects of local anesthetic toxicity occur by interference with sodium conductance. Ventricular tachycardia and fibrillation may occur. The toxicity with bupivacaine is of longer duration and, therefore, harder to treat. Diazepam has no place in the treatment of the cardiac effects of local anesthetic toxicity but is helpful in the treatment of CNS toxicity. *(1:1004; 99:3)*

241. **(B)** The use of the priming principle to hasten the onset of action of muscle relaxants uses divided doses with a time interval that is thought to be optimal at 4 minutes. The method is not consistent in giving good intubating conditions. Another problem is that one must wait for the time to elapse. During this time, the sensitive patient may have trouble swallowing and controlling the airway. There is one report of a patient aspirating during this period. *(1:201; 102:1)*

242. (C) Drug elimination may occur by metabolism or excretion and is usually complete after 5 half-lives. Elimination is slower than distribution. *(1:68; 102:2)*

243. (E) Vecuronium effects in the infant are complex. Although the ED$_{50}$ is the same as in adults, infants have a greater sensitivity to the drug. The volume of distribution of vecuronium in the infant is larger, and the drug lasts longer. *(1:904; 102:2)*

244. (C) When using an infusion of a muscle relaxant, monitoring is important during the entire period. It is important to maintain the first twitch of the train-of-four to make sure there is not an overdose. Volatile anesthetics affect the level of relaxant needed. Mixing atracurium in Ringer's lactate solution may hasten Hofmann degradation. *(75:357; 102:4)*

245. (B) Phenylephrine is used to treat the cyanotic episodes of tetralogy of Fallot. The vasoconstriction counteracts the right-to-left shunt. It also increases the pulmonary artery occlusion pressure. Cardiac output may be decreased by the reflex bradycardia that is seen. The dose is 50 to 150 μg in an adult. *(15:265; 104:3)*

246. (C) Aminophylline is a beta agonist and a phosphodiesterase inhibitor. Since it causes an increase of cyclic AMP, it can be an inotropic drug, but it is seldom used for this. Aminophylline is not a catecholamine nor an adrenergic drug. *(15:267; 104:4)*

247. (E) Halothane sensitization of the heart is increased with hypoxemia and hypercarbia. This effect is abolished by both alpha and beta blockers and by calcium channel blockers. *(15:45; 75:202)*

248. (E) The question is asked: How much epinephrine can I use? The references give a good regimen to keep in mind. Although this is not guaranteed to avoid problems, it gives a good guideline to follow. The dose that is allowable for use with isoflurane is even greater. *(1:332; 75:202)*

249. (B) The decrease of cerebral metabolic rate is most profound with isoflurane. It is linked with the cerebral electric activity in that seizure activity will lead to increases in metabolic rate. The dose is important. Only when isoelectricity is reached is the metabolic rate stable with dosage. *(1:1268; 75:298)*

250. (A) Halothane decreases blood pressure by decreasing cardiac output, isoflurane by decreasing peripheral vascular resistance, and enflurane by vasodilatation and decreased contractility. Halothane does not have as great an effect on heart rate as has isoflurane. *(1:650; 75:301)*

251. (D) Nitrous oxide increases blood pressure when it is given with halothane. Nitrous oxide increases pulmonary vascular resistance. When given with opioids, nitrous oxide causes decreases in cardiac output. When given with isoflurane, the blood pressure increases because of the increase in systemic vascular resistance. *(1:658; 75:302)*

252. (A) If you read the two references, you will note a difference in the answer. Hudson, in the book edited by Barash et al, states that the halogenated hydrocarbons decrease hepatic blood flow but that nitrous oxide has little effect. In Miller's text, Maze states that liver blood flow is increased by isoflurane and that nitrous oxide (with hyperventilation) will decrease the flow. *(1:1202; 75:144)*

253. (E) All of the drugs cited are considered safe for the patient with malignant hyperthermia. The amide local anesthetics have been reported to be a triggering agent, but most today believe that they are not a problem. Drugs that increase the heart rate may make diagnosis difficult, since one of the first signs is a tachycardia. *(1:1981; 75:462)*

254. (A) Increasing the dose of pancuronium to twice its ED$_{95}$ will shorten the onset of the block. This method is used by some to achieve more rapid intubating conditions. If this is done, you must be aware of the other effects: long effect, more profound block, and the heart rate increases that are dose related. *(75:347)*

255. (E) Halothane breaks down into trifluoroacetic acid, chloride, fluoride, and bromide ions. *(1:713; 75:326)*

256. (E) Physostigmine is an interesting drug that has many uses in reversing drug effects. Since it can penetrate the blood–brain barrier, it is able to counteract the acetylcholine effects in the brain. *(1:962; 75:194)*

257. (C) The benzodiazepines are not equal in effectiveness in amnesia. They are all metabolized in the liver. There is little cardiovascular depression seen. Respiratory depression and respiratory arrest have been seen in some patients. This is a particular risk in the elderly. *(1:810; 75:488)*

258. (E) Digoxin is an inotrope with an effect to cause bradycardia. The mechanism involves the function of sodium-potassium ATPase. Calcium will potentiate the effects of digoxin. *(1:516; 75:207; 105:358)*

259. (A) Digitalis toxicity is manifest as nausea and vomiting, visual disturbances, prolonged P-R interval, and arrhythmias, especially multifocal PVCs. A bradycardia is common. *(1:516; 75:207; 105:358)*

260. (C) Histamine release causes a tachycardia and hypotension. Erythema is common, and there is a decreased peripheral vascular resistance. In addition, there may be wheezing and increased airway pressures as a result of bronchospasm. *(1:912; 75:348)*

261. (C) The cardiomyopathy seen with doxorubicin may be seen long after the chemotherapy has been discontinued. The side effect is dose dependent and is evaluated by echocardiography. Patients who are concurrently receiving radiation therapy may have more problems with the cardiac effects. *(1:324; 15:490; 75:425)*

262. (B) Esmolol is an ester that is broken down by an esterase that is distinct from the one that breaks down succinylcholine. Therefore, there should be no prolongation of the effect with the use of succinylcholine. Esmolol is of short duration. The drug can be used to blunt the effect of intubation. *(15:287; 75:211)*

263. (E) Doxapram is a centrally acting analeptic that acts through the carotid body. This drug is not of use in coma that is drug induced. It has been touted to be of use in the patient who is still hypoventilating postoperatively, but that is a dangerous use. If a patient is not ventilating adequately, reversal of muscle relaxants or artificial ventilation is the treatment that should be employed. *(15:518)*

264. (D) The patient has all the symptoms of the central anticholinergic syndrome that may follow the ingestion of jimson weed. The typical symptoms of "blind as a bat, red as a beet, hot as a hare, and mad as a hatter" are due to antimuscarinic effects of drugs that can pass the blood–brain barrier. Physostigmine also can pass the blood–brain barrier and will counteract the effects. Administration of this drug will treat all of the symptoms and the CT scan, aspirin, and sponge baths will not be necessary. *(75:194)*

265. (C) Coverage of steroid therapy at the time of surgery is important to avoid stress reactions. The theory has been to give larger doses to avoid problems. At the present time, smaller doses are recommended and are based on the anticipated stress of the operative procedure. A dose at induction, through the case, and for 24 hours is now used for those who are having procedures with moderate to major stress. (See also the discussion in Chernow's lecture for the 1988 ASA meeting, reference 108.) *(1:266; 15:407; 75:1200)*

266. (E) The patient who has been on steroids is at risk of having a reaction and should be covered. The patient may get by without any trouble at all, but the risk of giving the steroids is less than the risk of the stress reaction. Smaller doses suited to the procedure should be used. *(1:266; 15:407; 75:1200)*

267. (E) A patient with the presented symptoms may be having an anaphylactic reaction. Your first reaction should be to stop the suspected offender. The treatment is to ensure oxygenation, to improve the relative volume status, and to improve the blood pressure. Antihistamines also may be administered. *(75:1385)*

268. (E) Tachyphylaxis, the tolerance to a drug that develops with only a few doses, is seen with all the drugs noted. *(15:3; 75:159,181)*

269. (A) Mannitol is filtered at the glomerulus. It is an osmotic diuretic and will acutely increase the blood volume. It may be a hazard in congestive failure, since the blood volume may be increased, making the failure worse until the diuresis takes effect. *(1:1571; 15:429; 75:1085)*

270. (E) Mannitol is relatively contraindicated in congestive heart failure, since the blood volume is increased transiently. In renal failure, the kidneys may not be able to excrete the fluid. In the two neurosurgical diagnoses, the contraindication pertains to the shrinking of the normal brain tissue, allowing the masses to expand. *(1:1571; 15:430)*

271. (A) The alpha$_1$ receptors are stimulated by norepinephrine, causing vasoconstriction. The receptors will be blocked by labetalol. The bronchioles are not affected by alpha$_1$ receptors. *(1:273,963; 15:629; 75:179)*

272. (A) The beta$_2$ receptors are stimulated by isoproterenol and are blocked by esmolol. Stimulation of these receptors will increase glycogenolysis. Vasodilatation results from stimulation. *(1:273,963; 15:629; 75:179)*

273. (E) Magnesium deficiency may occur as muscle spasm, arrhythmia, or CNS irritability. It should be suspected in the chronic alcoholic and in anyone who is nutritionally deprived. *(1:1321; 15:541; 75:960)*

274. (D) The opioids produce unconsciousness at high dosage, but it is important to recognize that unconsciousness is not guaranteed. The pupils are constricted. The opioids are not good amnestic drugs. The nausea and vomiting seen are mediated through the central nervous system in the area postrema. *(1:745; 15:69; 75:258)*

275. (A) The known drug abuser may have a full stomach due to the slower emptying time of the gastrointestinal tract. This population has a higher incidence of AIDS and hepatitis, and precautions must be taken. The need for anesthetic agents will be increased. *(1:768; 75:411)*

276. (B) Clonidine is a centrally acting sympathetic inhibitor and may be of use in the patient having withdrawal symptoms. Propranolol may be helpful for the same reasons. The other two options are both agonist–antagonist combinations and are likely to precipitate withdrawal. *(1:329; 75:411)*

277. (B) Cyanide toxicity must be avoided in the use of sodium nitroprusside. Captopril given before the nitroprusside is started has been shown to be effective in decreasing the amount needed to give the desired hypotension. Patients more at risk are those who are nutritionally deprived because of a deficiency of vitamin B_{12}. Miller cites the safe dose as under 0.5 mg/kg/hour. *(1:1954; 75:218; 106:3)*

278. (A) Vecuronium is not dependent on renal excretion for elimination from the body. The other options, penicillin, gallamine, and digoxin, are heavily influenced by renal excretion, and this must be taken into consideration in prescribing the dose. *(1:1649; 107:3)*

279. (C) The patient with hyperthyroidism should be adequately prepared preoperatively. If an emergency procedure must be performed, agents that cause a tachycardia should be avoided, since it makes it more difficult to follow the heart rate as a sign of the hyperthyroidism. Ketamine and pancuronium fall into this category. *(1:273; 108:228)*

280. (E) The coronary steal and its significance are still being debated. In effect, there must be a stenosed vessel and flow increase across the stenosis, with a resulting pressure drop across the stenosis. If the pressure stays constant, the distal flow to the collaterals supplied will decrease. The discussion by Merin and Buffington addresses the significance of this mechanism. Their conclusion is that isoflurane may lead to increased ischemia but that most patients can tolerate the agent if carefully managed. *(1:1541; 109:2)*

281. (D) Corticorticoids used for the treatment of asthma should be of the glucocorticoid type, since no mineralocorticoid effect is desired. The onset time is measured in hours. No drug should be used until the therapeutic ratio has been considered, but the advantage of steroids usually outweighs the disadvantage. Giving the drug by inhalation route does not decrease the onset time. *(110:2)*

282. (E) All of the drugs listed are antidysrhythmics or can be used for ventricular arrhythmias. Magnesium sulfate is not a drug that is used often, but in arrhythmias that are resistant to therapy, it may be life-saving. *(1:480; 111:6)*

283. (C) The mechanism of sodium nitroprusside is by dilatation of the resistance vessels, whereas that of nitroglycerin is by dilatation of the capacitance vessels. The mechanism of trimethaphan is by ganglionic blockade and isoflurane by dilatation of the peripheral vasculature. *(1:1954; 106:6)*

284. (D) When the halogenated hydrocarbons are used in sufficient dose to provide deliberate hypotension, the perfusion pressure decreases and myocardial blood flow decreases. There is loss of autoregulation. Seizure activity is seen with enflurane, not halothane. *(1:1952; 106:6)*

285. (D) The patient with renal failure needs decreased dosage of thiopental due to less protein binding leading to more unbound fraction available. Combinations of potent opioids and tranquilizers may lead to hypotension because of decreased cardiovascular reserve. Succinylcholine may lead to increases in potassium in a patient who is already at risk from hyperkalemia. It is generally thought that the anesthetic course is smoother with an inhalation agent such as isoflurane. *(1:1648; 107:6)*

286. (E) The inhalation agents and thiopental are all appropriate for the patient with asthma. It is important that the anesthesia be deep enough before airway instrumentation is attempted. At the usual induction doses of thiopental, bronchospasm is likely. If one takes enough time to allow the patient to be well anesthetized and administers lidocaine before intubation, bronchospasm usually is averted. *(110:4)*

287. (C) Reserpine and theophylline increase the production of cerebrospinal fluid. Acetazolamide, a carbonic anhydrase inhibitor, decreases production. Production is also decreased by digoxin through inhibition of the sodium-potassium pump. *(112:133)*

288. (E) Ionization of a drug is important in the drug's function, since charged particles do not cross membranes well. The ionization is a function of the pH and the pKa. *(15:8; 75:1218)*

289. (B) The activity of thiopental is affected by the high fat/blood coefficient. The adipose tissue is capable of taking up large amounts of thiopental. This fact is only important if a large amount is given. If a sleep dose is administered on induction and no more is given, it is of little importance. *(15:105)*

290. (D) Isoflurane is a good choice, since there is less metabolism of the agent. The initial bolus should be given based on the lean body mass. Previous ideas of prolonged emergence due to volatile agents leaching out of tissues for prolonged periods have been disproved. Equilibration between tissues and blood does occur. *(15:105; 75:1122)*

291. **(E)** All of the options may have an effect on the amount of intravenous drug needed for induction. The hypovolemic patient has a greater effect, and the elderly need less. Younger patients may require more. Hepatic disease may affect the dose need by protein binding. Other drugs that are being taken may affect the dose by enzyme induction or other drug interactions. *(15:108; 75:244)*

292. **(C)** The principal disadvantages of methohexital are pain on injection and involuntary muscle movements. Hiccoughs are frequent. The pH is high, and the solubility is not low. *(1:1901; 15:108; 75:244)*

293. **(D)** Patients with acute intermittent porphyria void urine that turns dark after standing. They have a positive Watson-Schwartz test. They also have a positive porphobilinogen, which is pathognomic of the disease. *(140:571)*

294. **(D)** The principal reason for the termination of drug effect with methohexital is redistribution. This drug is metabolized more than thiopental, but redistribution is the chief mechanism of terminating effect. The pH is high, and the fat solubility is high. *(1:803; 15:104; 75:231)*

295. **(E)** Injection of thiopental is followed by a rapid decrease of concentration in the central pool with a subsequent rise in the viscera. Following the rise in the viscera is the concentration rise in the lean tissues, such as muscle. The adipose tissues gradually build up a concentration after that. *(1:803; 15:104; 75:231)*

296. **(A)** The vessel-rich group includes those organs that receive the bulk of circulation. It includes the heart, kidneys, and the central nervous system. Muscles are not included. *(1:59; 15:7; 75:140)*

297. **(B)** The same dose of thiopental is not appropriate for all patients. An understanding of the diagram is important to the proper use of intravenous medications. A patient in shock will have an increased effect of thiopental. The patient who is anxious and has an increased cardiac output will have a faster redistribution, and the effect will be shorter. *(1:67; 75:144; 114:43)*

298. **(C)** Tissue perfusion is important. In the shock patient there is vasoconstriction, and the amount of thiopental going to the brain is relatively greater. Cerebral blood flow is preferentially maintained. *(1:67; 75:144; 114:42)*

299. **(C)** Dissociative anesthesia is noted by the presence of open eyes and occasional muscle movement. Movement is not a sign of inadequate dose. Muscle tone may be increased in dissociative anesthesia. *(1:815; 15:134; 144:1127–1128)*

300. **(D)** The administration of ketamine causes an increased systolic blood pressure, an increased diastolic blood pressure, an increased heart rate, and an increased cardiac output. *(1:815; 15:134; 144:1129)*

301. **(A)** Ketamine anesthesia is associated with open eyes at adequate level of anesthesia, diplopia in the postoperative period, and nystagmus. Lacrimation usually is not seen. Intraocular pressure levels are controversial. Some have found that there is an increase, which others have not confirmed. *(1:816)*

302. **(A)** Ketamine causes a depression of the medial thalamic nuclei. There is a retention of visceral sensation and maintenance of respiratory rate and tidal volume. The gag reflex is protected in most cases. However, cases of aspiration have been reported, and the patient with a need for airway protection should have it. *(1:814; 15:137; 75:236)*

303. **(D)** The emergence sequelae that are seen with ketamine include delirium and dreaming, which may be unpleasant in only about 10% of cases. These effects are more common in women. The recovery room treatment of these patients should be a leave-alone attitude. Nursing should not include a stir-up regimen but careful observation to ascertain that the patients are exchanging air well. The unpleasant dreams and emergence problems can be minimized by premedication. *(1:816; 15:140; 75:246)*

304. **(C)** Local anesthetics block conduction by blocking pores in the cell membrane. The local anesthetics do not depolarize the membrane. The drugs exist as salts. *(1:998; 15:156; 75:372)*

305. **(E)** Local anesthetics are affected by the pH of the surrounding tissue. The basic component of the salt penetrates the nerve membrane in the process of impulse blockade. Inflamed tissue has a lower pH, and the drugs do not function as well. Buffering the solutions is said to improve the activity. *(1:998; 15:156; 75:372)*

306. **(E)** All of the options are true concerning the duration of activity of the drugs. Adding epinephrine to a drug that is already of longer duration has less effect in prolonging the activity. *(1:1000; 15:151)*

307. **(E)** The toxicity of the local anesthetic drugs can be altered by adjusting the options cited. Limiting the dose, injecting over a longer period of time, and avoiding sites of high vascularity when possible will lessen the risk of toxicity. *(1:1000; 15:151; 75:390)*

308. **(B)** An allergic reaction to lidocaine from a multidose vial may be caused by the drug or its preservative. A reaction to lidocaine will not be reason to avoid procaine, since they are in two different groups. Although one assumes that the reaction is to the preservative, one cannot administer a second dose of lidocaine with impunity. *(15:158; 75:388)*

309. **(A)** Apnea at the end of the procedure is probably not due to thiopental, since it should be completely redistributed by that time. Low Pco$_2$ levels due to hyperventilation could explain it, as could prolonged effect from succinylcholine. Patients who have received echothiophate may not be able to break down the succinylcholine. Narcotic depression from the premedication could also be a cause. *(1:1854; 15:218; 75:1056)*

310. **(A)** In trying to determine the cause, a nerve stimulator can be used to assess the level of muscle relaxation. The Pco$_2$ can be assessed by blood gases. A narcotic antagonist may be administered to determine if narcotic effect is present. Allowing a patient to be unventilated for a period of time is hazardous, since hypoxia may occur during this time. The CO$_2$ will rise about 4 torr/minute in the apneic patient. *(75:475)*

311. **(D)** Once you have established that there is no twitch, the only course to take is to ventilate the patient as long as is necessary. In this patient, who may be awake but paralyzed, it is important to give some sedation and make people aware that she may be awake. *(1:885)*

312. **(B)** This reaction is not seen daily but is not uncommon. It may follow succinylcholine and may be due to a pharyngeal reflex. It has not been attributed to thiopental. Although intense sialorrhea may follow endoscopy, it is not common after intubation unless succinylcholine has been used. *(43:447; 46:1716)*

313. **(B)** This condition is usually self-limiting, and there is no need to cancel the procedure or to resort to tracheostomy. The patient should be observed, and there should be some resolution of the swelling before the endotracheal tube is removed. *(43:447; 46:1716)*

314. **(E)** The resting membrane is −90 mV and is due to the difference in the intra- and extracellular potassium. The membrane potential is dependent on the permeability of the membrane. The potential changes rapidly with depolarization. *(75:34)*

315. **(B)** Myoglobinemia may occur after a single dose of succinylcholine and is more common in children. It is not necessarily harmless, since there may be renal failure due to the deposition of the myoglobin in the kidneys. Myoglobin is released from skeletal muscle, not smooth muscle. *(1:1726; 15:179; 26:824; 43:447)*

316. **(C)** Succinylcholine may lead to prolonged apnea in a pregnant patient because of the decreased levels of cholinesterase. This is described often in the literature, but it may be more theoretical than real, since the blood volume is also increased at term. The higher volume of distribution will counteract the effect of the succinylcholine to some degree. A normal dibucaine number is higher, ie, 80, which is the percent of inhibition of normal plasma cholinesterase by dibucaine. Succinylcholine does not affect the motility of the uterine muscle and does not cross the placenta until higher doses are reached. *(1:1711; 15:177; 75:344)*

317. **(A)** Succinylcholine effect may be prolonged in the patient on echothiophate eyedrops and in those exposed to organophosphate insecticides. The patient with liver disease may have low cholinesterase levels. A patient who has a heterozygous atypical pseudocholinesterase should have no problem with succinylcholine. *(1:916; 15:176; 75:343,473)*

318. **(A)** A nondepolarizing block will be reversed by an anticholinesterase drug. Signs of a nondepolarizing block include a fade with the train-of-four, fade with tetanic stimulation, and posttetanic facilitation. *(1:876; 15:182; 75:580)*

319. **(A)** In a study reported by Hill (reference 75, page 364), the lithium potentiated the block by pancuronium and succinylcholine but not the block of gallamine or D-tubocurarine. The reason for the difference is difficult to explain. *(15:355; 75:364)*

320. **(E)** The release of acetylcholine is due to ionic conditions, eg, the presence of calcium. Magnesium ions have the opposite effect. The intensity of the depolarization and the duration of the depolarization are also important. The resting level of the membrane is important. Hyperpolarization of the membrane results in a greater release of acetylcholine. *(1:841; 148:22)*

321. **(A)** The hemodynamic response to a relaxant will be altered by depth of anesthesia. A patient deeply anesthetized may have a more pronounced vasodilatation and more sympathetic blockade. Surgical stimulation may lead to more sympathetic stimulation. Blood volume changes may make the effect of the relaxants more pronounced (in hypovolemia) or less pronounced (hypervolemia). The sex of the patient should have no effect. *(1:896)*

322. **(A)** The presence of myoglobinemia is not a usual reaction to succinylcholine injection nor is profound bradycardia. The muscle pain that is noted is usually in the trunk area. The rise in potassium is well documented. *(9:916)*

323. **(C)** Heart rate changes seen with succinylcholine are usually a decrease in the heart rate in children due to the parasympathetic preponderance in the child. The second dose may lead to profound bradycardia. Drugs with a vagotonic property, eg, sufentanil, may accentuate the bradycardia. In the adult, the change may be a tachycardia, and there is usually a rise in blood pressure. Some of the blood pressure increase may be attributable to response to tracheal intubation. *(1:918; 75:344)*

324. **(C)** The increase in intragastric pressure is well documented. Regurgitation may occur if the pressure exceeds 25 cm H_2O. Any condition that relaxes the esophageal sphincter, eg, hiatus hernia, will predispose to regurgitation. Atropine will not block the pressure rise, but pretreatment with curare will. *(1:921; 15:179; 75:345)*

325. **(E)** Atracurium is easily antagonized. It is broken down by hydrolysis, although the principal mechanism of breakdown is Hofmann elimination. There are minimal cardiovascular side effects, especially if the injection is slow in order to mitigate the histamine release. *(15:199; 75:350; 84:1)*

326. **(C)** The development of dual block follows a stage of tachyphylaxis. It is both time and dose dependent. It may occur with doses as low as 2 to 4 mg/kg. It is difficult to detect clinically. *(15:175; 75:357; 158:216)*

327. **(A)** The motor endplate cholinergic receptor is not the only site of action of acetylcholine. The receptor is activated by acetylcholine but also may be activated by similar molecules, such as succinylcholine. It is refractory to further depolarization for a short interval after activation. *(1:843; 15:174; 75:342)*

328. **(A)** Cholinergic receptor site activation is the cause of some of the side effects of muscle relaxants, but histamine release is not due to this mechanism. *(1:843; 15:174; 75:342)*

329. **(B)** Histamine release is followed by bronchospasm in some cases and by upper chest erythema. Hypotension is usually seen along with a tachycardia. *(1:912; 15:374; 75:342)*

330. **(A)** The drugs neostigmine, pyridostigmine, and physostigmine form a chemical complex at the esteratic site of the acetylcholinesterase molecule. In contrast, edrophonium forms an electrostatic bond at the anionic site and has hydrogen bonding at the esteratic site. *(15:218)*

331. **(B)** Plasma cholinesterase has no known physiologic function and is not specific for succinylcho-

line. The enzyme can be inhibited by hexafluorenium, and this was a strategy to make it last longer. It is antagonized by echothiophate. *(1:916)*

332. **(E)** Succinylcholine is relatively contraindicated in all of these cases, but factors that must be taken into consideration are the extent of burn, time of the burn, and the amount of muscle wasting. In most cases, another method is available to provide relaxation, and my policy is that if I have to consider the problems, I use another drug. *(1:919)*

333. **(D)** The hypotensive effect of D-tubocurarine becomes increasingly apparent as doses greater than 0.3 mg/kg are administered, especially if given as a single dose. The tachycardia due to pancuronium is less if the dose is kept below 0.05 mg/kg. If sufficient gallamine is given to provide relaxation, there will be a tachycardia. Finally, metocurine has much less cardiovascular effect than does D-tubocurarine. *(1:908)*

334. **(A)** It is important to remember that muscle relaxant requirements vary markedly from patient to patient. Therefore, the dosage must be carefully individualized by incremental administration and with careful monitoring by a nerve stimulator. *(102:4)*

335. **(C)** The peak effect of neostigmine is at 10 to 15 minutes. Adequate reversal is more important in the patient with renal disease, since complete excretion of the drug may not have taken place. The peak effect of atropine is about 5 minutes, and its onset is faster. This matches the onset time of edrophonium. The best indicator of full recovery is not the assessment of a single twitch height but the lack of fade with the train-of-four. *(1:928; 15:224)*

336. **(C)** Succinylcholine is more prolonged when administered by infusion, since a larger dose usually is given. The relaxation cannot be readily antagonized. There is a great variation in the effects from patient to patient. The onset of a desensitization does not necessarily prolong the block. *(1:916; 75:346)*

337. **(E)** There is a great deal of interaction with other drugs and patient conditions. This is another reason why patients should be monitored when relaxants are administered. *(1:896; 75:363)*

338. **(C)** The action of pancuronium is modified by deep halothane anesthesia, which will potentiate the relaxant effect. The prior injection of atropine will decrease or eliminate the cardiovascular effect of pancuronium. Previous injection of succinylcholine will increase the action of pancuronium. The site of administration will have little or no effect. *(1:913; 75:348)*

339. **(A)** Pyridostigmine has a longer duration of action and a greater dependence on the kidneys for excretion. The onset of action is slower. In general, there is little advantage in the use of pyridostigmine. *(6:928)*

340. **(B)** The patient with myasthenia gravis has weakness in the muscles of the cranial group and is very sensitive to nondepolarizing muscle relaxants. These patients do not normally have any neurologic defects, and their disease varies in the amount of paralysis present. *(1:2279; 75:441; 148:99)*

341. **(C)** Dual block usually follows a period of tachyphylaxis. It may not develop immediately, and the onset may follow a dose as small as 2 to 4 mg/kg. The block may respond to anticholinesterases, but this treatment is fraught with the possibility of free succinylcholine being present. If this is the case, the block will be potentiated. *(1:924; 158:217)*

342. **(B)** Patients with the Eaton-Lambert syndrome have a sensitivity to both depolarizing and nondepolarizing relaxants. The block is not readily reversed. Resection of the tumor does effect a cure. *(1:933; 75:442; 158:238)*

343. **(B)** Procaine and other local anesthetics inhibit the release of acetylcholine. Therefore, they potentiate nondepolarizing drugs and prolong the action of succinylcholine. This effect is important to bear in mind when administering anesthesia to a patient who is receiving lidocaine for its antidysrhythmic effect. *(1:931; 15:193; 158:240)*

344. **(A)** The muscle spasm seen with myotonia is not aggravated by procainamide but is relieved. Succinylcholine will lead to spasm, and the spasm is not relieved by curare. Quinine will relieve the spasm. *(1:933; 75:345; 158:240)*

345. **(C)** Curare is potentiated by respiratory acidosis. This may be a reason for difficult reversal. Renal disease may also lead to prolonged blockade. Gallamine reversal is not faster with respiratory acidosis. A patient with a high blood flow will have a shorter block than one with a low blood flow. *(1:925; 15:195)*

346. **(D)** Gallamine may be administered with thiopental. The increase in heart rate is mediated by the autonomic nervous system. The excretion is by the kidneys. The duration is shorter than that of curare. *(1:911; 2:698; 15:191)*

347. **(A)** The effects of neostigmine include bradycardia, sweating, and skeletal muscle stimulation. The bladder is stimulated to contract. *(1:928; 2:731; 15:222)*

348. **(E)** Tetanus is a rare disease, but we may be consulted for the treatment. The muscle spasm may be treated by diazepam, and relaxation may be needed for artificial ventilation. Labetalol may be employed to control the sympathetic overactivity. If pancuronium is used, it may lead to hypertension and increased heart rate; therefore, some recommend that it not be used. *(6:340)*

349. **(E)** Assessing the depth of anesthesia is more complicated than in the past. Instead of looking at the size of the pupils and the depth of respiration, one now must consider many factors and take all into consideration. All the options must be assessed. *(1:415; 75:308)*

350. **(B)** Drug antagonism occurs when two drugs have effects that tend to counteract one another. This may occur by combination, as in the case of heparin–protamine interaction, or they may compete for the same receptor site, as with muscle relaxants and acetylcholine. *(1:70; 15:3; 47:47; 75:161)*

351. **(D)** Additive effect refers to a combined effect that is the algebraic sum of the individual actions. If a drug prolongs the effect of another drug, the effect is potentiation. Some may describe this as a variation of additive effect. *(1:70; 15:3; 47:47; 75:161)*

352. **(E)** Drug interaction may take place by all of the mechanisms noted. For this reason, it is important to know all of the medications the patient may be taking. *(47:47)*

353. **(B)** In the graph, the blood level of drug A falls to very low levels between doses. Drug B shows increasing levels over a period of time. *(1:67; 190:48)*

354. **(D)** The graph shows that drug B is not completely eliminated before the second dose is given. The relative size of the dose cannot be determined from the diagram, but the doses are the same. The half-life of drug A is not long. *(1:67; 190:48)*

355. **(B)** Factors affecting the initial uptake include the cardiac output and the amount of alveolar ventilation. Temperature is not a factor in modern vaporizers, and the age of the patient has no direct effect. *(1:629; 75:295; 190:335)*

356. **(C)** The change of concentration, or the knee of the curve, is dependent on the blood gas solubility and the concentration of the agent. The vaporizer and the temperature are not of importance. *(1:630; 75:296; 190:335)*

357. (E) The rate at which a certain partial pressure is reached in the blood is dependent on all of the factors listed. The important factor is to keep a high gradient in the alveolus to encourage uptake into the blood, and then to keep a high gradient at the blood–tissue interface. *(1:630; 75:296; 190:332)*

358. (C) The alveolar concentration of a gas is independent of lung volume. The type of soda lime is not important. Both alveolar ventilation and uptake by the blood will affect the concentration. *(1:630; 75:296; 190:333)*

359. (A) Uptake of an agent is dependent on the passage across the alveolar membrane. The Ostwald coefficient is an expression of the solubility of an agent that has an effect on the uptake. Cardiac output also is important. The type of system does not affect the uptake. *(1:630; 75:296; 190:333)*

360. (B) The administration of halothane may decrease respiratory resistance through a beta agonistic effect. The effect on the bronchioles is not direct. The anesthetic effect also contributes to the decrease in resistance. Halothane may not always cause a decrease in resistance. *(1:672,673; 75:302)*

361. (A) The sympathetic stimulating effect of nitrous oxide is present in young, healthy volunteers. It may not be present in the patient on gangliolytics. It also may have little effect in the old and the debilitated, both patient populations where a stimulating effect would be helpful. The combination of halothane and nitrous oxide may not have any advantage over halothane alone. *(1:658; 49:284; 75:302)*

362. (B) When nitrous oxide is added to halothane, there is a sympathetic stimulating effect seen. This may antagonize halothane to some degree. The effect is seen early in the anesthesia and at light levels. The sympathetic stimulation causes vasoconstriction. *(1:658; 49:284; 75:302)*

363. (C) The circulatory effects of halothane include ganglionic blockade and reduced total peripheral resistance. The contractile force of the ventricle is decreased, and the cardiac output is reduced. *(1:655; 48:766)*

364. (B) The circulatory effects of halothane are due to multiple factors. The classic article by Price and Price showed, in dogs, little effect at 0.5% and about the same at 1% and 2%. The effects are due to action on the heart, the ganglia, and peripheral resistance. *(1:655; 48:767)*

365. (A) Enflurane causes electroencephalographic changes that may be interpreted as minor motor

seizures. The seizures are more common in the hypocapnic patient. There is no increase in seizures in the patient with established epilepsy. *(1:302,1269; 75:298)*

366. (B) MAC-BAR is the anesthetic concentration that blocks adrenergic response to a surgical stimulus. It will block reaction to tracheal intubation. The concentration is higher than MAC. It is not necessary to carry most patients at that deep a level of anesthesia. *(1:574; 75:298,308)*

367. (D) If nitrous oxide is added to an enflurane anesthetic, there is less depression of cardiovascular measurements than would be seen with enflurane alone. This is due to the sympathetic stimulation seen with nitrous oxide. *(1:659; 75:303)*

368. (B) The cuff on the endotracheal tube is an air-containing space, and will respond to exposure to nitrous oxide as any other air-containing space. If the cuff is filled with nitrous oxide, there will be no gradient and no inflow of nitrous oxide. *(1:639)*

369. (B) When nitrous oxide is administered to patients with coronary artery disease, there is a decrease in blood pressure and ventricular contractility. The LVEDP is increased, and the cardiac output will decrease. *(1:657; 75:302)*

370. (B) Beta receptors prepare the body for emergencies by increasing the cardiac output, dilating the bronchioles, increasing glucose, and increasing insulin release. *(1:951; 75:179)*

371. (E) Beta blockers have a wide therapeutic usefulness, and many patients are using them. The newer blockers have more specific effects, and there are fewer side effects in their use. *(1:971; 75:179)*

372. (E) As alluded to in the answer to Question 371, there are side effects to contend with in the use of beta blockers. In most of the diseases in the options, the sympathetic nervous system has been mobilized to compensate for the pathology. Blocking the compensatory effects may precipitate further problems. In the patient with peripheral vascular disease, further vasoconstriction may follow treatment. The diabetic patient may have hypoglycemia that interferes with the established insulin regimen. *(1:973; 15:288)*

373. (B) Metoprolol is a selective beta$_1$ adrenergic blocker. It inhibits the inotropic and chronotropic effects of isoproterenol and does not inhibit the vasodilator effects of that drug. *(15:286)*

374. (C) Propranolol causes hypoglycemia, as does insulin. Isoflurane has little effect on blood sugar, al-

though the stress of surgery should cause an increase. *(15:288; 75:1141)*

375. **(B)** One of the side effects of digitalis is gynecomastia. This is due to the steroid base. Another side effect is dizziness. Digitalis is not associated with hunger but may cause nausea. Alopecia is not a side effect. *(50:945; 105:358)*

376. **(E)** The aim of therapy with digitalis is to increase contractility and to control tachyarrhythmias. By moving the patient's hemodynamic profile to a better curve, higher stroke volume is possible with lower filling pressure. *(117:1911)*

377. **(C)** In patients who have heart disease secondary to their pulmonary disease, the treatment should be directed primarily at the correction of the pulmonary disease. The use of digitalis in patients who have cor pulmonale tends to produce arrhythmias. *(117:1912)*

378. **(B)** Administration of digitalis leads to increased contractility and a longer P-R interval. The heart rate decreases. Oxygen consumption will decrease if the failing heart is allowed to pump more efficiently. The oxygen consumption will increase if digitalis aggravates or causes arrhythmias. *(50:720)*

379. **(A)** The effectiveness of digitalis is affected by the thyroid status; hyperthyroid states are more resistant. Acid-base and electrolyte status also are important. Concomitant drugs have little effect. *(50:943)*

380. **(D)** Propanidid is a nonbarbiturate induction agent. It is an intravenous agent that is short acting and has no hepatotoxic effect. *(1:821; 15:144)*

381. **(A)** Diazepam is a benzodiazepine that has specificity for the limbic system. For this reason, it is effective in patients with local anesthetic toxicity. It is a poor analgesic. Diazepam causes anterograde amnesia but does not have good retrograde amnesic effects. *(1:812; 15:125)*

382. **(B)** Intravenous ethanol is mostly of historical importance, although it is probably still used occasionally. Its effects are sedative and diuretic. There is little effect on the cardiovascular system. It may lead to increased blood sugars. *(47:499)*

383. **(C)** The neuroleptic state is characterized by amnesia and analgesia. The reflexes are depressed, including the gag reflex in some patients. The patient is in a state resembling catalepsy—appearing awake but unaware of the environment. *(1:760,770; 15:351)*

384. **(C)** Intravenous morphine in large doses does not cause cardiac instability. Even with large doses, the patient may be awake. Catecholamine release is seen. If the morphine is given alone, there is cardiac stability. In the presence of nitrous oxide, the stability may not be apparent. *(1:760,771)*

385. **(B)** Ketamine anesthesia is characterized by analgesia and cardiovascular stimulation. The gag reflex is not always present. Respirations are not depressed. *(1:815; 15:136)*

386. **(E)** The patient who has been taking large doses of amphetamines presents problems from the standpoint of anesthetic requirements and altered compensatory mechanisms. These patients may have depleted catecholamine reserves. Temperature aberrations are not uncommon. Venous access is complicated by frequent occurrence of angiitis. *(75:246)*

387. **(E)** The narcotic addict has numerous problems related to the addiction. There is a danger to the addict and to the anesthesia provider in terms of hepatitis and AIDS. *(1:768)*

388. **(B)** The patient on MAO inhibitors should have a drug-free interval if that is possible. Effects of many drugs may be exaggerated. Meperidine should be avoided, as should drugs that are releasers of histamine. The main concern is instability of the cardiovascular system. *(1:331; 75:209)*

389. **(A)** The hypotension that is associated with morphine administration is not due to cardiac depression at the dose used in clinical practice. It is due to direct vasodilatation and to the effect of histamine. Increased vagal stimulation also is seen. *(1:754; 75:258)*

390. **(D)** The hypotension occasionally seen with fentanyl administration is due to bradycardia. There is no direct effect on the vessels or on the myocardium. *(1:754; 75:258)*

CHAPTER 5

Physics and Chemistry
Review

The consideration of basic physics is included in the study of anesthesiology, since so many of our activities involve physical principles. When we consider the anesthesia machine with its gases, regulators, and flowmeters, our monitors, intravenous fluids, respiratory gases, and the circulatory system, we can see the importance of physics to our practice.

Principles of biochemistry also are of importance and span the many areas of pharmacology, metabolism, and fluid and electrolytes. Many of these questions are covered in other areas.

The physics of compressed gases should be reviewed. The cylinder in common use on the anesthesia machine is the E size cylinder. The oxygen cylinder contains the gas in a compressed state with a pressure of 2000 psi. Nitrous oxide cylinders contain the gas in a liquid state with a pressure of 750 psi. As oxygen is used, the pressure decreases in the cylinder, and one can estimate the remaining amount from the pressure. With nitrous oxide, the pressure is maintained at the same level as long as any liquid is remaining in the cylinder. Only when the liquid is expended does the pressure decrease.

The gas in the cylinder must pass through a regulator to have the pressure reduced to a level that is useful in practice. The regulator is based on a pressure–area relationship to change the pressure as it leaves the cylinder to be presented to the flowmeter.

The flowmeter measures the gas being delivered using the principle of a variable orifice. The gas flow depends on the pressure drop across the constriction, the size of the annular opening, and the physical characteristics of the gas.

Flow characteristics are important in the delivery of gases, in breathing, and in the delivery of blood and fluids. Laminar flow is characterized by streamlined alignment of the flow, with the central part of the stream being the fastest, since there is less friction. Viscosity is a major determinant of laminar flow. Turbulent flow, on the other hand, is characterized by an erratic pattern, with the production of many eddy currents. Density is a major determinant in turbulent flow.

The Bernoulli principle and the Venturi effect have many medical applications, especially in respiratory therapy devices. These devices depend on the fact that as gas or liquid moves through a constriction of a tube, the velocity increases. This, in turn, causes a decrease in pressure, and entrainment can occur. Atomizers use this principle. The same principle can cause entrainment of air into intravenous lines.

The major gas laws should be reviewed. Many of the questions pertaining to the gas laws are in Chapter 1. They are equally important in the use of the anesthesia machine and respiratory therapy.

The physics of vaporizers should be reviewed, since it affects the delivery of anesthetic vapors. Most modern equipment is compensated for flow and temperature. Vapor pressure is the measure of the partial pressure created in a closed container by the molecules that escape from the liquid and that are in equilibrium with the liquid. The vapor pressure may be increased if the system is heated. The heat of vaporization of a liquid is the number of calories needed to convert 1 g of liquid into a vapor.

The use of electronic principles in the production and use of monitors is constantly growing. The use of transducers is constantly increasing. A transducer is a device that converts a measured parameter into an electrical signal that can be measured. Blood pressure and temperature are examples. The electrocardiogram measures an electrical signal; therefore, no transducer is needed.

Other principles in use include the Doppler principle, which is now used for measurement of blood pressure and for detecting air embolism, among other uses. The principle states that a wave train reflected from a moving surface will undergo a change in frequency.

The great increase in electronic monitoring and invasive monitoring have together increased the electrical hazards to the patient. Many hospitals no longer have operating rooms with conductive floors, since there are no explosive anesthetics in use. Explosions and static electricity have been replaced with the hazard of microshock. Microshock, that measured in the range of microamperes, is a hazard to the patient with indwelling catheters that are direct routes into the heart. Ten microamperes is the maximum allowable leakage current for medical equipment.

Questions

DIRECTIONS (Questions 1 through 28): Each of the numbered items or incomplete statements in this section is followed by answers or by completions of the statement. Select the ONE lettered answer or completion that is BEST in each case.

1. The statement that equal volumes of gases at the same temperature and pressure contain equal numbers of molecules is

    (A) Houssay's law
    (B) Avogadro's number
    (C) Lavoisier's law
    (D) Avogadro's hypothesis
    (E) Magill's hypothesis

2. As a person ascends to an altitude of 10,000 feet

    (A) atmospheric pressure remains the same
    (B) inspired oxygen pressure remains the same
    (C) inspired carbon dioxide decreases
    (D) alveolar carbon dioxide and water vapor pressure are constant.
    (E) alveolar oxygen pressure increases

3. The premise that "a wave train reflected from a moving surface will undergo a change in frequency" is the basis of

    (A) the electrocardiogram
    (B) the Doppler effect
    (C) cardiac output monitors
    (D) the pacemaker
    (E) ballistocardiography

4. The oxygen tanks on an anesthesia machine are

    (A) G tanks
    (B) M tanks
    (C) E tanks
    (D) D tanks
    (E) B tanks

5. If three containers each contain 22.4 L of oxygen (at standard pressure and temperature), nitrous oxide, and ether vapor, their weights will

    (A) be equal
    (B) vary according to the molecular weights
    (C) vary according to how many moles are contained
    (D) be dependent on the size of the container
    (E) vary inversely with the density

6. The number of calories required to raise the temperature of 1 g of a substance by 1°C is

    (A) the kilocalorie
    (B) the specific heat
    (C) the standard temperature
    (D) equal for all liquids
    (E) equal for all metals

7. The latent heat of vaporization

    (A) is equal for all liquids
    (B) is independent of the temperature
    (C) varies with the temperature of the liquid
    (D) is very low for solids
    (E) for water is 1 calorie/cm^3

8. In the graph shown, each side of the container holds gases with a pressure of 760 mm Hg. If the dividing wall were perforated to allow diffusion

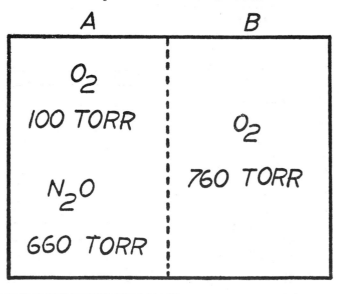

138

(A) O_2 would diffuse from A to B
(B) no diffusion would occur
(C) O_2 would diffuse from A to B and from B to A
(D) N_2O would diffuse from A to B
(E) N_2O would not diffuse across the membrane

9. If a liquid at a given temperature is in a closed container, equilibrium is reached when the number of vapor molecules leaving the liquid equals the number reentering it. This vapor pressure will change under all the following conditions EXCEPT if

(A) the temperature is raised
(B) the container is opened
(C) it is allowed to stand for 2 hours
(D) the container is compressed
(E) the container is cooled

10. Poiseuille's law refers to the flow of

(A) electrons in space
(B) liquid in relation to height
(C) gas in a closed system
(D) liquid in relation to the diameter of a tube
(E) water in relation to the pressure

11. The Bernoulli theorem states that

(A) pressure and volume in a pipe are related
(B) pressure and temperature in a pipe are related
(C) velocity of flow and lateral pressure are related
(D) the velocity of a gas is related to flow
(E) the velocity of a gas is related to its temperature

12. A mechanism used to reduce the pressure of a gas as it rises from a compressed gas cylinder to a usable, nearly constant pressure is

(A) a gauge
(B) a flowmeter
(C) an indicator
(D) a regulator
(E) a ball valve

13. Identical syringes are fitted with needles of different bores. The internal diameters of the needles are in the ratio of 1:2. The same force is applied to the plungers. The volume ejected in unit time is

(A) not related to the needle size
(B) 8 times greater through the large needle
(C) 16 times greater through the large needle
(D) 20 times greater through the large needle
(E) 32 times greater through the large needle

14. If a nitrous oxide tank is contaminated with water vapor, ice will form on the cylinder valve as a result of the

(A) latent heat of vaporization

(B) specific heat
(C) vapor pressure
(D) low pressure of the nitrous oxide
(E) ambient temperature

15. In the graph shown, the intravenous tubing regulators are placed distally in B and proximally in A. If a small hole is present in the tubing distal to the drip chamber, air embolus

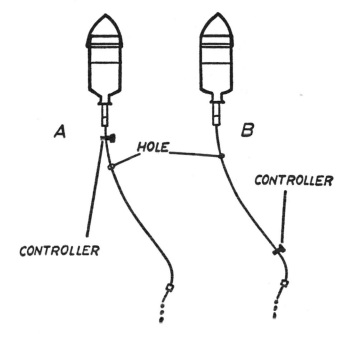

(A) is possible in A and B
(B) is possible in A
(C) is possible in B
(D) is not possible in A or B
(E) may occur, but there will not be enough air to be fatal

16. The maximum acceptable leakage current is

(A) 10 microamperes
(B) 10 amperes
(C) 100 microamperes
(D) 1 ampere
(E) 100 amperes

17. Alternating current (AC) delivered at a rate of 60 cycles per second

(A) is uncommon in the United States
(B) is the ideal current from a physiologic standpoint
(C) is avoided in medical appliances
(D) is in the ideal range to cause ventricular fibrillation
(E) will not cause cardiac irregularities unless it is perceptible

18. Contact with a current of 16 milliamperes produces a let-go current, meaning that

    (A) a person cannot hold the wire
    (B) the current causes paralysis of the body
    (C) the body is thrown away from the contact
    (D) a person cannot let go of an energized wire
    (E) a person cannot let go because of strong extensor contraction

19. Combustion accompanied by a self-propagating flame is referred to as

    (A) an explosion
    (B) spontaneous combustion
    (C) the heat of combustion
    (D) a deflagration
    (E) reduction

20. The reaction between oxygen and another molecule is called

    (A) oxidation
    (B) reduction
    (C) combustion
    (D) detonation
    (E) flaming

21. A reaction that removes electrons from a molecule is

    (A) oxidation
    (B) combustion
    (C) detonation
    (D) deflagration
    (E) flame propagation

22. Adiabatic compression refers to

    (A) compression of gas under water
    (B) compression of gas under a vacuum
    (C) compression of gas under hyperbaric conditions
    (D) compression of a gas at very low temperature
    (E) a compression process without heat loss to the outside

23. A device used to minimize voltage leaks is the

    (A) voltage regulator
    (B) conductive floor
    (C) three-prong plug
    (D) explosion-proof plug
    (E) ohm meter

24. The unit of resistance is the

    (A) ohm
    (B) ampere
    (C) volt
    (D) milliampere
    (E) microampere

25. The aerobic conversion of 1 mole of glucose

    (A) yields 2 moles of ATP
    (B) is less efficient than anaerobic conversion
    (C) involves the Krebs cycle
    (D) converts glucose to lactate
    (E) is the only pathway for energy production

26. Epinephrine causes an elevation in blood glucose by

    (A) direct action on the cell
    (B) action directly on glycogen
    (C) the action of cyclic AMP
    (D) action of growth hormone
    (E) increased production of insulin

27. The substrate for energy production is

    (A) water
    (B) carbon dioxide
    (C) ATP
    (D) glucose
    (E) oxygen

28. All of the following hormones require production of cyclic AMP as a second messenger EXCEPT

    (A) dopamine
    (B) thyroid hormone
    (C) glucagon
    (D) vasopressin
    (E) ACTH

DIRECTIONS (Questions 29 through 50): For each of the items in this section, ONE or MORE of the numbered options is correct. Choose the answer

    A if only 1, 2, and 3 are correct,
    B if only 1 and 3 are correct,
    C if only 2 and 4 are correct,
    D if only 4 is correct,
    E if all are correct.

29. Specific gravity

    (1) of air is 1
    (2) applies only to solids
    (3) describes a ratio of weight of one substance to a similar volume of water or air
    (4) describes mass per unit volume

30. The density of a gas

    (1) determines its flow through an orifice
    (2) is related to the explosive potential
    (3) is important in turbulent flow
    (4) is independent of temperature

31. Microshock hazard is increased in patients

    (1) with a pacemaker in place
    (2) who are in rooms with isolation transformers
    (3) with a central venous line in place
    (4) in mechanically operated beds

32. The Venturi tube shown in the diagram

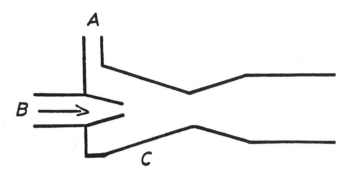

(1) is the basis for injector systems
(2) to be effective must open out gradually distal to the constriction C
(3) has a delivery gas that is denoted by B
(4) has an entrained gas denoted by A

33. Operating rooms use an isolated power supply because

(1) it affords added protection against high-amperage electrocution
(2) grounding cannot occur
(3) there is less hazard of fire and explosion
(4) leakage cannot occur

34. Heat loss from the body occurs by

(1) conduction
(2) radiation
(3) convection
(4) evaporation

35. Leakage current is

(1) harmless
(2) of the direct current (DC) type
(3) always at levels within safety limits
(4) unintentional flow of current from the internal wiring of a device

36. Safety rules of importance to anesthesiologists are contained in a publication(s) of the

(1) National Fire Protection Association (NFPA)
(2) American Society of Operating Room Design
(3) Joint Commission on Accreditation of Healthcare Organizations (JCAHO)
(4) American Association of Anesthesia Hazard Surveyors

37. The flow rate of fluid flowing smoothly through a tube is

(1) proportional to the pressure gradient
(2) proportional to the fourth power of the radius of the tube
(3) inversely proportional to the viscosity of the fluid
(4) proportional to the temperature of the tube

38. Helium and oxygen have similar viscosities but markedly different densities. This difference will be apparent

(1) across the entire breathing cycle
(2) more at low flow rates
(3) only in vitro; it has no practical application
(4) more at high flow rates

39. A transducer is a device used to

(1) convert a nonelectric parameter to an electric signal
(2) measure heart voltages in the electrocardiogram
(3) measure temperature using the thermistor
(4) measure electrical activity in the electroencephalograph

40. Turbulent flow is

(1) characterized by irregular lines of flow
(2) characterized by parallel lines of flow
(3) noted at branches, obstructions, or roughness of the conduit
(4) proportional to volume flow

41. Pulse oximeters

(1) are based on Beer's law
(2) will not read carboxyhemoglobin
(3) will read methemoglobin
(4) provide a heart rate but do not need pulsatile flow

42. A rectifier is a device that

(1) varies the amperage flowing to an appliance
(2) changes the resistance in an electrical circuit
(3) allows an electrical device to be grounded
(4) converts alternating current (AC) to direct current (DC)

43. The solubility of nitrogen in the body is important in

(1) breathing at high altitudes
(2) air embolus in a patient receiving nitrous oxide
(3) compression disease (caisson disease)
(4) a patient with pneumothorax who receives nitrous oxide

44. The current from a typical wall outlet

(1) has a frequency of 60 cycles/second
(2) has a constant polarity
(3) has a frequency of 60 hertz
(4) always flows in one direction

45. Ohm's law involves

    (1) the ampere
    (2) the ohm
    (3) the volt
    (4) a generator

46. The viscosity of a fluid

    (1) depends on its density
    (2) affects its specific gravity
    (3) does not affect resistance to flow
    (4) is the intrinsic property that affects its laminar flow

47. High-frequency positive-pressure ventilation (HFP-PV) accomplishes alveolar ventilation by

    (1) hyperinflation
    (2) convection
    (3) increased pressure of the gases
    (4) improved gas diffusion

48. Breathing through an endotracheal tube of markedly inadequate size will lead to

    (1) increased intrathoracic pressure
    (2) negative intrathoracic pressure
    (3) mediastinal shift
    (4) pulmonary edema

49. A nitrous oxide tank contains gas at a pressure of 750 psi. When the last drop of liquid nitrous oxide evaporates

    (1) the pressure will fall rapidly
    (2) the pressure will be zero
    (3) the pressure will remain at 750 psi until the tank is empty
    (4) the rate of pressure fall is dependent on the rate of flow

50. The second-messenger concept of hormone action involves

    (1) the action of a hormone at the cell membrane
    (2) the production of cyclic AMP
    (3) the initiation of biochemical reactions by cyclic AMP
    (4) ATP as the source of cyclic AMP

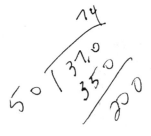

Answers and Explanations

1. **(D)** The statement that 1 mole of anything contains an equal number of molecules is Avogadro's hypothesis. The number, 6.023×10^{23} is Avogadro's number. The other options are not pertinent. *(51:4; 75:102)*

2. **(D)** Carbon dioxide is a function of body metabolism and therefore will remain essentially constant. Water vapor is essentially dependent on body temperature, and therefore it also will remain constant. Levels of both of these gases may be altered by the hyperventilation that usually accompanies the ascent to altitude. *(51:84; 129:582)*

3. **(B)** Doppler technology is being used to an increasing degree in medicine. It is not used in the usual electrocardiogram or in cardiac output monitors. Pacemakers are electrical generators. Ballistocardiography is based on detection of the motion produced by the heart beat. *(1:91; 75:107)*

4. **(C)** Gas cylinders are designated by letters from A to M. The size increases as one advances in the alphabet. *(170:1)*

5. **(B)** At normal temperature and pressure, 1 mole of a gas occupies 22.4 L. Therefore, the weight of these containers would vary according to the molecular weight of the gases. *(51:4)*

6. **(B)** The number of calories required to raise the temperature of 1 g of a substance by 1°C is its specific heat. The specific heat varies for different substances. *(51:18; 75:516)*

7. **(C)** The heat of vaporization is dependent on the temperature. The colder the liquid, the more calories needed to vaporize a given amount of liquid. The heat of vaporization for water is 540 calories/g. For halothane, it is 35 calories/g. *(1:125; 51:29–31; 75:516)*

8. **(D)** A gas will diffuse from a place where it is at a high partial pressure to a place where it is at a low partial pressure. This is the reason nitrous oxide diffuses into air-containing pockets. *(1:84; 51:69; 75:114)*

9. **(C)** The vapor pressure is subject to change with increases in temperature, since more molecules will leave the liquid. If the container is opened, the space above the liquid will be expanded, and it will take longer for equilibrium to be reached. If the container is compressed, more molecules will be in the liquid phase (as in a soda bottle). *(1:125; 51:69)*

10. **(D)** Poiseuille's law refers to the flow of liquid in relation to the diameter of a tube. The flow through a tube will be proportional to the driving pressure. The resultant flow is further modified by resistance. *(1:89,2342; 75:99)*

11. **(C)** The Bernoulli theorem states that the velocity of flow and lateral pressure are related. If a liquid is flowing through a pipe, the lateral wall pressure decreases if the flow velocity increases. *(1:79; 75:97)*

12. **(D)** The mechanism to reduce pressure of a gas to a useful pressure is a regulator. A gauge is a device to measure the pressure. The flowmeter is a device to measure the flow being delivered. A ball valve is a device to allow flow in one direction only. *(170:43)*

13. **(C)** Since the internal radii are in a ratio of 1:2, the volume ejected in that time will be 16 times greater through the larger needle because the resistance is related to the radius to the fourth power. *(1:89; 75:98)*

14. **(A)** The nitrous oxide tank contains a liquid, and in order for it to become vaporized, heat must be supplied. As the cylinder is opened, heat is removed from the cylinder and from the air in the immediate vicinity. The temperature falls, causing condensation. *(1:125; 51:96; 75:516)*

15. **(B)** When the drip controller is placed distally, a back pressure is present throughout the entire tubing. This prevents any entrainment of air. *(51:189)*

16. **(A)** The maximum acceptable leakage current is 10 microamperes. This is a small current, but it does not take a great amount of current to cause ventricular fibrillation in a patient with lines directly into the heart. There was little discussion of leakage current until it became technically possible to place lines into the heart and pacemakers became commonplace. *(1:111; 75:628)*

17. **(D)** Our typical 60 cycle AC is in the ideal range to cause ventricular fibrillation. It is not possible to avoid this type of current unless direct current (DC) is supplied. One need not feel the current for it to be detrimental. *(1:111; 75:628)*

18. **(D)** The let-go current means that a person cannot let go of an energized wire. A current of this magnitude causes flexion contractions. *(1:111; 75:628)*

19. **(D)** Sudden combustion with a self-propagating flame is a deflagration. An explosion is a sudden release of energy, in this case due to combustion. These terms are old and are of little import today. However, even though we have stopped using explosive agents and conductive floors are not universally used, others are bringing explosive substances into the operating room. Our neurology technicians try to bring large cans of collodion into the operating room to fix the leads on the patient for evoked potential monitoring. The aroma of ether is reminiscent. We still must be watchful. *(51:306)*

20. **(A)** The reaction of oxygen and another molecule is oxidation. This causes the loss of hydrogen or loss of electrons. The reverse process is reduction. *(51:287)*

21. **(A)** See answer to Question 20. *(75:146; 129:237)*

22. **(E)** Adiabatic compression refers to the compression of a gas without heat loss to the outside. The term has no reference to the presence of a vacuum or to the temperature at which the compression takes place. *(51:384; 75:103)*

23. **(C)** A three-prong plug allows instruments to be grounded, thereby providing a path for leakage current. Conductive floors are (were) used to prevent buildup of static electricity. An explosion-proof plug makes the electrical connection without causing a spark. *(75:634; 171:82–84)*

24. **(A)** The ohm is the unit of resistance. The ampere is the unit of current. The volt is the measure of electrical pressure. *(75:123)*

25. **(C)** Aerobic conversion of glucose involves the Krebs cycle. This system is more efficient than anaerobic metabolism, although both pathways may function. The Krebs cycle produces 4 moles of ATP per mole of glucose. The system converts glucose to pyruvate. *(75:968; 129:241)*

26. **(C)** Epinephrine and many other hormones act as messenger hormones, causing an increased production of cyclic AMP, which, in turn, creates biochemical reactions on the inside of the cell. Cyclic AMP is referred to as the "second messenger." *(1:2294; 75:181; 129:293)*

27. **(D)** The substrate for energy production is glucose. The other options, ATP and oxygen, are needed for the reaction. Water and carbon dioxide are products of the reaction. *(1:2294; 75:181)*

28. **(B)** Thyroid hormone does not require the production of cyclic AMP to function. Thyroid hormone does increase the activity of the sodium-potassium ATPase in the cell membrane. All of the other options require cyclic AMP. *(1:2299; 75:182; 129:34)*

29. **(B)** The specific gravity describes a ratio of the weight of a unit volume of one substance to a similar volume of water, in the case of solids or liquids, or of air in the case of gases. Both substances must be compared at the same conditions of temperature and pressure. Mass per unit volume is density. *(75:771)*

30. **(B)** The density of a gas determines its rate of flow through an orifice. Density is not related to the explosion potential. Density is important to turbulent flow. It is not independent of temperature. *(51:162,192; 75:100)*

31. **(B)** Any direct entry into the heart is a pathway for microshock. Mechanical beds should have no electrical hazard. Isolation transformers serve to protect the patient from ungrounded equipment. *(1:111; 75:628)*

32. **(E)** The Venturi tube is the basis of injector systems. The gradual opening distal to the constriction maintains the increased flow through the constriction. Two gases are noted in the diagram: the delivery gas B and the entrained gas A. *(1:79; 51:223–227; 75:97)*

33. **(B)** An isolated power supply affords protection against macroshock. Grounding can still occur. There is less hazard of fire with an isolated circuit. Leakage current can still occur. *(1:108; 75:637; 171:84)*

34. **(E)** Heat loss in the operating room occurs by evaporation, by convection, by radiation, and by conduction. Heat loss is not a big problem during short cases in adults, but in the longer procedures in an infant, it may be critical. *(75:110; 129:208)*

35. **(D)** Leakage current is the unintentional flow of current from the internal wiring of a device. It may present problems to the patient with direct lines to the heart. The current may be harmful at levels over 10 microamperes. It may be alternating current (AC). *(1:111; 75:636)*

36. **(B)** Safety regulations are in publications from the NFPA and the JCAHO. *(75:643)*

37. **(A)** The flow rate through a tube of a smoothly flowing liquid is proportional to the pressure gradient and the fourth power of the radius. There is an inverse relationship to viscosity. The temperature of the tube is not involved. *(1:89; 51:165)*

38. **(D)** At low flow rates, viscosity effects dominate, but at high flow rates, the effect of density is predominant. In the asthmatic and the patient with croup, helium may help ventilation. *(1:1444; 51:205)*

39. **(B)** A transducer converts a nonelectric parameter into an electrical signal that can be recorded. Temperature is such a parameter. Electrocardiograms and electroencephalograms measure electrical signals and, therefore, do not need transducers. *(171:22–23)*

40. **(B)** Turbulent flow is characterized by irregular lines of flow. It is mainly noted at branches, obstructions, and roughness of the tubes. Parallel lines of flow are seen with laminar flow. *(1:89; 75:99)*

41. **(B)** Pulse oximeters are based on technology that follows Beer's law, which relates the concentration of a solute to the intensity of light transmitted through the solution. The oximeter will read both carboxyhemoglobin and methemoglobin. In the currently used pulse oximeters, a pulsatile waveform is needed, since they analyze the pulsatile component of absorbance. *(1:174; 75:119)*

42. **(D)** A rectifier converts AC to DC by use of a one-way valve that allows only current passing in one direction to go through. *(171:13)*

43. **(E)** The solubility of nitrogen is important in high-altitude breathing and in compression disease. The problems encountered with nitrous oxide and pneumothorax are also functions of solubility. *(51:245)*

44. **(B)** The wall current has a frequency of 60 hertz which is 60 cycles/second. It is alternating current. *(75:627; 171:12–13)*

45. **(A)** Ohm's law involves the ampere, the ohm, and the volt. A generator is not involved. *(1:89; 75:625)*

46. **(D)** The viscosity of a fluid is an intrinsic property that affects its laminar flow characteristics. It is not dependent on density and does not affect its specific gravity. It does affect resistance to flow. *(1:87; 75:97)*

47. **(C)** HFPPV accomplishes ventilation by convection and improved gas diffusion. It does not cause hyperinflation, and there is little pressure increase *(75:933; 172:796)*

48. **(C)** Breathing through a small endotracheal tube leads to negative intrathoracic pressure. This may upset the very delicate balance in forces within the capillary and lead to pulmonary edema. This may happen in a very short time. *(51:267; 100:508)*

49. **(D)** When the last drop of nitrous oxide evaporates, the pressure fall will depend on the size of the tank and the rate of flow. *(51:100; 75:105)*

50. **(E)** All of the options are true. *(75:181 182; 129.33)*

PART II
Clinical Science

CHAPTER 6

Regional Anesthesia
Review

The use of regional anesthesia varies throughout the country. Some institutions do little regional anesthesia; others do little except for obstetrics. On the other hand, some do a majority of their procedures under regional block. Most of these differences are due to physician preference. The technique requires a knowledge of the anatomy, an experience with regional anesthesia, and the ability to work with the patient and the surgeon to make the anesthetic a success. Dissatisfaction on the part of any of the participants will make the experience unpleasant.

You should review the local anesthetics, the mechanisms of their action, the doses, and complications.

SPINAL ANESTHESIA

Spinal anesthesia is used primarily for procedures involving the lower abdomen and lower extremities. It involves the injection of a local anesthetic into the subarachnoid space. The anesthesia is due to the effect of the local anesthetic on the spinal nerve roots and the dorsal root ganglia. The smallest fibers are affected first. Nerve function loss with the onset of anesthesia follows the order of autonomic, superficial pain, temperature, vibratory, motor power, and touch.

The spinal needle in the midline approach passes through the skin, the subcutaneous tissue, the supraspinous ligaments, the intraspinous ligaments, the ligamentum flavum, the epidural space, and the dura mater. Other anatomic features that are important are the natural curves of the spine, the lumbar curve having the most effect on the spinal anesthetic.

The drug is deposited into the cerebrospinal fluid. The factors that have an effect on the level of anesthesia are the volume of the drug, the baricity of the drug, the position of the patient, and the speed of injection. Once injected, the drug diffuses into the spinal fluid and bathes the nerve roots. Its action is terminated by absorption into the systemic circulation. The action can be prolonged by the addition of a vasoconstrictor.

The cardiovascular effects of spinal anesthesia include bradycardia due to blockade of the sympathetic fibers, allowing the vagal effects to be predominant. Hypotension may occur, especially in the patient who is hypovolemic and in the pregnant patient who develops the supine hypotensive syndrome. This is due to pressure on the inferior vena cava decreasing venous return. Cardiac output is decreased.

The respiratory effects are proportional to the height of the blockade. If the anesthesia is high, blockade of the intercostal muscles may decrease ventilation and the ability to cough. A very high spinal will affect the ability to use the diaphragm. Respiratory failure will ensue.

The sympathetic block causes unopposed parasympathetic activity that contracts the bowel. This may be advantageous to the surgeon for bowel surgery.

The contraindications to spinal anesthesia are nervous system disease, eg, brain tumor with increased cerebrospinal fluid pressure, infection at the injection site, coagulation defects with bleeding disorders, and severe hypovolemia. In addition, spinal anesthesia should not be used in the patient who refuses to have this technique performed. The use of spinal anesthesia in the patient with multiple sclerosis also bears some discussion. This disease has cycles of remissions and exacerbations. An exacerbation occurring coincident with a surgical procedure may be attributed to the anesthesia technique. For this reason, I avoid spinal anesthesia in these patients.

EPIDURAL ANESTHESIA

Epidural techniques have become very popular in the past decade because of the ability to use a continuous technique and the popularity of the technique for obstetrics.

The epidural space extends from the foramen magnum to the coccyx. It is a potential space, and it is found by one of two techniques, the loss of resistance or the hanging drop method. Since larger amounts of local anesthetic are used for epidural techniques, the importance of being certain that one has not entered the subarachnoid space should be obvious.

The spread of the local anesthetic in the epidural space is influenced by the amount injected but little by the position of the patient. Age and height have little affect on spread. The higher level in the pregnant patient is due to venous congestion caused by the pressure of the gravid uterus on the inferior vena cava. There is evidence also that the pregnant patient is more sensitive to the effects of local anesthesia.

The physiologic effects of epidural anesthesia are similar to those of spinal anesthesia.

The one complication not shared with spinal anesthesia is that of postspinal puncture headache. This is seen in the epidural patient only after accidental puncture of the dura. The typical patient with postspinal puncture headache is a young woman who complains of a frontal or occipital headache, worse in the sitting position and relieved by the recumbent position. There may be tinnitus or ocular signs associated with it. Treatment consists of fluids, analgesics, and bedrest. If the headache is persistent, an epidural blood patch should be used.

PERIPHERAL NERVE BLOCKADE

The numerous techniques employed for peripheral nerve blockade should be reviewed. You should be familiar with techniques for blockade of the major nerves as well as sympathetic ganglion blocks.

The intravenous regional technique (Bier block) should be reviewed along with its indications and contraindications.

Since most of these blocks require large amounts of local anesthesia, you must be aware of the treatment of toxicity reactions.

Questions

DIRECTIONS (Questions 1 through 25): Each of the numbered items or incomplete statements in this section is followed by answers or by completions of the statement. Select the ONE lettered answer or completion that is BEST in each case.

1. The gasserian ganglion is associated with the

   (A) second cranial nerve
   (B) third cranial nerve
   (C) fifth cranial nerve
   (D) seventh cranial nerve
   (E) ninth cranial nerve

2. The superior laryngeal nerve lies

   (A) superior to the hyoid bone
   (B) deep to the hyoid bone
   (C) immediately above the notch of the thyroid cartilage
   (D) between the great cornu of the hyoid bone and the superior cornu of the thyroid cartilage
   (E) deep to the cricothyroid membrane

3. If a line is drawn around the neck at the level of the lower border of the cricoid cartilage, it will mark the level of the transverse process of the

   (A) second cervical vertebra
   (B) third cervical vertebra
   (C) fourth cervical vertebra
   (D) fifth cervical vertebra
   (E) sixth cervical vertebra

4. The tubercle of Chassaignac is the eponym for the

   (A) horn of the hyoid bone
   (B) anterior portion of the cricoid
   (C) transverse process of the sixth cervical vertebra
   (D) tip of the mastoid
   (E) medial portion of the clavicle

5. The axillary approach to the brachial plexus

   (A) carries the risk of pneumothorax
   (B) uses the axillary artery as a landmark

   (C) is made from the lateral aspect of the arm
   (D) uses the pectoralis minor insertion as a landmark
   (E) is the preferable route if there is an infection in the axilla

6. In the drawing below, the structure labeled B is the

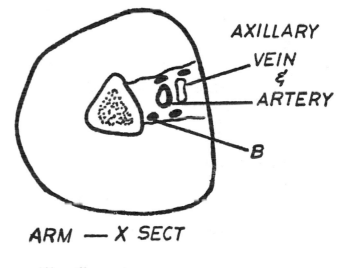

ARM — X SECT

   (A) axillary artery
   (B) axillary vein
   (C) radial nerve
   (D) ulnar nerve
   (E) median nerve

7. Anatomic points of note in intercostal blocks include

   (A) the intercostal nerves serve only the thoracic area
   (B) the intercostal nerve runs above the rib
   (C) each intercostal nerve gives off a lateral cutaneous branch
   (D) the intercostal innervation runs from the vertebral column posteriorly to the nipple line anteriorly
   (E) the abdominal innervation is easily anesthetized by blocking two adjacent nerves

8. When performing a caudal block

   (A) the needle enters through the sacral hiatus
   (B) anomalies are seldom encountered
   (C) the patient should be kept flat
   (D) the patient should be asked to keep his or her heels together
   (E) small volumes of agent are needed, since the volume of the canal is only 8 to 12 ml

9. The stellate ganglion

   (A) is a fusion of the inferior cervical and first thoracic ganglia
   (B) is closer to the apex of the lung on the left than on the right side
   (C) is primarily a parasympathetic ganglion
   (D) lies at the level of the fifth cervical vertebra
   (E) may be blocked with little danger of complications

10. When doing a digital nerve block

    (A) large volumes of agent should be used to increase the chance of success
    (B) epinephrine should always be used to secure a long block
    (C) the nerve can be blocked by injecting only on the medial side of the digit where the nerve courses
    (D) the course of the nerve lies close to the dorsum of the finger
    (E) one must remember that the digital arteries are terminal arteries

11. Postspinal headaches are

    (A) more frequent with large-bore needles
    (B) not lessened by the use of a Whittaker 22-gauge needle
    (C) aggravated by the supine position
    (D) noted immediately
    (E) relieved in 12 hours by an epidural blood patch

12. A patient has a hand-shoulder-arm syndrome following a stroke that resulted in left hemiparesis. You are asked to perform a nerve block to relieve this. You would use a

    (A) left deep cervical block
    (B) rib block
    (C) left axillary block
    (D) right stellate ganglion block
    (E) left stellate ganglion block

13. The pain of carcinoma of the pancreas can be blocked by

    (A) celiac ganglion block
    (B) rib block
    (C) lumbar block
    (D) stellate block
    (E) aortic plexus block

14. Postoperative nerve deficits following regional anesthesia may be due to all of the following EXCEPT

    (A) epinephrine 1:200,000 added to lidocaine
    (B) positioning
    (C) multiple sclerosis
    (D) orthopedic casts
    (E) surgical trauma

15. The dermatome level at the nipple line is

    (A) T-4
    (B) T-6
    (C) T-10
    (D) S-1
    (E) L-1

16. The dermatome level that supplies the inguinal area is

    (A) T-4
    (B) T-6
    (C) T-10
    (D) S-1
    (E) L-1

17. The dermatome level that supplies sensation to the heel is

    (A) T-4
    (B) T-6
    (C) T-10
    (D) S-1
    (E) L-1

18. The dermatome level of the xiphoid is

    (A) T-4
    (B) T-6
    (C) T-10
    (D) S-1
    (E) L-1

19. The dermatome level corresponding to the umbilicus is

    (A) T-4
    (B) T-6
    (C) T-10
    (D) S-1
    (E) L-1

20. In performing a spinal puncture by the lateral approach, all of the following are true EXCEPT that

    (A) it is necessary to flex the spine
    (B) the needle penetrates the ligamentum flavum
    (C) the lateral or sitting position is satisfactory
    (D) the needle does not penetrate the interspinous ligament
    (E) the needle enters between the laminae

21. The first function to be lost on onset of spinal anesthesia is

    (A) touch
    (B) motor power
    (C) temperature
    (D) vibration
    (E) autonomic activity

22. A spinal anesthetic is said to be fixed when

    (A) it begins to wear off
    (B) positional changes no longer affect the level
    (C) ephedrine is administered for hypotension
    (D) epinephrine is added to the solution
    (E) sodium bicarbonate is added to the solution as a buffer

23. When an anesthetic agent is injected into the subarachnoid space, it

    (A) immediately leaves the space
    (B) is adherent to the nervous tissue and no longer present in the cerebrospinal fluid
    (C) is detectable in the fluid up to the point of the anesthesia wearing off
    (D) remains pooled at the base of the spinal foramen
    (E) enters into a chemical reaction with the cerebrospinal fluid

24. When administering a local anesthetic

    (A) large fibers are blocked first
    (B) myelinated fibers are blocked first
    (C) pain fibers are blocked first
    (D) myelinated motor fibers are blocked first
    (E) small unmyelinated fibers are easiest to block

25. When a spinal anesthetic becomes fixed, it is due to

    (A) adsorption of the agent to the nerve
    (B) loss of the agent from the subarachnoid space by absorption
    (C) equalization of the specific gravity of the agent and cerebrospinal fluid
    (D) loss of agent through the foramina
    (E) the short action of the agent

DIRECTIONS (Questions 26 through 50): For each of the items in this section, ONE or MORE of the numbered options is correct. Choose the answer

    A if only 1, 2, and 3 are correct,
    B if only 1 and 3 are correct,
    C if only 2 and 4 are correct,
    D if only 4 is correct,
    E if all are correct.

26. The sensory innervation of the exterior part of the nose includes the

    (1) infratrochlear nerve
    (2) infraorbital nerve
    (3) external nasal nerve
    (4) supraorbital nerve

27. The relationship of the femoral nerve in the inguinal area is that it lies

    (1) superficial to the inguinal ligament
    (2) lateral to the femoral artery
    (3) medial to the femoral vein
    (4) lateral to the lacunar ligament

28. A caudal block may fail as a result of

    (1) injection of solutions that are too dilute
    (2) injection of insufficient volume
    (3) perforation of the rectum
    (4) wide foramina, which allow the local anesthesia to seep out

29. When performing a lumbar puncture, the spinal needle passes through the

    (1) supraspinal ligament
    (2) interspinal ligament
    (3) ligamentum flavum
    (4) pia mater

30. The addition of 10% dextrose to a spinal anesthetic

    (1) decreases the baricity
    (2) increases the specific gravity of the solution relative to the cerebrospinal fluid
    (3) causes a higher level when the patient is sitting
    (4) allows the solution to gravitate toward the dependent portion

31. Contraindications to spinal anesthesia include

    (1) hypervolemia
    (2) cardiac decompensation
    (3) erythocytosis
    (4) neurologic disease

SUMMARY OF DIRECTIONS

A	B	C	D	E
1, 2, 3 only	1, 3 only	2, 4 only	4 only	All are correct

32. The sensory distribution of the hand includes the

    (1) dorsum of the thumb: radial nerve
    (2) dorsum of the middle finger: median nerve
    (3) dorsum of the fifth finger: ulnar nerve
    (4) volar surface of the fifth finger: ulnar nerve

33. Circumcision performed under regional block requires the infiltration of the

    (1) shaft of the penis
    (2) glans penis
    (3) foreskin in a circular manner
    (4) base of the penis

34. Anesthesia for surgery on the medial malleolus requires block of the

    (1) femoral nerve
    (2) obturator nerve
    (3) sciatic nerve
    (4) inguinal nerve

35. The landmark(s) for a sciatic nerve block is (are) the

    (1) lumbosacral joint
    (2) greater trochanter
    (3) tip of the coccyx
    (4) posterior superior iliac spine

36. An epidural block

    (1) does not cause spinal headache unless the dura is punctured
    (2) has a greater risk of drug overdose than does a spinal block
    (3) depends on volume to attain level
    (4) depends on the baricity of the agent to attain level

37. In performing a supraclavicular block

    (1) the musculocutaneous nerve frequently is missed
    (2) there is a hazard of pneumothorax
    (3) the long thoracic nerve is blocked
    (4) the first rib is an important landmark

38. Structures lying on the lateral aspect of the antecubital space anteriorly include the

    (1) radial nerve
    (2) median nerve
    (3) musculocutaneous nerve
    (4) ulnar nerve

39. Structures lying medially on the anterior aspect of the wrist include the

    (1) median nerve
    (2) ulnar nerve
    (3) radial nerve
    (4) ulnar artery

40. When administering a spinal anesthetic, the solution and technique to be used are influenced by the

    (1) duration of anesthesia desired
    (2) intraabdominal pressure of obesity
    (3) height of the patient
    (4) sex of the patient

41. The position of the patient is important in administering a spinal. Which of the following statements is (are) correct?

    (1) a patient in the sitting position will have a lower block if the solution is hypobaric and the patient remains erect
    (2) the normal lumbar lordosis limits the spread of solution in a supine patient
    (3) flexion of the patient in the lateral position will increase intraabdominal pressure and give a lower level
    (4) flexion of the thighs on the abdomen in a supine patient limits the cephalic spread of a hyperbaric solution

42. Factors that influence the frequency of pulmonary complications include

    (1) age of patient
    (2) skill of anesthetist
    (3) condition of patient
    (4) anesthetic agent or technique

43. After a spinal anesthetic has been administered, the patient should be immediately observed for

    (1) evidence of block level
    (2) evidence of hypotension
    (3) respiratory insufficiency
    (4) spinal headache

44. A 26-year-old woman gave birth under spinal anesthesia. The following day, she complained of a severe headache, and, on examination, there was internal strabismus. These symptoms are

    (1) unrelated to her anesthesia
    (2) related to her anesthesia but will clear with treatment
    (3) due to overhydration
    (4) due to loss of cerebrospinal fluid pressure and abducens paralysis

45. The epidural space

(1) extends from the base of the skull to the coccyx
(2) contains the spinal cord
(3) is traversed by spinal nerves
(4) contains a plexus of veins

46. Which of the following statements is (are) correct when comparing spinal to peridural anesthesia of equal degree:

(1) hypotension is less profound with spinal anesthesia
(2) there is a greater loss of peripheral resistance with peridural anesthesia
(3) there are few systemic effects of the local anesthesia with peridural anesthesia
(4) systemic effects of epinephrine are more evident with peridural anesthesia

47. The ulnar nerve

(1) lies dorsal to the axillary artery in the proximal arm
(2) lies in the groove of the lateral condyle at the elbow
(3) lies adjacent to the flexor carpi radialis at the wrist
(4) gives sensation to the fifth finger and part of the fourth finger

48. The level of anesthesia resulting from subarachnoid injection of an agent is directly proportional to the

(1) concentration of the drug
(2) speed of the injection
(3) specific gravity for hyperbaric solutions
(4) volume of the fluid injected

49. Undesirable aspects of spinal anesthesia include

(1) poor control
(2) respiratory embarrassment
(3) hypotension
(4) decreased vagal activity

50. After spinal anesthesia

(1) heart rate increases
(2) venous pressure falls
(3) cardiac output increases
(4) venous return decreases

Answers and Explanations

1. **(C)** The gasserian ganglion is associated with the fifth (trigeminal) cranial nerve. *(1:2106; 2:903; 75:790)*

2. **(D)** The superior laryngeal nerve lies between the great cornu of the hyoid bone and the superior cornu of the thyroid cartilage. This nerve can be blocked to provide airway anesthesia for laryngoscopy or bronchoscopy. *(2:313; 75:797)*

3. **(E)** The lower border of the cricoid cartilage is at the same level of the tubercle as the sixth cervical vertebra. This tubercle is an important landmark for doing a stellate ganglion block. *(75:880)*

4. **(C)** The tubercle referred to in preceding questions is referred to as Chassaignac's tubercle. *(1:2090; 2:904)*

5. **(B)** The major landmark for performing an axillary block is the axillary artery. The approach is from the medial aspect of the arm. There is no risk of pneumothorax, which is an advantage over the supraclavicular approach. The muscle inserting in the area is the pectoralis major. An infection in the axilla is a contraindication to the block. *(1:1029; 75:801–802)*

6. **(C)** The radial nerve is the structure identified. It lies in a posterior and lateral position relative to the landmark artery. The ulnar nerve lies posterior to the artery. The median nerve lies anterior. *(75:802)*

7. **(C)** The intercostal nerves serve the abdomen and the thorax. Running under the rib, the nerve gives off a lateral cutaneous branch near the midaxillary line and an anterior cutaneous branch near the sternum. If abdominal surgery is to be performed, the lower six to eight intercostals should be blocked. *(1:1049; 75:804; 173:40)*

8. **(A)** The needle for the caudal block enters through the sacral hiatus. Anomalies in the sacral region are frequent. The patient should be prone, with the hips on a pillow and the toes pointed in. Even though the caudal canal is of low volume, there is leakage through the foramina, requiring injection of a larger volume. *(1:1101; 75:784; 173:36)*

9. **(A)** The stellate ganglion is a fusion of the inferior cervical and first thoracic ganglia. The apex of the lung is closer on the right than the left. The ganglion is a sympathetic ganglion. It lies at the level of the seventh cervical vertebra. The block has complications, including pneumothorax, intravascular injection, and subarachnoid injection. *(75:807)*

10. **(E)** When doing a digital nerve block, one must remember that the digital arteries are terminal arteries. Ischemia must be prevented; therefore, epinephrine and large volumes are avoided. The nerves lie closer to the palmar side of the hand. *(173:40)*

11. **(A)** Postspinal headaches are less frequent with small-bore needles and with the 22-gauge Whittaker needle. The typical headache must be posturally dependent, being relieved by the supine position and aggravated by standing. It is relieved immediately by an epidural blood patch. *(1:1708; 75:778; 174:60)*

12. **(E)** In the past, stellate ganglion blocks were part of the treatment for acute strokes. In the case presented, the symptoms are later in the course. This is treated with a stellate ganglion block on the ipsilateral side of the symptoms. *(2:912)*

13. **(A)** The pain of carcinoma of the pancreas is treated with a celiac ganglion block. This block provides anesthesia for the abdominal viscera. It does not block the pelvic viscera. The other blocks listed are not helpful in carcinoma of the pancreas. *(1:2094; 75:808)*

14. **(A)** Postoperative nerve deficits following anesthesia are rare. Epinephrine is not a known cause. There are many causes, including positioning and preoperative neurologic disease. *(1:1056; 174:59)*

15. **(A)** *(1:1065; 75:760)*

16. **(E)** *(1:1065; 75:760)*

17. **(D)** *(1:1065; 75:760)*

18. **(B)** *(1:1065; 75:760)*

19. **(C)** The dermatome levels are important in assessing the extent of the block. One must know the level of block needed and then adjust dosage and position to achieve that level. *(1:1065; 75:760)*

20. **(A)** It is not necessary to flex the spine when using the lateral approach. For this reason, it is a good approach for the pregnant patient and those who would have trouble flexing. The block can be done in the sitting or lateral position. The needle does not penetrate the interspinous ligament but does penetrate the ligamentum flavum. The needle enters between the laminae. *(1:1071; 75:765)*

21. **(E)** The first function to be blocked by a spinal anesthetic is autonomic function. These nerves are of small diameter and are exposed to the local anesthetic. The next sensation to be blocked is temperature, followed by pain, tactile sensation, motor power, and proprioception. *(1:1080; 2:863; 75:768)*

22. **(B)** The spinal anesthetic may be said to be fixed when change of position no longer affects the level. This may be due to adsorption of the drug onto the nerve, loss of agent, or dilution to an extent that no further movement of the agent takes place. *(1:1078)*

23. **(C)** Once an anesthetic is injected into the subarachnoid space, it can be detected until the block wears off. There is no chemical reaction with the cerebrospinal fluid. Some of it may leave the space. *(2:871; 131:217; 175:6)*

24. **(E)** The small unmyelinated fibers are the easiest to block. Blockade depends on the size of the nerve as well as the exposure to the agent. *(175:7)*

25. **(C)** When one injects a local anesthetic into the subarachnoid fluid, it will diffuse until the specific gravity of the agent and the cerebrospinal fluid have become equal. At that time, no further movement of the agent will take place. (See also answer to Question 23.) *(175:6)*

26. **(A)** The infratrochlear nerve, the infraorbital nerve, and the external nasal nerve all serve the external part of the nose. The supraorbital nerve is not involved. *(75:791)*

27. **(C)** The femoral nerve lies lateral to the femoral artery and lateral to the lacunar ligament. The femoral vein lies medial to the artery. *(1:1038; 75:824)*

28. **(E)** Caudal anesthesia can be difficult because of anomalies, incorrect technique, and insufficient volume. Since the foramina may allow some of the agent to escape, more volume must be used. *(1:1101; 75:784)*

29. **(A)** The needle does not pass through the pia mater, the covering immediately investing the spinal cord. It does pass through the supraspinal ligament, the interspinal ligament (unless the lateral approach is used), and the ligamentum flavum. *(1:1070; 2:859; 75:757)*

30. **(C)** The addition of dextrose to the agent makes it heavier than the cerebrospinal fluid. The baricity is increased. If the patient is sitting, the block will be lower, since the agent will gravitate toward the dependent portion of the subarachnoid space. *(1:1077; 75:771)*

31. **(C)** Many of the contraindications to spinal anesthesia are relative. Cardiac decompensation is a contraindication because the heart cannot compensate for changes that will occur with peripheral dilatation. On the other hand, the peripheral dilatation may decrease the afterload and, therefore, decrease the decompensation. The presence of neurologic disease is also a contraindication to the use of spinal anesthesia. This is especially true if the disease involves the spinal cord, is not fully developed, or is cyclic, such as multiple sclerosis. *(1:1083; 75:762)*

32. **(E)** The sensory distribution of the hand is correct for all of the options. *(75:802)*

33. **(D)** Nerve block of the penis for circumcision requires a circular block at the base of the penis. It is not necessary to block the glans, the shaft, or the foreskin. *(75:811,1107)*

34. **(B)** A sciatic–femoral block may be used for procedures below the knee that do not require the use of a tourniquet. The obturator nerve and the inguinal nerve need not be blocked. *(1:1040)*

35. **(C)** The landmarks for a sciatic block are the greater trochanter and the posterior superior iliac spine. A line is drawn between the two, and at its midpoint, a line is drawn about 4 cm caudally. That is the site of injection. Another technique uses the sacral hiatus as a landmark. *(1:1041; 75:813)*

36. **(A)** An epidural block does not cause headache if the dura has not been violated. There is a greater risk of drug toxicity, since larger doses are used.

The level is dependent on the volume of drug injected. *(1:1086,1099; 75:776)*

37. **(C)** In doing a supraclavicular block, the first rib is an important landmark. If one stays on the rib, pneumothorax is less likely. The musculocutaneous nerve is blocked. The long thoracic nerve is not blocked. *(1:1029; 75:799)*

38. **(B)** The radial nerve and the musculocutaneous nerve lie on the lateral aspect of the antecubital space anteriorly. The median nerve and the ulnar nerve are medial. *(1:1032,1033; 75:803)*

39. **(C)** The ulnar nerve and ulnar artery lie medially on the anterior aspect of the wrist. The median nerve lies in the central part of the wrist, and the radial nerve lies laterally. *(1:1033; 75:803)*

40. **(A)** A spinal anesthetic will vary with the duration of the agent, the presence of increased abdominal pressure, and the height of the patient. The sex of the patient has no effect. *(75:771; 131:231)*

41. **(C)** A patient in the sitting position will have a higher block if a hypobaric agent is used. The lumbar lordosis limits the spread of the solution in a supine patient. Flexion of the patient will increase intraabdominal pressure and give a higher block. If the legs are flexed on the abdomen, the lumbar curve will be flattened, and the cephalic spread of a hyperbaric solution will be limited. *(131:234)*

42. **(A)** Factors that affect the frequency of pulmonary complications are age of the patient, skill of the anesthetist, and the condition of the patient. The agent or technique is not important. *(175:129)*

43. **(A)** The patient must be observed in the postoperative period for spinal headache, but this is not something that occurs immediately. Immediately after performing a block, it is important that the patient be observed closely for the level of anesthesia and its consequences. *(131:224; 1:1081–1082)*

44. **(D)** The symptoms of spinal headache combined with cranial nerve palsy demand immediate treatment. *(2:884; 131:244)*

45. **(E)** The epidural space extends from the base of the skull to the coccyx. The space envelops the spinal cord and is traversed by the spinal nerves. There is a large plexus of veins that may be easily punctured. *(1:1063; 75:759; 131:229)*

46. **(C)** Hypotension is more profound with spinal anesthesia. Peripheral resistance decreases to a greater degree with epidural anesthesia. Since more drug is used for epidural anesthesia, more systemic effects are to be expected. The systemic effects of epinephrine are more likely. *(1:1096; 75:769; 131:231)*

47. **(D)** The ulnar nerve lies inferior to the axillary artery in the proximal arm and lies in a groove on the medial aspect of the elbow. The nerve lies adjacent to the flexor carpi ulnaris at the wrist. The ulnar nerve gives sensation to the fifth finger and part of the fourth finger. *(75:802–803; 131:245)*

48. **(E)** When a drug is injected into the subarachnoid space, the level of anesthesia is proportional to the concentration of the drug, more concentrated drugs providing more intense block for longer periods. The specific gravity of a drug will affect the extent of a block. A rapid injection will cause a higher level of blockade. A higher volume will produce a higher block. *(75:771)*

49. **(A)** Undesirable effects of spinal anesthetics include poor control, respiratory embarrassment if the block is too high, and hypotension. Vagal activity is increased, since the sympathetic system is blocked. *(75:777)*

50. **(C)** After spinal anesthesia, the heart rate decreases due to the preponderance of vagal activity. The venous pressure and venous return fall due to vasodilatation. Cardiac output decreases due to the decreased venous return and decreased heart rate. *(75:768, 777)*

CHAPTER 7

General Anesthesia
Review

In spite of the fact that anesthesia has been used for many years, the exact mechanism of its effect is still unknown. Many theories have been proposed, but none is the predominant theory today. Most believe that some membrane effect is most likely and that there is not a specific receptor involved.

There is a large body of knowledge concerning the uptake and distribution of volatile agents. Eger has a book on the subject, and there is a section in each of the major texts.

In order for a volatile agent to reach the brain, it must be taken up by the blood as it passes through the lung. The amount of uptake is dependent on the pressure gradient between the alveolus and the blood; the higher the gradient, the more the uptake.

The alveolar pressure (tension) is affected by the amount of anesthetic agent brought to the alveolus and the amount removed. An increased inspired tension of the anesthetic and an increase in the minute volume of ventilation will increase the tension. The rate of removal also is important. If the cardiac output is low or if the agent is relatively insoluble, the tension will remain elevated. Changes in any of these will change the tension. Therefore, if the inspired tension is low, the minute volume low, the cardiac output high, or the solubility high, an effective tension gradient cannot be developed, and the onset of anesthesia is slower.

During administration of a volatile agent, the alveolar tension rises rapidly and then more slowly. The more soluble the agent, the less rapidly the tension rises. The arterial tension rises as the alveolar tension rises until an equilibrium is reached. The arterial tension is distributed to the vessel-rich group, including the brain, and anesthesia ensues. The other organs follow. During a prolonged procedure, all tissues will approach equilibrium with the agent. At the end of the procedure, the agent will be removed from the body in a similar manner.

The second gas effect is important in the induction of anesthesia with a volatile agent. This requires the administration of two gases simultaneously. In the typical case, nitrous oxide and halothane are administered together. Nitrous oxide, the first gas, is taken up by the bloodstream in a large amount that leads to a concentration of the second gas and an augmentation of its uptake. The second gas is halothane. Nitrous oxide, although it is relatively insoluble, is taken up in large amounts (up to 1500 ml/minute) because it is delivered in high concentration.

At the end of the procedure, the reverse takes place, and nitrous oxide leaves the bloodstream in great amounts when the administration is stopped. The rapid transfer of nitrous oxide from the blood to the alveolus will dilute the alveolar oxygen and carbon dioxide and may lead to hypoxemia and lack of stimulus to breathe. Oxygen should be administered and the patient's ventilation assisted during this period.

The concept of minimum alveolar concentration (MAC) should be reviewed. This is the concentration of anesthetic that will prevent the response of 50% of subjects to a painful stimulus. It is affected by age, simultaneous administration of nitrous oxide, temperature, and many drugs. Inhalational agents are considered to be additive in their effects.

MAC values for agents (in oxygen) are:

Nitrous oxide	104
Halothane	0.77
Isoflurane	1.15
Enflurane	1.7
Sevoflurane	1.71

A lower number represents a more potent anesthetic.

Various signs of anesthesia have been described in the past as guides to the depth of anesthesia. With the advent of injectable induction agents and the use of muscle relaxants and drugs that affect the autonomic nervous system, these signs are less dependable. Probably the most dependable sign of depth of anesthesia is a change in breathing, since that is less dependent on the autonomic nervous system.

Questions

DIRECTIONS (Questions 1 through 10): Each of the numbered items or incomplete statements in this section is followed by answers or by completions of the statement. Select the ONE lettered answer or completion that is BEST in each case.

1. A patient with obstructive lung disease has an altered anesthetic induction with an insoluble agent because of

   (A) decreased cardiac output
   (B) increased perfusion
   (C) increased P_{CO_2}
   (D) uneven ventilation
   (E) decreased minute volume

2. Depth of anesthesia with inhalational agents is primarily due to

   (A) rate of ventilation
   (B) potency of the anesthetic agent
   (C) age of the patient
   (D) concentration of the agent in the brain
   (E) cardiac output

3. The term MAC refers to

   (A) minimal anesthetic concentration
   (B) anesthesia sufficient to prevent movement in response to a painful stimulus in 100% of subjects
   (C) a measurement not affected by age
   (D) measurement that is pertinent only with thiopental
   (E) minimal alveolar concentration

4. Signs of light anesthesia include all of the following EXCEPT

   (A) eyelid movement
   (B) pupillary constriction
   (C) forehead wrinkling
   (D) sweating
   (E) slight limb movement

5. Stage I anesthesia can be characterized by all of the following EXCEPT that

   (A) there are no planes: the patient passes quickly through stage I to stage II
   (B) there is a plane of sedation
   (C) there is a plane of amnesia
   (D) there is a plane of analgesia
   (E) the patient remains conscious

6. As a patient becomes more deeply anesthetized, the last sense to disappear is

   (A) smell
   (B) vision
   (C) pain
   (D) discomfort
   (E) hearing

7. A patient with mild to moderate systemic disturbance, eg, essential hypertension, would be classified as ASA physical

   (A) class I
   (B) class II
   (C) class III
   (D) class IV
   (E) class V

8. The tension of a gas in solution is equivalent to

   (A) partial pressure
   (B) solubililty
   (C) molecular weight
   (D) temperature
   (E) blood/gas coefficient

Questions 9 and 10

A 32-year-old woman is admitted for a radical mastectomy. Her medications include chlorpromazine, oxyphenisatin (Dialose Plus), and papaverine. Her anesthesia is maintained with halothane. During the procedure, it is necessary to administer 2 units of red cells and penicillin. Three days postoperatively, she develops weakness, fever, and jaundice, with abnormal liver enzymes.

9. Possible causes of her condition include all of the following EXCEPT

   (A) chlorpromazine
   (B) oxyphenisatin
   (C) papaverine
   (D) halothane
   (E) penicillin

10. Her condition continues to deteriorate and develops into massive hepatic failure with necrosis. This occurs

    (A) once in 10,000 general anesthetics
    (B) once in 10,000 general anesthetics with halothane
    (C) once in 100,000 general anesthetics
    (D) much less with cyclopropane
    (E) much less with ether

DIRECTIONS (Questions 11 through 18): For each of the items in this section, ONE or MORE of the numbered options is correct. Choose the answer

    A if only 1, 2, and 3 are correct,
    B if only 1 and 3 are correct,
    C if only 2 and 4 are correct,
    D if only 4 is correct,
    E if all are correct.

11. The factor(s) of importance in determining alveolar tension of an anesthetic is (are)

    (1) ventilatory input
    (2) circulatory uptake
    (3) concentration effect
    (4) body temperature

12. General anesthetics act

    (1) in the reticular formation
    (2) by depressing spinal cord transmission
    (3) by depressing excitatory transmission
    (4) by enhancing excitation

13. The MAC value for halothane is

    (1) highest in the young
    (2) decreased at age 70 or older
    (3) decreased at lowered body temperature
    (4) decreased by administration of 70% nitrous oxide

14. Emergence from anesthesia with halothane

    (1) is not affected by the length of the anesthetic
    (2) is affected by the cardiac output
    (3) is less prolonged than emergence from nitrous oxide
    (4) can be demonstrated with alveolar curves that are the inverted patterns of uptake curves

15. The current theories of anesthesia suggest that anesthetics

    (1) act at a specific receptor
    (2) depress excitatory transmission
    (3) depress release of neurotransmitters
    (4) are active in the reticular activating system

16. A patient with a pulmonary embolus has

    (1) a prolonged induction with a soluble agent
    (2) slow induction as a result of decreased respiratory rate
    (3) an induction with an insoluble agent that is little changed from normal
    (4) a prolonged induction owing to an increase in shunt

17. The second gas effect

    (1) has its maximum effect early in an anesthetic
    (2) applies only to anesthetic gases
    (3) requires a respiratory gas or anesthetic agent that can be concentrated
    (4) requires that the administered concentration of halothane be changed

18. Diffusion hypoxia

    (1) is due to a large volume of nitrous oxide in the lungs
    (2) is due to dilution of alveolar carbon dioxide
    (3) is due to oxygen displacement
    (4) occurs only in the first 5 to 10 minutes of recovery

Answers and Explanations

1. **(D)** The patient with chronic obstructive lung disease has a difficult induction due to ventilation/perfusion mismatching. There is not usually decreased cardiac output. The increased P_{CO_2} does not directly affect the uptake of the agent. Decreased minute volume is not a factor. *(1:636; 75:1410)*

2. **(D)** The concentration of an agent in the brain is the determinant of the depth of anesthesia. The amount that gets to the brain is dependent on the amount of ventilation, the potency, and the cardiac output. Some agents may have greater effect in patients of different ages. *(1:417,625; 75:295)*

3. **(E)** The term MAC refers to minimal alveolar concentration. It is measured as an anesthetic concentration sufficient to prevent movement in response to a painful stimulus in 50% of the subjects. It is affected by age. The dose of thiopental is not measured in this way, since it is not an inhalation agent. *(1:554; 75:297)*

4. **(B)** Pupillary dilatation is one of the signs of light anesthesia. Eye movement is a better determinant of depth. The various eye signs and breathing patterns that were described for ether are not useful today, since we use intravenous inductions and muscle relaxants. *(75:307,308; 131:180)*

5. **(A)** In the stages of anesthesia described, there are planes within the stages. The stages are moot points unless one gives the induction agent so slowly that the various stages are seen. *(75:307)*

6. **(E)** This is an important point, since we have all heard operating room personnel say things that they would not want the patient to hear. Since hearing is the last sense to be lost, the patient may be aware of the operating room sounds longer than we think. *(75:308; 190; 175)*

7. **(B)** A patient with a moderate disease that is not incapacitating would be ASA physical class II *(1:365; 75:307,308)*

8. **(A)** The tension of a gas in solution is equivalent to the partial pressure of that gas. The solubility, the molecular weight, and the blood/gas coefficient are not related. Temperature is related but only because it affects the amount of gas that can be in solution. *(47:558)*

9. **(E)** Penicillin does not cause jaundice. All of the other options may be associated with jaundice. When asked to review a chart of a patient with postoperative jaundice, it is important to note all of the medications the patient has received in the recent past. Most would not mention a laxative that was not prescribed. *(192:1333; 193:83)*

10. **(A)** The National Halothane Study found that 1 in 10,000 anesthetics was associated with massive hepatic failure. There was also a significant occurrence with both ether and cyclopropane. *(131:127; 194:121)*

11. **(A)** Ventilation, cardiac output, and concentration effect all affect the alveolar tension of the anesthetic gas. Body temperature is not a factor. *(1:626; 75:295)*

12. **(E)** General anesthetics act by many different mechanisms. No specific mechanism is known that explains all of the effects of a given agent. *(1:585; 75:285)*

13. **(E)** The MAC value is highest in the very young child and decreases as one gets older. It is also decreased by lower body temperature. Nitrous oxide in 70% concentration decreases the MAC for a given agent. *(1:570; 75:298)*

14. **(C)** Emergence from anesthesia is affected by cardiac output, since the circulation to the lung affects the gradient between the alveolar capillary and the alveolus. The alveolar curve is the inverted pattern of induction with a few minor differences. Emergence will be longer with a longer anesthetic. Emergence from nitrous oxide is shorter. *(1:642; 75:311)*

15. **(C)** Current theories of anesthesia suggest that there is a depression of excitatory transmission. The agents are thought to be active in the reticular activating system. There is not thought to be a specific receptor, since the various agents have different chemical structures. Release of neurotransmitters is not thought to be inhibited. *(1:585; 75:285)*

16. **(B)** The patient with a pulmonary embolus represents a situation with ventilation in excess of perfusion. With relatively insoluble anesthetics, uptake from the perfused alveoli removes only a small fraction of the anesthetic brought to the lungs by ventilation. There is, therefore, little difference between inspired and alveolar partial pressure, either in the perfused or nonperfused lungs. However, with the soluble agents, high uptake continues to remove a substantial portion of inspired anesthesia for a long time, and the concentration in the perfused lung remains considerably lower than that inspired. The concentration in the unperfused lung equals the inspired concentration, with the result that the alveolar–arterial difference remains high for an extended period of time, leading to a prolonged induction. *(1:634)*

17. **(B)** The second gas effect can apply to any gases. The maximum effect in anesthesia is early in the course of the anesthetic. One of the gases must be capable of being concentrated. There is not a requirement of change in the concentration of halothane. *(1:631; 75:296)*

18. **(E)** Diffusion hypoxia is due to an outpouring of nitrous oxide, which displaces oxygen and dilutes carbon dioxide, thus leading to less stimulus to breathe. *(1:644; 2:129)*

CHAPTER 8

Complications of Anesthesia
Review

Webster defines a medical complication as "a condition coexistent with and modifying a primary disease." In the context of anesthesia, these conditions are modifications of expected outcomes; eg, a drug is administered, and the result is unexpected in effect or extent.

Some problems are unavoidable. There are idiosyncratic reactions to drugs that are not known or expected. There are patient variations in anatomy or physiology, unknown beforehand, that affect our techniques and drugs.

Some problems are known and expected but are accepted as a risk of the procedure. These must be explained to patients, since they are the ones at risk. A patient with loose or prominent teeth and a difficult airway is an example. Postoperative nausea and vomiting is another example.

There are problems that are described in the literature and that should be known. The onset of hyperkalemia after the administration of succinylcholine to the patient with quadriplegia is a problem that should be known, and the precipitating drug should be avoided. Before this problem was described and studied, the complication was in the category of the "unavoidable." It is important to recognize a complication when it occurs. Only by analyzing the problem and finding its cause can it be avoided the next time.

In recent years there has been a concerted effort to study how complications and incidents occur. Our equipment and approach have been studied, and changes have been recommended. Anesthesia safety has become an important topic. Standards have been developed to provide the safest environment for our patients.

There are differences of opinion concerning complications and causation. Some believe that all problems are due to error; others believe that some are unavoidable. Is each death that occurs under anesthesia due to human error? Deaths occur every day, in the young and old, that are unexplained. If the same deaths occurred on the operating table, we would have to explain them.

There are many texts and articles written on complications. No one can be expected to know all of the possible complications, but one can be expected to remain current with the present knowledge.

This review will consider only three areas of complications: trauma, the nervous system, and equipment.

TRAUMA

Anesthesia may result in injuries to the patient from many sources. Damage to the dentition can occur as a result of poor technique of intubation or unavoidable difficulties in intubation. Each of us is not equally skillful in laryngoscopy. One may have a problem that another would not. That does not mean that one of us is negligent.

Nosebleeds may be the result of trauma from an endotracheal tube or from suction catheters. A careful history and examination may avert some of these. A patient with a history of nasal polyps should not have a nasal intubation, nor should the patient with a low platelet count or coagulation defects.

Careful positioning of the patient will avoid some injuries under anesthesia. Nerve palsies and pressure spots should be anticipated and steps taken to avoid them. Most patients do well in the supine position, but when we move to another position, problems may occur. Each position has its own set of concerns: the prone position with eye damage, the lateral position with brachial plexus injury, and the lithotomy position with nerve damage due to flexion or pressure.

Merely changing to a second position has led to loss of monitors and intravenous and arterial lines and extubation of the trachea. The move calls for a coordinated effort on the part of all participants.

Retractors may distort the anatomy and lead to changes in circulation and ischemia. Although these are not under our direct control, it is incumbent on us to keep a watchful eye on the surgical field to warn others of problems. Members of the surgical team may lean on the patient and cause damage. The smaller patient is especially at risk.

Electrical burns are a constant threat to the patient in the operating rooms with electrocautery. These units must be in good repair, and any alarms must be investigated. I have seen a surgeon ignore an alarm only to have the anesthetist receive an electric shock from the stool on which she sat. A working knowledge of the electrical system in the operating room, with isolation circuits and fault detectors, is necessary.

NERVOUS SYSTEM

Complications involving the nervous system vary from the patient with a nerve palsy to the patient who does not awaken at the end of the procedure. Nerve palsies may be due to traction, to pressure, or to direct damage to the nerve. In some cases, the injury was already present and was made manifest by the procedure. A careful history is helpful. In addition, electromyography may be helpful in sorting out the cause.

Some drugs may cause direct damage to the nerve and should be avoided. The recent publicity concerning 2-chloroprocaine is an example. In other cases, drug switching has been reported. A drug has been accidentally injected into the subarachnoid space in place of another drug. Careful labeling and reading of labels will avert some of these problems.

Malignant hyperthermia is a prototype of the unexpected, life-threatening event during a procedure. In retrospective histories, some of the patients may be viewed as at risk. In others, the onset is completely unexpected. Since this is a well-known complication, every anesthesiologist should have a plan in mind by which to approach the treatment when the syndrome becomes evident. Careful monitoring and planning should avoid fatal outcomes in most of these patients.

Awareness during a surgical procedure is another complication that can be avoided in almost all cases. We must be alert to the problem and its treatment. In some procedures, it is not possible to maintain anesthetic levels of drugs and preserve circulatory function. Resuscitation should be carried out and anesthesia restored as soon as possible. Amnestic agents may be administered in the interim.

ANESTHESIA EQUIPMENT

One of the most fertile fields for human error is in the use of anesthesia equipment. Technology has advanced to a point where there should be less problems, but the same technology has brought its own hazards. The number of monitors has mushroomed, and the number of alarms has expanded with them. Watching the patient is relegated to secondary importance by some people.

Careful equipment checks must be carried out each day. If equipment is not functioning, it should be replaced. The components that require calibration should have calibration performed each day. Such simple devices as thermometers may lead to unneeded interventions if they are not calibrated. A systematic approach should be used to check the machine. Such an approach is described in many manuals and textbooks.

Since the anesthesia machine is one of the important elements of our work, it behooves each of us to understand how the machine works and to make sure it is in working condition. Temporizing measures have no place in the maintenance of machines.

Each of us will have complications occur in the provision of anesthesia to our patients. It is important that we anticipate those that can be expected, react to those that do occur, and avoid all that we can. Maintaining our education will help greatly.

Questions

DIRECTIONS (Questions 1 through 41): Each of the numbered items or incomplete statements in this section is followed by answers or by completions of the statement. Select the ONE lettered answer or completion that is BEST in each case.

1. If nitrous oxide is administered at a constant concentration, the uptake into the bloodstream in milliliters per minute will

    (A) be constant
    (B) increase with time
    (C) decrease with time
    (D) depend on temperature
    (E) be independent of concentration

2. After induction of anesthesia, an armored tube is inserted into the patient's trachea, and the cuff is inflated. However, it is not possible to ventilate the patient, even with high pressure. Which of the following is NOT a possible cause of this?

    (A) anesthesia machine is not connected to wall outlet
    (B) herniation of cuff
    (C) intraluminal herniation
    (D) impingement of the tip against the trachea
    (E) kinking

3. The most common eye injury sustained under anesthesia is

    (A) corneal perforation
    (B) conjunctivitis
    (C) uveitis
    (D) corneal abrasion
    (E) retinal artery thrombosis

4. A patient who develops a corneal abrasion during anesthesia should be treated with all of the following EXCEPT

    (A) an eye patch
    (B) a topical anesthetic to relieve pain
    (C) an antibiotic ointment
    (D) a cycloplegic
    (E) a mydriatic

5. The most common time for untoward anesthetic incidents to occur is

    (A) preinduction
    (B) induction
    (C) middle of procedure
    (D) end of procedure
    (E) after procedure

6. A patient is undergoing a mediastinoscopy when there is a sudden loss of pulse and pressure wave being monitored at the right wrist. The mediastinoscope is withdrawn, with resumption of vital signs. The most likely cause of the problem is

    (A) cardiac arrest
    (B) superior vena cava obstruction
    (C) air in the mediastinum
    (D) compression of the innominate artery
    (E) vagal stimulation

7. A patient with rheumatoid arthritis has a cricothyroid membrane puncture to facilitate intubation. This procedure

    (A) is harmless
    (B) is contraindicated in a patient with a bleeding diathesis
    (C) is contraindicated in a patient with respiratory failure
    (D) should be followed by intentional coughing to keep the airway open
    (E) should be performed with the largest needle feasible

8. Complications of cricothyroid membrane puncture include all of the following EXCEPT

    (A) subcutaneous emphysema
    (B) bleeding
    (C) pneumothroax
    (D) hoarseness
    (E) bronchial tear

9. If a patient is given ketamine, 2 mg/kg IV, and is allowed to breathe spontaneously, blood gas results will show

(A) no change from control
(B) P_{O_2} change but normal P_{CO_2}
(C) P_{CO_2} change but normal P_{O_2}
(D) abnormal P_{O_2} and P_{CO_2}
(E) low P_{CO_2}

10. Drugs useful in the treatment of anaphylaxis include all of the following EXCEPT

(A) atropine
(B) cortisone
(C) propranolol
(D) epinephrine
(E) diphenhydramine

11. If 700 ml of 5% alcohol solution (mistaken for lactated Ringer's solution) is administered to a woman immediately before delivery, you could expect

(A) no effect on mother or child
(B) drowsiness in the mother but no effect on the fetus
(C) a profound effect on mother and child
(D) a syndrome in the child of microcephaly, growth retardation, and multiple congenital abnormalities
(E) a transient alcohol level in the fetus that will be near zero by the time of delivery

12. Hypoxia secondary to oxygen failure may be due to all of the following EXCEPT

(A) a cracked flowmeter
(B) transposition of pipes during construction
(C) failure of the reducing valve
(D) an accidental change of flowmeter setting
(E) a shift of the oxyhemoglobin dissociation curve

13. A high-volume, low-pressure cuff

(A) may not prevent aspiration
(B) has more tendency to leak fluids in patients on controlled ventilation
(C) will protect from aspiration if filled to specifications
(D) is better if vaginations are present along the wall
(E) will seal better in patients who are breathing spontaneously

14. A patient with upper gastrointestinal tract bleeding is intubated with a high-volume, low-pressure cuff endotracheal tube. There is blood present in the tracheal aspirate each time she is suctioned. The most likely cause of this is

(A) tracheoesophageal fistula
(B) tracheal bleeding
(C) a bleeding diathesis

(D) aspiration of regurgitated blood
(E) burst cuff on endotracheal tube

15. If a patient has been receiving propranolol and requires reversal of a nondepolarizing relaxant, you should

(A) expect no difficulty with heart rate
(B) carefully monitor heart rate
(C) expect a tachycardia to become apparent
(D) proceed without atropine
(E) never reverse a muscle relaxant in a patient receiving propranolol

16. Sulfhemoglobin

(A) can be converted to hemoglobin by methylene blue
(B) is an effective oxygen carrier
(C) cannot be converted to hemoglobin
(D) is converted to hemoglobin by phenacetin
(E) is not associated with cyanosis

17. A patient was admitted for treatment of injuries suffered in an auto accident. After induction of anesthesia with thiopental and maintenance of anesthesia with halothane, nitrous oxide, and oxygen, the blood was noted to be very dark. The nitrous oxide was turned off, but there was no improvement. Vital signs were normal. There were good breath sounds bilaterally, and the P_{O_2} of arterial blood was 331 torr. The cause of the dark blood may be all of the following EXCEPT

(A) carbon monoxide
(B) positional compromise of venous drainage of the operated site
(C) sulfhemoglobin
(D) methemoglobin
(E) ingestion of phenacetin

18. Measures to avoid anesthesia mishaps include

(A) thorough knowledge of equipment
(B) appropriate vigilance aids
(C) organized workspace
(D) equipment maintenance
(E) all of the above

19. The differential diagnosis of cyanosis during or immediately following anesthesia includes all of the following EXCEPT

(A) asphyxia from diffusion anoxia
(B) central respiratory stimulation
(C) upper respiratory tract obstruction
(D) atelectasis
(E) respiratory paralysis from high spinal

20. The most common cause of anesthetic disasters is

(A) aspiration pneumonia
(B) halothane hepatitis

(C) circulatory instability
(D) malignant hyperthermia
(E) hypoxemia

Questions 21 through 23

A 26-year old woman was admitted in premature labor. An intravenous drip was started with 10% alcohol in 5% dextrose in water. In spite of 1000 ml of this solution, labor progressed and delivery was imminent. The patient refused regional anesthesia. She had no food or drink for 10 hours.

21. If a general anesthetic becomes necessary

    (A) anesthesia under mask is acceptable
    (B) the patient should be considered to have an empty stomach
    (C) the patient must be treated as a full-stomach patient
    (D) a gas induction should be used
    (E) an intravenous induction should be used

22. Previous therapy with intravenous alcohol is important in the conduct of anesthesia because

    (A) alcohol may affect the depth of anesthesia
    (B) the patient may require more anesthesia
    (C) alcohol may cause problems with the veins
    (D) alcohol is a secretagogue
    (E) alcohol causes high pH gastric secretions

23. If this patient aspirates gastric contents, treatment should consist of all of the following EXCEPT

    (A) intubation
    (B) suctioning
    (C) pulmonary lavage
    (D) high F_{IO_2}
    (E) artificial ventilation as necessary

Questions 24 through 26
Please refer to the following figure:

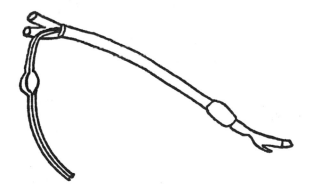

24. The tube in the figure is

    (A) a Macintosh tube
    (B) a Guedel tube
    (C) a Carlens tube

(D) an Adriani tube
(E) a Waters tube

25. The tube is designed to do all of the following EXCEPT

    (A) give one-lung anesthesia
    (B) bronchspirometry
    (C) hook the carina
    (D) have tube extension into the right bronchus
    (E) have a cuff to seal off the left bronchus

26. A double-lumen tube is used for anesthesia in patients with

    (A) asthma
    (B) bronchiectasis
    (C) emphysema
    (D) pneumonia
    (E) oat cell carcinoma

27. Nasotracheal intubation has a higher incidence of

    (A) sinusitis
    (B) sore throat
    (C) vocal cord injury
    (D) subglottic stenosis
    (E) arytenoid cartilage injury

28. Umbilical vessel catheterization may result in all of the following EXCEPT

    (A) rupture of the bladder
    (B) arteriovenous fistula
    (C) infection
    (D) thrombophlebitis
    (E) hepatic necrosis

29. The internal jugular approach for placement of central venous catheters

    (A) is free of complications
    (B) is done without benefit of landmarks
    (C) has a high incidence of pneumothorax
    (D) is especially fraught with difficulty in obese patients
    (E) provides a straighter course into superior vena cava

30. Percutaneous catheterization of the internal jugular vein may result in all of the following complications EXCEPT

    (A) hematoma
    (B) ascites
    (C) chylothorax
    (D) cardiac arrythmias
    (E) bleeding

31. In a patient with a known vena cava syndrome

    (A) at least two large-bore catheters should be place before induction
    (B) an internal jugular central venous line is necessary
    (C) intravenous lines should not be used in the upper extremities
    (D) tracheal intubation may be performed with a large tube
    (E) induction is facilitated by the head-down position

32. A 16-year-old girl with Hodgkin's disease is admitted for a staging procedure. She has massively enlarged hilar nodes. During the procedure, she develops conjunctival edema, facial swelling, and difficult ventilation. A diagnosis of superior vena caval syndrome is made. The following step should be taken

    (A) extubate to eliminate the tube as a source of irritation
    (B) pull the tube back to avoid the area of possible hilar compression
    (C) give intravenous fluids rapidly, using the central venous pressure line
    (D) advance the tube carefully to the position of best ventilation
    (E) remove 500 ml of blood to relieve congestion

33. A 5-month-old infant is anesthetized for correction of an eye condition. There are loud breathing noises noted after intubation with a 4.0-mm tube but no retraction, and good chest excursion is noted. The noise fades slowly, and then there is complete obstruction of the airway. The most probable cause is

    (A) a kinked endotracheal tube
    (B) bronchospasm
    (C) dislodged tube
    (D) inspissated secretions plugging the tube
    (E) a failure in the anesthesia machine

34. A 71-year-old male is admitted with a complaint of hoarseness and sore throat. On indirect laryngoscopy, a supraglottic mass is noted with edema of the cords. He is scheduled for a direct laryngoscopy under general anesthesia. The approach to this procedure should be

    (A) kept simple, since it is a short procedure
    (B) induction, paralysis, and laryngoscopy
    (C) induction, paralysis, intubation, and laryngoscopy
    (D) paralysis, intubation, induction, and laryngoscopy
    (E) to establish an airway before any medication is given or instrumentation done

35. You are working in a newly renovated operating room. After induction of anesthesia with thiopental, you deliver a mixture of nitrous oxide and oxygen, each at 2 L/minute. The nitrous oxide is turned off before intubation, and the patient becomes cyanotic. Flushing with oxygen does not help. The problem that must be ruled out is

    (A) the patient may be obstructed
    (B) the patient may have had a heart attack
    (C) the patient may be febrile
    (D) the oxygen and nitrous oxide lines may have been switched
    (E) there is no flow from the machine

36. The one check that is mandatory to detect the problem in Question 35 is

    (A) check for tightness of the circuit
    (B) check tanks for fullness
    (C) have a functional oxygen analyzer
    (D) check endotracheal tube for patency
    (E) check flush valve on machine

37. All of the following are complications of tracheostomy EXCEPT

    (A) infection of the tracheobronchial tree
    (B) tracheal erosion
    (C) arytenoid cartilage damage
    (D) stomal structure
    (E) plugged tube

38. Chronic exposure to anesthetic gases has been linked to all of the following disease states EXCEPT

    (A) spontaneous abortion
    (B) congenital abnormalities in children of operating room personnel
    (C) cancer
    (D) emphysema
    (E) liver disease

39. Efforts to scavenge gases have led to the development of equipment that may present its own hazards. Problems reported with scavenging systems include all of the following EXCEPT

    (A) negative airway pressure
    (B) positive end-expiratory pressure
    (C) obstructed circuits
    (D) pneumothorax
    (E) decreased functional residual capacity

Questions 40 and 41

A premature, 1300-g infant is born of a diabetic mother. The child is depressed, with an Apgar score (at 1 minute) of 2, and he became apneic on suctioning. Glucose is reported as 48 mg/100ml

40. The treatment should consist of all of the following EXCEPT

(A) oxygen
(B) radiant heat
(C) intubation
(D) glucose
(E) bicarbonate

41. The normal serum glucose in a newborn is

(A) 10 to 20 mg/100ml
(B) 20 to 30 mg/100ml
(C) 40 to 60 mg/100ml
(D) 60 to 70 mg/100ml
(E) 80 to 90 mg/100ml

DIRECTIONS (Questions 42 through 76): For each of the items in this section, <u>ONE</u> or <u>MORE</u> of the numbered options is correct. Choose the answer

A if only <u>1, 2, and 3</u> are correct,
B if only <u>1 and 3</u> are correct,
C if only <u>2 and 4</u> are correct,
D if only <u>4</u> is correct,
E if <u>all</u> are correct.

42. In the patient with an acute injury at the C4-5 level, you would expect

(1) a major loss of diaphragmatic power
(2) no breathing
(3) grossly impaired alveolar ventilation
(4) disturbance of heart rate

43. To ascertain proper placement of the endotracheal tube, the

(1) cords should be visualized
(2) tube should been seen to pass between the cords
(3) thorax should be auscultated
(4) end-tidal carbon dioxide should be detected on the monitor

44. Tracheal stenosis is a serious complication of long-term ventilation. It can be avoided best by the use of

(1) hourly cuff deflation
(2) minimal leak
(3) frequent suctioning
(4) low-pressure cuff

45. Bacteremia may be hazardous for those with heart lesions or prosthetic valves. If an operative procedure is required

(1) the patients should always be anesthetized under mask
(2) oral intubation is more likely to cause bacteremia than is nasal intubation
(3) intubation is not a source of bacteremia
(4) nasotracheal intubation should be avoided if possible

46. A patient has right-sided internal jugular catheterization done while under anesthesia. Complications that may occur include

(1) hematoma
(2) arrhythmias
(3) air embolism
(4) chylothorax

47. The needle used for nerve block is more likely to break if

(1) it is inserted into the skin to the hub
(2) its direction is changed without withdrawal to the subcutaneous tissue
(3) it has been bent previously
(4) it has a security bead

48. Amniotic fluid embolus is associated with a very high mortality. If the patient survives the first embolic insult, other problems that must be anticipated include

(1) severe headache
(2) bleeding diathesis
(3) paralysis
(4) renal failure

49. The usual presentation of amniotic fluid embolus is one of

(1) pallor
(2) coma
(3) hypertension
(4) respiratory distress

50. Administering humidified gases and mist therapy to a patient may result in

(1) lung infection
(2) loss of heat
(3) water load
(4) increased airway resistance

51. If a patient is known to have a mediastinal mass and there is difficulty ventilating the patient during the procedure even with an endotracheal tube in place, factors that must be considered include

(1) malposition of the endotracheal tube
(2) compression of the bronchus
(3) kinking of the tube
(4) mucous plug

SUMMARY OF DIRECTIONS				
A	B	C	D	E
1, 2, 3 only	1, 3 only	2, 4 only	4 only	All are correct

Questions 52 and 53

A 27-year-old woman is anesthetized with thiopental, enflurane, nitrous oxide, and oxygen for laparoscopy. She is placed in a steep Trendelenburg position after insertion of the trocar, and carbon dioxide is insufflated. There is sudden onset of hypotension.

52. This may be due to

   (1) CO_2 embolism
   (2) hemorrhage
   (3) compression of the inferior vena cava
   (4) position

53. The immediate step(s) to be taken is (are) to

   (1) flatten the table
   (2) inform the surgeon
   (3) administer lidocaine
   (4) turn off the nitrous oxide

54. Patients with acromegaly are more prone to airway obstruction because of

   (1) thickening of the vocal cords
   (2) laryngeal stenosis
   (3) large tongue
   (4) receding chin

55. Problems associated with disposable rebreathing circuits include

   (1) indentation with resulting increased resistance
   (2) kinking
   (3) cracks in the system
   (4) increase of laminar flow characteristics

56. A cachectic 27-year-old woman is undergoing anesthesia for carcinoma of the cervix. Blood loss required the use of blood transfusion under pressure via two large-bore cannulae. During this time, arterial pressure decreased from 90 torr to 75 torr systolic. The reason(s) for this drop in pressure may be

   (1) anesthetic overdose
   (2) acidosis
   (3) cardiac arrhythmia
   (4) hypocalcemia

57. Hypocalcemia occurring during blood transfusion

   (1) follows rapid transfusion
   (2) is of no clinical significance
   (3) is aggravated by hypothermia
   (4) need not be treated

58. Humoral substances responsible for the manifestations of anaphylaxis include

   (1) histamine
   (2) epinephrine
   (3) slow-reacting substance (SRS-A)
   (4) methylxanthine

59. Anaphylaxis occurring during anesthesia

   (1) always begins with laryngeal edema
   (2) always includes laryngeal, circulatory, and respiratory symptoms
   (3) is always of short duration
   (4) must always be treated vigorously

60. Complications of nasotracheal intubation include

   (1) sinusitis
   (2) nosebleed
   (3) nasal necrosis
   (4) broken teeth

61. Hypoxia secondary to oxygen failure may be due to

   (1) depletion of the oxygen cylinder
   (2) insufficient opening of the cylinder to permit free flow of gas
   (3) failure of gas pressure
   (4) failure to open the valve of the system

62. When performing an epidural block

   (1) failure to aspirate spinal fluid is assurance that the dura has not been punctured
   (2) the dura is punctured in about 2% of attempts
   (3) if aspiration is negative, a test dose is not necessary
   (4) a test dose is the most important diagnostic measure to ascertain dural puncture

63. Methemoglobinemia results from

   (1) congenital enzymatic defect
   (2) ingestion of nitrites
   (3) aniline dyes
   (4) aspirin therapy

64. Methemoglobin

   (1) results from oxidation of hemoglobin iron to the ferrous state
   (2) cannot be converted to hemoglobin
   (3) is an effective oxygen carrier
   (4) is usually the result of medication

65. Pneumothorax associated with surgery may

   (1) be spontaneous
   (2) follow tracheostomy more commonly in adults than in children

(3) follow attempts at subclavian catheterization
(4) be associated with decreased ventilatory pressure

66. Pneumothorax may be due to

(1) alveolar rupture
(2) injury to the fascial planes of the neck
(3) connection between the distal airway and the pleural space
(4) a break in the parietal pleura

67. Factors that predispose to aspiration include

(1) old age
(2) debilitation
(3) alcoholic stupor
(4) impaired swallowing function

68. The patient with a full stomach

(1) should have regional anesthesia to protect against aspiration
(2) can have light general anesthesia with no danger of aspiration
(3) should be intubated in the head-down position
(4) should remain intubated until the reflexes have returned

69. Redundant mild cases of croup following intubation should be treated with

(1) high humidity
(2) low oxygen atmosphere
(3) cooling of body temperature
(4) fluid restriction

70. Subglottic edema in children may be prevented by

(1) gentle intubation
(2) use of an anesthetic cream on the tube
(3) use of a sterile endotracheal tube
(4) use of steroid cream on the tube

71. A 60-year-old female was admitted with a large goiter and a history of hoarseness. An incidental finding on the chest x-ray was tracheal deviation, with questionable narrowing of the tracheal lumen. The thyroid was removed with some difficulty, and at the end of the procedure, the patient was breathing spontaneously. Immediately after extubation, breathing was labored and retraction was noted Causes of this may include

(1) recurrent laryngeal nerve injury
(2) laryngospasm
(3) tracheal collapse
(4) bronchospasm

72. At the end of a procedure for teeth extraction, the patient is crowing on ventilation. This

(1) may signify complete laryngospasm
(2) may be relieved by gentle assistance to ventilation
(3) will require administration of succinylcholine
(4) may signify partial glottic closure

73. A patient may achieve too great a depth of anesthesia if ventilation is increased with

(1) nitrous oxide
(2) enflurane
(3) cyclopropane
(4) isoflurane

74. Nitrous oxide

(1) is less soluble than nitrogen
(2) movement into an air-containing cavity leads to an increase in volume
(3) diffuses into an air-containing cavity at a slower rate than the egress of nitrogen
(4) movement into an air-containing cavity leads to an increase in pressure

75. The prerequisites for an explosion in the operating room include

(1) an explosive gas, not necessarily an anesthetic
(2) a supply of oxygen
(3) a relatively confined space
(4) a source of ignition

76. Sources of explosive gases may occur from

(1) ether anesthesia
(2) bladder fulguration
(3) use of collodion in the operating room
(4) large bowel gases

Answers and Explanations

1. **(C)** Since nitrous oxide is a relatively insoluble agent, the uptake will decrease over time as equilibrium is reached. The uptake is dependent on concentration, being greater with a higher concentration. *(1:629; 131:130)*

2. **(A)** There are many causes of ventilatory problems during a procedure. It is important to have an approach in mind when this type of situation occurs. Not having the machine connected will not cause the problem, although it may be associated with serious problems. *(43:133; 197:710–711)*

3. **(D)** The most common eye problem under anesthesia is corneal abrasion. It is important to have the eyes protected at all times. Corneal abrasion may occur in any position, although it is more common if the head is draped. Retinal artery thrombosis is a very serious problem, usually caused by pressure on the eyes. *(43:345; 198:465)*

4. **(B)** Corneal abrasions are very painful and should be adequately treated. The use of topical anesthesia is not recommended by all authors because of its tendency to retard regeneration of the corneal epithelium. In addition, if a topical anesthetic is placed in the eye and the patient rubs the eye as he or she emerges from anesthesia, further damage may be incurred. In some references, the use of local anesthesia is still recommended. *(1:1858; 43:346; 75:1062; 196:465)*

5. **(C)** The most common time for incidents to occur is in the middle of the procedure. Vigilance is important at all times during the procedure. The work of Cooper et al has given us some new insights into the problems with our equipment and our approach to providing anesthesia. *(197:402)*

6. **(D)** Compression of the innominate artery may cause a problem, since the blood pressure and the pressure trace may not be apparent. This presents a problem in diagnosis, since the patient may have had a cardiac arrest. For this reason, the surgeon should be notified immediately. Air in the mediastinum and superior vena cava obstruction should not have the same immediate effect. *(1:1432; 75:910, 932)*

7. **(B)** Cricothyroid membrane puncture either for topical anesthesia or for placement of a retrograde catheter to facilitate intubation may be of benefit. One must always ascertain that the patient has no difficulty with coagulation before it is performed. Intentional coughing following cricothyroid membrane puncture may lead to subcutaneous emphysema. Obviously, one should use the smallest needle compatible with good results. *(198:299)*

8. **(E)** Bronchial tear should not occur, since the bronchi are more distal. The other options are possible, especially hoarseness, and the patient should be warned that they may occur. *(198:300)*

9. **(D)** The references vary in the answer to this question. Reference 199 showed decreased oxygenation and increased carbon dioxide levels in the study patients, albeit a low number. Other references state that there is little or no change. The result has some age relationship, being more depressant in the elderly. The message is that ketamine cannot be depended on to stimulate ventilation. *(1:815; 75:237; 199:311)*

10. **(C)** Treatment of anaphylaxis is aimed at terminating the allergic reaction and dilating the bronchioles. Propranolol is not used because it may cause bronchial constriction due to its beta-blocking activity. *(75:495)*

11. **(C)** Alcohol has a depressant effect on the mother and her child. Fetal alcohol syndrome is not present after an acute episode as the one described. This question points out another potential problem, ie, that we often have fluids hanging and they may be opened at the time of an emergency to give the patient fluids. We must always check the contents before we administer them. *(200:603)*

12. **(E)** Anesthesia machines must be checked before use, since the oxygen path may be interrupted at many stages. Many of the leaks are hard to detect. These defects do not affect the oxyhemoglobin dissociation curve. *(170:289)*

13. **(A)** The high-volume, low-pressure cuff has been associated with cases of aspiration. The presence of vaginations decreases pressure but allows a track for fluids. The cuff is still helpful in protecting the trachea from injury but we must not think it is full protection from regurgitation. Other methods should be used with it, eg, nasogastric suctioning and antacids. *(43:218)*

14. **(D)** As discussed in the answer to Question 13, regurgitation may still occur. Although this is the most likely problem, the other causes should be ruled out. *(43:216)*

15. **(B)** One must carefully monitor heart rate, since there are reports of severe bradycardia with the combination of a cholinesterase inhibitor and propranolol. Atropine should be administered. It is not necessary to abstain from reversal, but one must proceed cautiously. *(1:502; 75:597)*

16. **(C)** Sulfhemoglobin cannot be converted to hemoglobin by methylene blue or any known medication. Sulfhemoglobin is not an effective oxygen carrier. Cyanosis may occur if it is present at levels as low as 0.5 g/dl. *(2:132; 43:501)*

17. **(A)** Carbon monoxide does not lead to cyanosis but to hemoglobin that is cherry red. The other hemoglobins are associated with cyanosis, and stagnant blood may apear cyanotic. *(1:2225; 75:1370)*

18. **(E)** All of these options are correct. The references given are necessary reading for those practicing anesthesiology. *(197:402; 201:51)*

19. **(B)** Central respiratory stimulation wil not lead to cyanosis. Diffusion anoxia may lead to cyanosis, as may obstruction of the airway. Atelectasis and respiratory paralysis may also cause cause compromise of oxygenation. *(1:1144; 43:186)*

20. **(E)** The most common cause of anesthetic disasters is hypoxemia. Hypoxemia is the endpoint of other problems, eg, esophageal intubation, low blood pressure, and machine problems. For this reason, it is important to monitor carefully and do machine checks carefully. *(201:4)*

21. **(C)** Alcohol is a secretagogue and may lead to high levels of gastric acid. This drug is of little use today in the obstetric patient, but alcohol is still in wide use by social drinkers. Patients with a history of alcohol intake must have antacids to neutralize the acid. *(184:289)*

22. **(D)** As discussed in the preceding answer, steps must be taken to avoid acid aspiration. Alcohol can affect the depth of anesthesia, since it is a sedative. *(75:410; 184:289)*

23. **(C)** Treatment of aspiration includes intubation, suctioning, high FIo₂ if needed, and artificial ventilation if needed. Pulmonary lavage is not useful unless there is particulate matter. Most studies have found that lavage is not useful and is potentially harmful. *(1:2043; 184:137)*

24. **(C)** The depicted tube is a Carlens tube, used for one-lung anesthesia and bronchospirometry. The tube extends into the right bronchus. The hook is used to catch the carina. *(1:1397; 75:919)*

25. **(E)** See answer to Question 24. *(1:1397; 75:919)*

26. **(B)** One-lung anesthesia is useful in patients with bronchiectasis to avoid soiling the down lung. It has no usefulness in asthma, carcinoma, emphysema, or pneumonia. *(1:1396; 75:918)*

27. **(A)** Sinusitis is more common with nasotracheal intubation due to blockage of the sinus drainage. This must be considered in the febrile patient who has a nasotracheal tube in place. Sore throat, vocal cord injury, subglottic stenosis, and arytenoid damage are of equal incidence with orotracheal intubation. *(1:537; 32:232)*

28. **(A)** Umbilical vessel catheterization may be of great help in the resuscitation of the newborn infant. There are some complications with the technique, and one must weigh the benefits against the risk before undertaking the procedure. Bladder rupture is not a risk. AV fistulas have been reported, as have portal vein thrombosis, infection, and hepatic necrosis. *(184:452)*

29. **(E)** Internal jugular cannulation is done with landmarks that are definite. There are risks with the procedure, including pneumothorax and bleeding. These should occur with low incidence with experienced operators. The vessels are more superficial in the obese, and the vessels should be easy to cannulate if the landmarks are followed. The right side gives a straight course to the superior vena cava. *(1:438; 75:571)*

30. **(B)** Ascites is not a risk of internal jugular catheterization. Bleeding and hematoma formation may occur. Arrhythmias may occur as the catheter enters the heart. Chylothorax is a risk if the left side is used due to damage to the thoracic duct. *(1:441; 75:576)*

31. (C) If the patient has a known superior vena cava syndrome, intravenous lines should be placed in the lower extremities. All efforts are made to facilitate drainage of the upper vessels; therefore, the patient should be head-up, upper body intravenous lines are avoided, and jugular lines are avoided. *(1:1435; 75:930)*

32. (D) Patients with hilar and mediastinal adenopathy can present very serious problems. In reference 75, there is a flow chart detailing the preoperative workup needed to avoid an anesthetic disaster. Many of these patients need only a biopsy, and that should be done under local anesthesia if possible. If a general anesthetic is needed, careful placement of the endotracheal tube is needed. Phlebotomy is not appropriate. *(1:1435; 75:930)*

33. (D) The time course favors the plugging by secretions. A child may buck when the tube is inserted or if the anesthesia becomes light. The secretions enter the tube, become dried out with the anesthetic gases, and then completely obstruct the tube. *(1:430; 75:556)*

34. (D) In any patient with hoarseness and a documented supraglottic mass, it is mandatory to estabish the airway before proceeding with the anesthesia. Any other approach is likely to make the airway maintenance difficult if not impossible. *(1:1871; 43:135)*

35. (D) Any time there is construction activity in an operating room suite, one must check the gases being delivered. The most common problems are with the patient, eg, obstruction or cardiovascular disease, but you must make sure the oxygen is getting to the patient. *(1:1144; 170:292)*

36. (C) A functional oxygen analyzer is mandatory to check the gases being delivered. All of the other checks are important, but an analyzer is a must. *(1:426; 170:151)*

37. (C) Arytenoid damage does not occur with tracheostomy. Infection may occur. Tracheal erosion may occur as a long-term problem. Stricture of the stoma may occur and require revision. The tube may be plugged with secretions. *(1:1875; 43:170)*

38. (D) Emphysema is not reported as a problem with anesthetic gases. Studies have shown an association with abortion, congenital abnormalities, cancer, and liver disease. This has not proven to be causative. Still we must protect the operating room personnel from unnecessary exposure by ensuring good scavenging. *(1:151; 75:69)*

39. (E) Scavenging systems that are poorly designed can lead to many problems. Systems must have provisions to prevent buildup and loss of breathing bag filling. The release of the scavenged gas also is important. In one hospital, the scavenged gas was evacuated very close to the hospital cafeteria. *(1:154; 170:265)*

40. (D) In the newborn infant, the glucose level is normally lower, the value normally being 30 mg/ml. Resuscitation wil require intubation, oxygen, heat, and bicarbonate. *(1:1735, 2373)*

41. (C) The glucose is lower in the newborn than the adult and lower in the premature than the full-term infant. *(1:2373; 202:3)*

42. (B) There would be no disturbance of heart rate unless hypoxemia occurred. The diaphragmatic innervation is by the phrenic nerve, which arises from cervical segments 3–5. This patient would have severe ventilatory problems. *(129:551)*

43. (E) Proper placement of the endotracheal tube is necessary to avoid ventilatory problems. The advent of the end-tidal carbon dioxide monitor has been a great advance. With this monitor, one can show that the tube placement is correct, whereas previously, we had several presumptive methods. Carbon dioxide demonstration is definitive. *(32:226; 75:554)*

44. (C) The use of a low-pressure cuff will decrease trauma to the trachea. Other techniques, eg, using a high-pressure cuff with a leak, frequent suctioning, and hourly deflation, are not as helpful. Frequent suctioning may cause more damage to the trachea. *(1:532; 32:256)*

45. (D) Nasotracheal intubation is a source of bacteremia. If such a tube is needed, it should be used, but if the procedure can be done safely without a nasotracheal tube, that should be done. The patient should receive prophylactic antibiotics as recommended by the American Heart Association. *(1:290; 75:1466)*

46. (A) Chylothorax should not occur with a right internal jugular cannulation. Air embolism may occur if air is allowed to enter the catheter. Hematoma is a possibility. Arrhythmias may occur if the catheter enters the heart and stimulates the sensitive areas of the right ventricle. *(1:441; 75:576)*

47. (A) Needles with security beads cannot be inserted to the hub and, therefore, are less likely to break. Needles should never be inserted to the hub. If a change in needle direction is attempted without

withdrawing it to the skin, the needle may be weakened. Bending weakens the needle. *(203:92)*

48. **(C)** There is a high mortality with the original insult of amniotic fluid embolus. The survivors are plagued by renal failure and coagulation problems. Headache and paralysis are not associated problems. *(184:174)*

49. **(C)** The usual presentation of amniotic fluid embolus is cyanosis, coma, hypotension, and respiratory distress. *(184:251)*

50. **(E)** Administration of humidified gases is of benefit to some patients. The risks are that the humidifier may become contaminated, that the body will have to expend heat to warm the humidified gases, that the patient will receive a water load, and that the airway resistance will increase. These are not insurmountable problems: the mist can be heated to avoid patient heat loss, the fluid load can be compensated for by decreasing other fluids, and contamination can be avoided with good technique. *(1:132; 75:536)*

51. **(E)** As discussed previously, tracheal compression is a big fear. One must also be prepared to rule out the more common problems, eg, mucous plug, kinking, and malposition. *(1:1436; 75:930)*

52. **(A)** The patient for laparoscopic examination may be hypotensive due to carbon dioxide embolus, hemorrhage, and compression of the vena cava. The position should not be a factor. *(43:181; 184:303; 204:143)*

53. **(C)** The onset of hypotension during laparoscopic examination should immediately call for the response of informing the surgeon so that any gas pressure may be relieved. Once that has been accomplished, the situation can be reevaluated to determine what other steps need to be taken. *(204:143)*

54. **(A)** Patients with acromegaly present problems for the anesthesiologist in addition to their large structures. The upper airway is different in that they have thickening of the vocal cords, often laryngeal stenosis, and macroglossia. The chin is prognathic. Intubation may be difficult. *(1:1606; 75:863)*

55. **(A)** When using disposable circuits, it is important to inspect the circuits before putting them into use. It is an increase not in laminar flow characteristics but in turbulent flow characteristics that causes the problems. Indentations, kinking, and cracks all have been reported. *(75:532; 205:744)*

56. **(E)** All of these options are possible causes of hypotension. Most of the time, transfusion is not associated with hypocalcemia. In reference 206, the rapid transfusion of citrated blood was accompanied by hypotension and documented low calcium levels. The levels returned to normal merely by slowing the transfusion. *(1:1345; 206:35)*

57. **(B)** Hypothermia will aggravate the problem of hypocalcemia by decreasing the rate of metabolic clearance of exogenous citrate. This is another good reason to warm blood when it is given rapidly. *(1:1345; 206:35)*

58. **(B)** Anaphylaxis is associated with the release of histamine and SRS-A. Epinephrine and methylxanthine are used to treat the attacks. *(1:298; 75:1384)*

59. **(D)** Anaphylaxis is treated immediately. It may begin with bronchospasm or an intense rash. The first symptom may be hypotension and no wheezing is heard. The duration may be prolonged. *(1:300; 75:1385)*

60. **(E)** Nasotracheal intubation has the usual possibility of broken teeth and, in addition, the problems of sinusitis, nosebleed, and nasal necrosis. *(43:166; 131:187)*

61. **(E)** Hypoxia due to delivery failure has many causes. The only way to protect our patients is to check carefully and monitor carefully. *(1:1144; 170:289)*

62. **(C)** The dura is punctured in epidural attempts about 2% of the time. A test dose is important in determining the placement of the catheter. Failure to aspirate fluid is not an absolute sign that the dura has not been punctured. *(1:1100; 43:103; 75:765)*

63. **(A)** Methemoglobinemia does not result from aspirin ingestion. It may be congenital or may follow the ingestion of nitrites or exposure to aniline dyes. *(2:132; 43:497)*

64. **(D)** Although methemoglobinemia may be congenital, most cases are due to medication or chemical substances. The iron transformation is to the ferric state. Methemoglobin is not an effective oxygen carrier. It can be converted to hemoglobin. *(2:132; 43:497)*

65. **(B)** Pneumothorax is more common in children. It should always be considered as a cause of problems if subclavian catheterization has been attempted immediately before surgery. Pneumothorax is associated with higher airway pressures. *(2:63; 43:173)*

66. **(E)** Pneumothorax may be due to all of the options. *(2:63; 43:173)*

67. **(E)** Aspiration may follow sedation, debility, impaired swallowing, or any factor that affects the ability to protect the airway. *(43:160; 75:1344)*

68. **(D)** Regional anesthesia does not guarantee that aspiration will not occur. The head-down position is not appropriate, since passive regurgitation is more likely to occur in that position. Once intubated, the patient should remain intubated until awake and able to protect the airway. *(43:160; 75:1344)*

69. **(B)** Posttraumatic croup should be treated with mist and reduction of fever. Oxygen should be provided as needed. Fluid restriction is not appropriate. *(43:169; 75:1296)*

70. **(B)** Subglottic edema may be prevented by a gentle intubation and the use of sterile tubes. The head should be kept still to prevent movement of the tube. The use of creams on the tubes has not been shown to be effective. *(43:169; 180:430)*

71. **(E)** All of these options may be correct. Nerve injury is common with difficult dissections. Laryngospasm may be present due to secretions or injury to the cord. Tracheal collapse may be present due to tracheomalacia. Bronchospasm may be a reason for the dyspnea due to airway sensitivity. *(2:992; 43:130)*

72. **(C)** The fact that the patient is crowing on ventilation means that the patient has partial glottic closure. With full glottic closure, the patient will have retraction but will not be moving air that would make any sounds. Gentle positive pressure will usually relieve the phonation. *(1:1860; 2:1130)*

73. **(C)** Enflurane and isoflurane are soluble agents and, therefore, will be affected by the increasing ventilation. The insoluble agents are not affected to the same degree. *(1:630; 75:296)*

74. **(C)** Nitrous oxide is 30 to 40 times more soluble than nitrogen in blood. Its movement into an air-containing cavity will lead to an increase in pressure and volume. *(1:638,640; 2:175)*

75. **(E)** *(2:240; 131:395; 170:314)*

76. **(E)** Our current practice is devoid of explosive agents. Many of the people practicing have never used explosive agents or had any training in the use of such agents. When others come into the operating room with explosive substances, no one knows how to react. We must ensure that the environment is free of combustible gases and solvents. *(2:240; 131:395; 171:314)*

CHAPTER 9

Obstetric Anesthesia
Review

The anesthetic management of the pregnant patient is unique in that both the patient and her baby are involved. The labor and delivery are the termination of a pregnancy, which has an effect on the anatomy and physiology of the mother. One must have a knowledge of the effects of the anesthetic management on both the mother and child. The first aim of any technique must be the safety of both.

During pregnancy there is a narrowing of the respiratory tract due to capillary engorgement. Nose breathing may be more difficult. After about the fifth month there are decreases in lung volumes, including expiratory reserve volume, residual volume, and functional residual capacity (FRC). Airway resistance decreases. There is an increase in ventilation that reaches a maximum in the first trimester but that extends to term. The hyperventilation at term is due to the presence of painful stimuli.

These changes in the airway make the parturient more susceptible to nasal trauma with instrumentation of the nose, whether by suction catheter, nasal airways, or endotracheal tubes. The decrease in FRC makes the patient more prone to hypoxia with apnea and to alkalosis with hyperventilation. The resulting alkalosis decreases the blood flow to the placenta and may lead to fetal hypoxia and fetal metabolic acidosis.

The circulatory system undergoes progressive changes during pregnancy. The cardiac output increases to 50% above normal. In the supine position, the cardiac output will fall because of the effects of the uterine weight on the vena cava. This obstructs venous return and may lead to the supine hypotensive syndrome.

During labor, the cardiac output increases with each uterine contraction due to the augmentation of circulation by blood squeezed from the uterus. This increases stroke volume and left ventricular work. Immediately after delivery, the cardiac output reaches its peak because of redistribution of flow.

These changes in the circulatory system must be considered in the development of an anesthesia plan. The normal circulatory system has compensatory mechanisms to provide for homeostasis. Our anesthesia must protect those protective mechanisms. A regional anesthetic may dilate the peripheral vessels, leading to hypotension. Vasopressors may be necessry to maintain venous return. In the postpartum period, vasodilatation occurs to compensate for the increased cardiac output. Administration of vasopressors at this time may lead to undesired increases in blood pressure.

The patient with a normal heart and cardiovascular system may have little difficulty with labor and delivery. The patient with heart disease may be stressed severely. Careful planning is necessary.

Other changes that occur with pregnancy include decreased gastric motility and incompetence of the gastroesophageal junction, leading to increased susceptibility to regurgitation and aspiration.

Uterine blood flow is decreased by maternal hypotension, by aortoiliac compression, and by uterine contractions. Any factor that causes further decreases in flow, eg, increase in the length or strength of contractions, hemorrhage, or hyperventilation, may aggravate an already tenuous situation, making fetal distress probable. Drugs administered to the mother and transferred across the placenta to the fetus may potentiate the harmful effects.

The plan for pain control and anesthesia must take into consideration fetal effects. The drugs should be given in doses necessary to provide the deisred effect without stressing the fetus. The administration should be timed to avoid fetal effects and prolongation of labor. Epidural techniques may be employed for their effects in labor and delivery.

Other techniques, including paracervical blocks, pudendal blocks, and local infiltration, may be employed by the obstetrician. The team caring for the patient must coordinate their efforts to avoid excess drugs and toxicity.

The three main techniques for pain control today are natural childbirth with the Lamaze training classes, epidural, and spinal anesthesia. All of these can and should involve us. The mother should understand our efforts to provide pain relief and an epidural block should not be viewed as a failure of the Lamaze classes.

You should carefully review spinal and epidural techniques, their indication, and contraindications. Complications of these techniques are important and should be reviewed.

Emergency procedures, eg cesarean section for prolapsed cord, placenta previa, and fetal distress, should be reviewed.

There are several good textbooks available on anesthesia for obstetrics. The comprehensive general texts have sections on obstetric anesthesia, but they are more cursory discussions. The annual refresher course at the ASA meeting always has a series of lectures concerning obstetric anesthesia.

Questions

DIRECTIONS (Questions 1 through 25): Each of the numbered items or incomplete statements in this section is followed by answers or by completions of the statement. Select the ONE lettered answer or completion that is BEST in each case.

1. An infant born with a heart rate of 70, a weak cry, good muscle flexion, poor reflexes, and a blue-pale complexion would be given an Apgar score of

   (A) 2
   (B) 4
   (C) 5
   (D) 6
   (E) 7

   ı ı 3 ı ı

Questions 2 and 3

Please refer to the following figure:

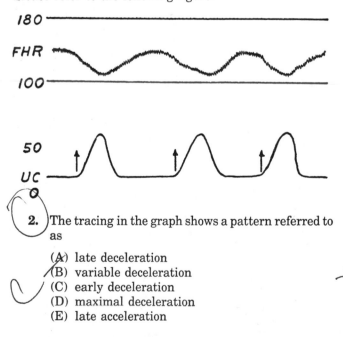

2. The tracing in the graph shows a pattern referred to as

   (A) late deceleration
   (B) variable deceleration
   (C) early deceleration
   (D) maximal deceleration
   (E) late acceleration

3. The type of heart rate tracing shown in the graph is usually associated with

   (A) cord compression
   (B) placental insufficiency
   (C) head compressions
   (D) acute fetal asphyxia
   (E) tetanic contraction

4. In the anesthetic management of a patient with preeclampsia, all of the following are important EXCEPT that

   (A) hypertensive crises may occur
   (B) the fetus usually is premature
   (C) convulsions may be imminent
   (D) oxygen consumption is decreased
   (E) inadequate pain relief may aggravate the hypertension

5. Preeclampsia is associated with

   (A) hypovolemia
   (B) hypernatremia
   (C) low hematocrit reading
   (D) hyperkalemia
   (E) hypotension

6. If internal podalic version is to be attempted

   (A) no anesthesia should be administered
   (B) perineal relaxation is most important
   (C) halothane and nitrous oxide may be used to provide optimum conditions
   (D) mask ventilation is desirable
   (E) muscle relaxation is not desirable

7. In the delivery of a breech presentation

   (A) narcotics should be avoided at all stages
   (B) oxygen should be avoided for fear of harming the fetus
   (C) pudendal and subarachnoid blocks may be used and still maintain the bearing-down reflex
   (D) relaxation of the perineum is important
   (E) a saddle block should be administered early

8. Regional anesthesia techniques that can be used for forceps deliveries include all of the following EXCEPT

   (A) bilateral pudendal block
   (B) paracervical block
   (C) subarachnoid block
   (D) caudal block
   (E) spinal epidural block

9. The usual blood loss with a normal delivery is

   (A) 100 ml
   (B) 200 ml
   (C) 600 ml
   (D) 800 ml
   (E) 1000 ml

10. Measures to prevent aspiration pneumonia include all of the following EXCEPT

    (A) administration of an antacid before delivery
    (B) rapid intubation
    (C) rapid induction
    (D) determination of the last time the patient has eaten
    (E) cricoid pressure

11. Postpuncture headache

    (A) is worse in the supine position
    (B) is of higher incidence following puncture with a 25-gauge needle
    (C) is more prevalent in nonpregnant patients
    (D) will be worse with a larger dural hole
    (E) is lessened if the patient is dehydrated

12. The usual blood loss with an uncomplicated vaginal delivery of twins or with cesarean section is

    (A) 400 ml
    (B) 600 ml
    (C) 800 ml
    (D) 1000 ml
    (E) 1200 ml

13. Prophylactic measures taken to prevent maternal hypotension following spinal anesthesia include all of the following EXCEPT

    (A) administration of 500 to 1000 ml of fluid before induction
    (B) lateral displacement of the uterus
    (C) head-down tilt immediately after injection
    (D) placing the patient on her side after block is established
    (E) infusion of vasopressor

14. In the Friedman curve shown in the graph, area C is the

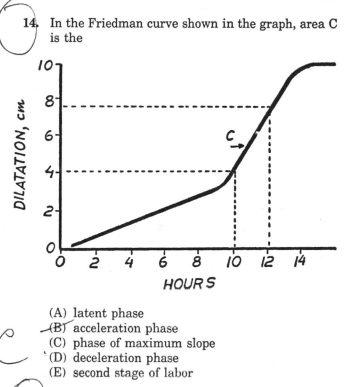

    (A) latent phase
    (B) acceleration phase
    (C) phase of maximum slope
    (D) deceleration phase
    (E) second stage of labor

15. If sedatives or narcotics are given to a woman in labor, they should be given in the

    (A) latent phase
    (B) acceleration phase
    (C) phase of maximum slope
    (D) deceleration phase
    (E) second stage of labor

16. The muscle power for spontaneous delivery is provided by the

    (A) abdominal muscles alone
    (B) perineal muscle
    (C) abdominal muscles and uterine muscles, the abdominal being dominant
    (D) abdominal muscles and uterine muscles, the uterine being dominant
    (E) abdominal and back muscles

17. The local anesthetic that attains the lowest fetal concentration relative to maternal concentration is

    (A) lidocaine
    (B) procaine
    (C) 2-chloroprocaine
    (D) mepivacaine
    (E) bupivacaine

Questions 18 and 19

Please refer to the following figure:

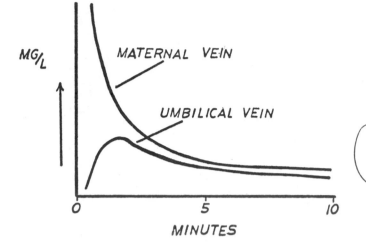

18. The graph shows the concentration of thiopental in maternal and fetal circulation. The maternal blood level

    (A) reaches equilibrium at 10 minutes
    (B) decreases rapidly and has a second peak at 5 minutes
    (C) bears no relationship to fetal levels
    (D) falls rapidly and attains an equilibrium with the fetal circulation
    (E) remains essentially equal

19. From the graph shown, one can project that

    (A) little thiopental enters the fetal circulation for 5 to 7 minutes
    (B) the larger the dose of thiopental, the higher the amount that will cross to the fetus
    (C) maternal and fetal levels bear no relationship
    (D) at least 15 minutes is needed to attain equilibrium
    (E) the umbilical artery contains a higher concentration

20. Cholinesterase levels during pregnancy are

    (A) highest at term
    (B) unchanged from normal levels
    (C) decreased but not to significant levels
    (D) increased
    (E) decreased to a level at which prolonged apnea may follow the use of succinylcholine

21. During delivery, a lower dose of local anesthetic is required for regional anesthesia because

    (A) pregnant women have greater pain tolerance
    (B) the pain fibers are more superficial in the spinal canal

    (C) the epidural and subarachnoid spaces are larger
    (D) the epidural and subarachnoid spaces are decreased in size
    (E) maternal hyperventilation decreases pain

22. During parturition

    (A) cardiac output is decreased
    (B) cardiac output is increased
    (C) stroke volume is decreased
    (D) central venous pressure is decreased
    (E) cardiac output remains constant

23. The graph shows the change in cardiac output with pregnancy. The discrepancy in the two lines is due to the effect

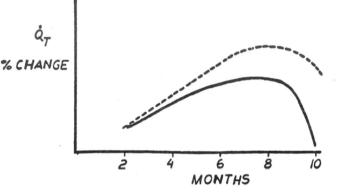

    (A) on respiration
    (B) on uterine blood flow
    (C) on venous return
    (D) of pressure on the aorta
    (E) on the central nervous system

24. The pregnant woman at term

    (A) shows no anatomic changes in the respiratory system
    (B) is primarily a nose breather
    (C) is primarily a mouth breather
    (D) is less susceptible to hypoxia
    (E) has decreased oxygen consumption

25. In a pregnant woman at term, you would expect an increase in all of the following values EXCEPT

    (A) functional residual capacity (FRC)
    (B) vital capacity
    (C) peak flow rate
    (D) lung compliance
    (E) inspiratory capacity

DIRECTIONS (Questions 26 through 50): For each of the items in this section, ONE or MORE of the numbered options is correct. Choose the answer

A if only 1, 2, and 3 are correct,
B if only 1 and 3 are correct,
C if only 2 and 4 are correct,
D if only 4 is correct,
E if all are correct.

26. Factors that may contribute to the hypotension seen with aortocaval compression include

(1) thiopental
(2) epidural block
(3) halothane
(4) hypervolemia

27. After a spinal anesthetic, the parturient woman becomes hypotensive. The drug(s) of choice for treatment is (are)

(1) norepinephrine
(2) methoxamine
(3) phenylephrine drip
(4) ephedrine

28. Gastric changes associated with pregnancy include

(1) decreased acid secretion
(2) decreased gastric emptying time
(3) downward displacement of the pylorus
(4) incompetence of the gastroesophageal sphincter

29. A woman has been in labor for 2 hours when her membranes rupture and the umbilical cord is prolapsed. Her treatment should include

(1) breech extraction or forceps extraction if the cervix is fully dilated
(2) knee-chest position
(3) constant monitoring of fetal heart tones
(4) immediate cesarean section if delivery is not imminent

30. The administration of meperidine (Demerol) to a parturient may lead to

(1) decreased Apgar scores
(2) decreased neonatal minute volume
(3) respiratory acidosis
(4) highest exposure in the fetus 2 to 3 hours after administration

31. Maternal changes associated with preeclampsia include

(1) increased cardiac output
(2) decreased renal blood flow
(3) decreased cerebral blood flow
(4) increased hepatic blood flow

32. Anesthesia for emergency cesarean section can be provided by

(1) general anesthesia
(2) local infiltration
(3) subarachnoid block
(4) spinal epidural block

33. In multiple deliveries, anesthetic considerations must include the fact(s) that

(1) the infants are usually postmature
(2) complications, such as prolapsed cord, are more frequent
(3) the first infant has a higher incidence of complications
(4) the mother has a higher incidence of complications

34. Serious risks of general anesthesia in obstetric patients include

(1) aspiration pneumonia
(2) depression of the newborn
(3) impaired uterine contractility
(4) hemorrhage

35. Halothane is not often used in obstetrics because

(1) it is not of sufficient solubility to give fast relief
(2) it is not a good analgesic
(3) of its liver toxicity
(4) it produces myometrial depression even in low concentrations

36. Treatment of postspinal headache includes

(1) orders to keep NPO
(2) reassurance
(3) subarachnoid injection of the patient's blood
(4) codeine or aspirin

37. Serious complications from the use of local anesthetics in obstetrics can be avoided by

(1) using the lowest concentration of local anesthetic consistent with good results
(2) using the smallest volume of local anesthetic consistent with good results
(3) aspirating to ascertain that the needle is not in a vein
(4) avoiding the use of epinephrine

38. When compared to spinal anesthesia, epidural anesthesia

(1) permits less control
(2) causes more hypotension
(3) is more apt to cause spinal headache
(4) carries less risk of arachnoiditis

SUMMARY OF DIRECTIONS				
A	**B**	**C**	**D**	**E**
1, 2, 3 only	1, 3 only	2, 4 only	4 only	All are correct

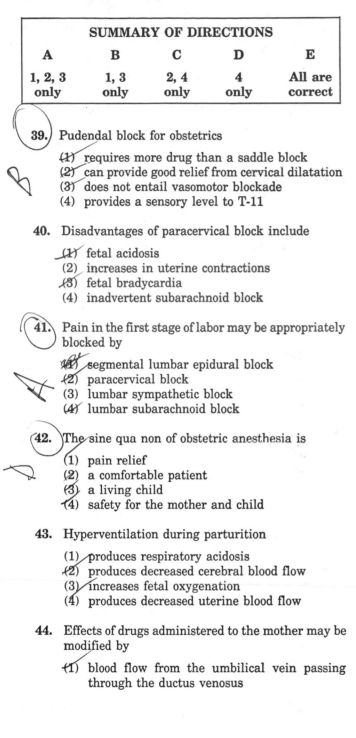

39. Pudendal block for obstetrics

   (1) requires more drug than a saddle block
   (2) can provide good relief from cervical dilatation
   (3) does not entail vasomotor blockade
   (4) provides a sensory level to T-11

40. Disadvantages of paracervical block include

   (1) fetal acidosis
   (2) increases in uterine contractions
   (3) fetal bradycardia
   (4) inadvertent subarachnoid block

41. Pain in the first stage of labor may be appropriately blocked by

   (1) segmental lumbar epidural block
   (2) paracervical block
   (3) lumbar sympathetic block
   (4) lumbar subarachnoid block

42. The sine qua non of obstetric anesthesia is

   (1) pain relief
   (2) a comfortable patient
   (3) a living child
   (4) safety for the mother and child

43. Hyperventilation during parturition

   (1) produces respiratory acidosis
   (2) produces decreased cerebral blood flow
   (3) increases fetal oxygenation
   (4) produces decreased uterine blood flow

44. Effects of drugs administered to the mother may be modified by

   (1) blood flow from the umbilical vein passing through the ductus venosus

   (2) hepatic drug uptake
   (3) dilution of blood in the right atrium
   (4) shunting across the foramen ovale

45. Inhalation agents pass through the placental membrane rapidly as a result of

   (1) rapid rate of diffusion
   (2) low fat solubility
   (3) low molecular weight
   (4) low concentration gradient

46. Placental circulation may be decreased by

   (1) uterine contractions
   (2) maternal hypotension
   (3) aortoiliac compression
   (4) hemorrhage

47. A normal pregnancy is associated with increased

   (1) minute volume
   (2) tidal volume
   (3) respiratory rate
   (4) ventilation only at term

48. The newborn infant

   (1) has a respiratory acidosis
   (2) has a high P_{CO_2}
   (3) is hypoxic
   (4) has a metabolic acidosis

49. The newborn infant who remains apneic

   (1) has an exaggerated acidosis
   (2) develops a P_{CO_2} rise of 10 mm Hg per minute
   (3) has a fall in pH of 0.1 unit per minute
   (4) can tolerate this condition without permanent damage

50. Proper resuscitation of the newborn requires

   (1) ambient temperature
   (2) suctioning
   (3) prone position
   (4) stimulation

Answers and Explanations

1. **(C)** The baby would get 1 point for heart rate, 1 for a weak cry, 2 for muscle tone, 1 for reflexes, and no points for color. *(1:1753; 75:1241; 184:354)*

2. **(C)** The pattern represented is that of early deceleration, in which the heart rate decreases with the onset of contraction, reaches the low point with the peak of contraction, and then returns to baseline as the uterus relaxes. In contrast, late decelerations start after the contraction is underway, and the low point occurs after the contraction is over. Variable decelerations are variable in shape and onset. *(75:1236; 184:339)*

3. **(C)** The early deceleration pattern is seen with fetal head compression, which leads to increased vagal tone. Cord compression leads to variable decelerations, whereas placental insufficiency leads to late decelerations. *(75:1235; 184:339)*

4. **(D)** In the patient with preeclampsia, the maternal metabolism is increased; therefore, the oxygen consumption is increased. Hypertensive crises may occur. The hypertension may be aggravated if adequate pain control is not provided. Convulsions are also a threat. The fetus often is premature. *(1:1713; 75:1235; 184:339)*

5. **(A)** In spite of the fact that patients may exhibit edema and weight gain, they are hypovolemic due to the vasoconstriction that is part of the disease. They have hypertension, hyponatremia, increased hematocrit (due to the vasoconstriction and hypovolemia), and hypokalemia. *(75:1229; 184:152)*

6. **(C)** If podalic version is to be performed, good uterine relaxation should be provided. This can be provided with halothane and nitrous oxide. Mask ventilation is not adequate. The patient needs uterine relaxation, not perineal relaxation. Muscle relaxation is not a requirement. *(184:286)*

7. **(D)** Relaxation of the perineum is important for the delivery of a breech presentation. Anesthesia should not be initiated too early, since it is important that the voluntary bearing-down efforts be preserved. Oxygen and pain control are important. An early saddle block is inappropriate. *(1:1716; 184:286)*

8. **(B)** A paracervical block is good for the first stage of labor, since it helps with the pain associated with cervical dilatation. A pudendal block will provide anesthesia for the second stage and is appropriate for low forceps delivery and episiotomies. A subarachnoid block, caudal block, or epidural block also is appropriate. *(1:1716; 75:1224; 184:286)*

9. **(C)** The usual blood loss for a normal vaginal delivery is 400 to 600 ml. *(1:1685)*

10. **(D)** The obstetric patient is treated as a patient with a full stomach, so the history of no recent food intake is not important. If a general anesthetic is needed, the patient should have antacids and rapid sequence induction with cricoid pressure. *(75:1226; 184:138)*

11. **(D)** The typical postspinal puncture headache is worse in the upright position and relieved by the recumbent position. It is more prevalent in the obstetric female. A smaller needle makes a smaller dural hole, and there is a lower incidence of headache. Dehydration aggravates the headache. *(1:1707; 75:778; 184:100)*

12. **(D)** The usual blood loss in an uncomplicated vaginal delivery of twins or in a cesarean section is 1000 ml. *(1:1685; 75:1227)*

13. **(C)** Methods to prevent maternal hypotension include fluid administration, lateral displacement of the uterus, placing the patient on her side, and infusion of a vasopressor. A head-down tilt will increase the level of the block and make the hypotension worse. *(1:1705; 75:778; 184:111)*

14. **(C)** The area labeled C is the phase of maximum slope. The first, relatively flat area is the latent

phase. This is followed by an acceleration phase, the phase of maximum slope, and then the deceleration phase. The second stage of labor follows. Knowing the normal progression of labor helps one to decide when to provide anesthesia. *(1:1705)*

15. **(C)** If analgesics and sedatives are given in the phase of maximum slope, they should not slow down the labor. If given too early in the latent phase, labor may be slowed. If delayed too long, the drugs are not as necessary and may have more effect on the fetus. *(1:1690; 184:121)*

16. **(D)** The muscle power is provided by both the uterus and the abdominal muscles. The uterine muscle is the more important. The perineal muscle does not have any effect in pushing the child through the birth canal. Relaxation of the perineum will help in the birth. *(2:1013; 189:22)*

17. **(C)** 2-Chloroprocaine is metabolized very rapidly; therefore, it does not attain a high concentration in the fetus. The other agents are broken down more slowly and are able to cross the placenta. *(1:1702; 75:1219; 184:74)*

18. **(D)** In the graph, the maternal blood level falls rapidly and reaches an equilibrium with the fetal circulation within 3 minutes. There is no second peak unless the drug dose is repeated. The fetal drug level rises rapidly as the maternal level decreases, an equilibrium is reached, and then the level in each slowly decreases. *(75:1222; 184:49)*

19. **(B)** From the graph, it is apparent that the higher the dose of thiopental, the higher the fetal level. This level is reached within 3 minutes. The umbilical concentration never exceeds the maternal concentration. *(75:1222; 184:49)*

20. **(E)** Succinylcholine is a drug frequently used in the obstetric patient. The cholinesterase level is decreased at term and may be decreased significantly. This may lead to prolongation of the effect. This complication is not often seen but should be considered when using the drug. *(75:387; 184:21)*

21. **(D)** Less local anesthetic is needed in the later stages of pregnancy, since the epidural space is decreased in size. This is due to the venous congestion caused by the weight of the uterus. In addition, there are studies showing that the nerves are more sensitive to the local anesthetics. This is thought to be a hormonal effect. *(75:777,1217; 131:222)*

22. **(B)** During parturition, the cardiac output is increased. This may be offset by the effects of the uterine weight on the vena cava, leading to de-

creased return and decrease in cardiac output. Central venous pressure increases. *(75:1216; 184:8,10)*

23. **(C)** There is an increase in cardiac output as pregnancy progresses until about the eighth month, at which time the increase is attenuated. When studying the cardiac output in the pregnant patient, one must know whether the study was made with the patient in the supine or lateral position. In the supine position, cardiac output will be decreased because of the weight of the uterus on the great veins of the abdomen. *(1:1684; 75:1216; 184:9)*

24. **(C)** The pregnant patient at term is a mouth breather, since nasal congestion and swelling make it more difficult to breathe through the nose. Placement of nasal catheters or airways may lead to bleeding. The FRC is decreased at term, making the patient more prone to hypoxia. There is an increase in oxygen consumption. *(1:1682; 75:1216; 184:11)*

25. **(A)** FRC decreases at term. Vital capacity increases by 5%, and there is an increase in peak flow rate, lung compliance, and inspiratory capacity. *(1:1682; 75:1216; 184:11)*

26. **(A)** Any drug or technique, such as thiopental, epidural block, or halothane, will contribute to the hypotension. Hypervolemia will counteract the problem. *(1:1687; 184:10,11)*

27. **(D)** Ephedrine increases the blood pressure without decreasing uterine blood flow. Drugs with pure alpha action will increase uterine resistance and decrease uterine bood flow. *(1:1705; 75:1237; 184:100)*

28. **(D)** Gastric changes seen with pregnancy include incompetence of the gastroesophageal sphincter, increased acid secretion, increased gastric emptying time, and upward displacement of the pylorus. These make the pregnant patient more susceptible to aspiration. *(1:1688; 75:1217; 184:12)*

29. **(E)** Prolapse of the umbilical cord is a true obstetric emergency. Steps should include all of the options. This can occur without warning, and one must always be prepared for such an emergency. *(208:489)*

30. **(E)** The administration of meperidine may lead to decreased Apgar scores due to fetal depression and decreased fetal minute volume. This may lead to respiratory acidosis. The highest exposure in the fetus is 2 to 3 hours after administration to the mother. This makes timing of the drug to the mother important. *(1:1695; 75:1222; 184:43,124)*

31. **(A)** Maternal changes seen with preeclampsia include increased cardiac output, decreased renal blood flow, and decreased cerebral blood flow. The

last two are reasons for some of the complications. Hepatic flow is decreased in the preeclamptic patient. *(1:1713; 75:1228; 184:152)*

32. **(A)** Anesthesia for an emergency cesarean section requires fast onset. Therefore, a spinal epidural block is not appropriate. Since time is of the essence in these situations, a room with all equipment is kept ready at all times. *(75:1225; 184:147)*

33. **(C)** The multiple delivery birth has the potential for many problems. The infants are frequently premature. Complications, such as prolapsed cord, are more frequent. The first infant has a lower incidence of complications. The mother also has a higher incidence of problems with multiple births. *(1:1225; 184:284)*

34. **(E)** All of these factors may be problems in the obstetric patient for general anesthesia. Steps must be taken to avert the problem when possible. In some patients, general anesthesia is the best approach. One must use the lowest dose of anesthesia possible and take steps to avoid aspiration. The possibility of hemorrhage must be borne in mind, and avoid those agents that might cause it if possible. *(1:1710; 184:145)*

35. **(C)** Halothane, although a good anesthetic agent in general, provides little analgesia and leads to depression of the uterus. This may be a positive characteristic in some procedures, but in most obstetric procedures, it is unwanted. The drug has been associated with liver problems, but that is not the reason for avoiding it in the obstetric patient. Halothane solubility is not a reason to avoid it. *(75:307, 1242; 184:55,56)*

36. **(C)** Treatment of a postspinal headache includes reassurance and analgesics. In addition, the patient should have fluids and, if necessary, an epidural not subarachnoid blood patch. *(1:1708; 75:778; 184:101)*

37. **(A)** Toxicity from local anesthetics can be avoided by using the lowest concentration and smallest volume possible. One should always aspirate to avoid intravascular injection. This is not foolproof. The use of epinephrine is helpful, since it delays absorption, and it also, when used in the test dose, gives an indication of intravascular injection. *(1:1005; 75:394; 184:68)*

38. **(D)** The epidural technique is less controllable and causes less hypotension than the spinal technique. There is much less risk of postspinal puncture headache. The incidence of arachnoiditis is decreased with the epidural approach. *(1:1709; 131:235; 184:102)*

39. **(B)** The pudendal block is useful for relieving pain for low forceps application and for episiotomy. It requires more drug than that used for a saddle block. There is no vasomotor blockade. The sensory loss is in the area of the perineum only. *(131:292; 184:113)*

40. **(B)** A paracervical block can lead to fetal bradycardia and subsequent fetal acidosis. The block does not affect uterine contractions. There is no risk of subarachnoid injection. *(1:1698; 184:113)*

41. **(A)** Pain in the first stage of labor may be blocked by all of the options, but a lumbar subarachnoid block is not appropriate at that stage of labor. A segmental epidural or paracervical block is appropriate, and a lumbar sympathetic block may be used. There is some evidence that this block may accelerate the first stage of labor. *(1:1698; 184:113)*

42. **(D)** There are many requirements of anesthesia for labor and delivery. None of these is as important as safety for both the woman and the child. This fact must be borne in mind with every intervention. *(184:133; 189:29)*

43. **(C)** Hyperventilation during delivery will lead to decreased cerebral blood flow and decreased uterine blood flow. A respiratory alkalosis will occur. Fetal oxygenation may be compromised. *(184:36,118)*

44. **(E)** These factors all protect the fetus from receiving the full effect of drugs administered to the mother. The blood is diverted or diluted at several spots, decreasing the drug concentration in the brain of the fetus. *(1:1691; 75:1220)*

45. **(B)** Inhalation agents pass through the placental membrane rapidly as a result of a rapid diffusion rate a high fat solubility, low molecular weight, and a high concentration gradient. *(1:1691; 75:1217; 184:39)*

46. **(E)** Placental circulation is decreased by uterine contractions. This is part of normal labor. If tetanic contractions occur, the fetal circulation may be seriously impaired. Hemorrhage may lead to maternal hypotension, which may decrease uterine blood flow. Aortoiliac compression may decrease uterine blood flow directly, and if vena cava compression occurs with it, the hypotension will aggravate the problem. *(184:31; 189:14)*

47. **(A)** Respiratory effects of pregnancy are noted early and are progressive during the pregnancy. Minute volume increases, as does tidal volume and respiratory rate. Hyperventilation begins very early, reaches its maximum at about the end of the first trimester, and remains elevated at term. *(75:1216; 184:14; 189:2)*

48. **(E)** The newborn infant is prone to respiratory problems, since he or she has acidosis on both metabolic and respiratory bases and is hypoxic. *(1:1730)*

49. **(A)** The newborn has an acidosis as noted previously. Any apnea at birth will aggravate this problem. Immediate resuscitation is mandatory, since the P_{CO_2} will rise rapidly and the pH will fall. *(1:1732)*

50. **(C)** Newborn resuscitation requires increased temperature, suctioning to remove meconium or other secretions, head-down position to facilitate drainage of secretions, and stimulation to encourage breathing. *(1:1734)*

CHAPTER 10

Pediatric Anesthesia
Review

The infant and child have many different physiologic and anatomic characteristics, which make them unique from a standpoint of anesthesia care.

Physiologically, the infant and child have a different cardiovascular system. The heart must be transformed from the fetal configuration with its shunts and high pulmonary pressure to the adult configuration with low right-sided pressure and closure of the shunts. In the process, it passes through a transitional configuration. There may be reversions to the fetal type circulation with changes in the environment. Hypoxia may cause the ductus to remain open or to reopen. The pulmonary vasculature undergoes changes in the early periods to change from a system of high pressures to a system of low pressures.

The hepatic enzyme systems are not mature at birth, and the infant cannot handle drugs in the same fashion as an adult. Lower levels of albumin may lead to less drug binding and greater effect from some drugs. Hyperbilirubinemia may be a problem early in life due to the inability of the liver to break down the larger amount of bilirubin presented to the liver.

The pulmonary system contains about 25 million alveoli at birth and continues development until the adult complement of 300 million is present. This usually occurs by age 8. The chest wall in the neonate has a different configuration. The ribs come off at almost right angles from the vertebrae, which makes it more difficult for the small infant to increase the intrathoracic volume. The adult thoracic cage, with its bucket-handle rib movement, can increase the volume easily. In addition, the neonate has a very pliable sternum that yields readily to the inspiratory forces. Retraction further decreases intrathoracic volume.

The upper airway and the relatively larger head cause additional compromise. In the supine position, the child is much more subject to obstruction as the head flexes on the neck. The nostrils are small, and the tongue has a tendency to be larger, making obstruction of the airway common, especially since the newborn is an obligate nasal breather.

The smallest part of the infant airway is at the level of the cricoid cartilage. A cuffed endotracheal tube is not necessary or desirable in the young child, since the cuff will occupy space that is better used with a larger internal diameter of endotracheal tube.

The nervous system of the infant is not fully developed, and many tracts will not be fully developed until adolescence. Still, the newborn, even the premature newborn, should have anesthesia for any painful procedure. We should approach the anesthetic needs of the newborn as we would an adult. If the infant cannot tolerate it, anesthesia should be reduced or discontinued while resuscitation is undertaken to restore stability. The anesthesia should be restored as soon as it is tolerated.

The blood volume of a full-term infant is 80 ml/kg. The newborn infant has a high hemoglobin concentration, but it decreases over the first 3 months because of low iron stores and decreased marrow activity. The physiologic anemia of the newborn is worse in the premature infant. It may be aggravated by the frequent blood sampling of the infant for laboratory tests. These children are in need of hemoglobin for oxygen-carrying capacity, just as are adults, and anemia is a risk factor for anesthesia complications.

Careful monitoring of blood loss is important to prevent hypovolemia during a procedure. This must be a constant process, not waiting until a certain number of sponges is used. To wait may allow the very small patient to lose a relatively large amount of blood before blood loss is assessed.

Anesthesia equipment designed specifically for the infant and child should be used when possible, and we should not rely on adaptations of adult equipment. The equipment dead space may be larger than the tidal volume of the infant. Various modifications of the Ayre's T-piece are in use today and are available as disposable products for use in infants and children. Dead space and resistance must be taken into account with all circuits.

Monitoring of the patient is most important. The availability of the pulse oximeter has been a great advance in the safety of pediatric anesthesia. The ability to obtain blood pressures in the small child by automated equipment also has been a big advance. Most operating rooms today monitor end-tidal CO_2 as well.

Temperature monitoring is very important, since the small child is at greater risk for hypothermia and hyperthermia. The operating rooms are cold, and the child may be exposed for long periods while venous access is obtained. Warming lights are necessary to prevent heat loss. At the other end of the spectrum is the hyperthermic child, and the decision must be made whether the increased temperature is due to environmental factors, intercurrent infection, or malignant hyperthermia.

The infant and child should be monitored by listening to heart tones with either an esophageal or a precordial stethoscope. Changes in heart tones with decreases in volume are readily apparent. The electrocardiogram is also monitored.

Special monitoring procedures, eg, urinary output and invasive arterial blood pressure, are used more often in children now and should be used when indicated.

Endotracheal tube placement may be critical in the small child. The ability to auscultate the lungs to ascertain the depth is not good in the smaller children, since the breath sounds are transmitted so easily. Depths of endotracheal tubes needed to place the tip in the mid-trachea are:

1 kg	7 cm
2 kg	8 cm
3 kg	9 cm

$$\frac{age}{2} + 12$$

In the older child, the formula of

$$12 + \text{one-half the age}$$

is a good method to determine the proper depth in centimeters. The size of the endotracheal tube may be determined by the formula

$$\frac{age}{4} + 4 \qquad \frac{(16 + \text{the age})}{4}$$

This should give a good fit with some leak. Posttraumatic croup is seen frequently in the recovery room. The child should be obseved to make sure that the croup is not progressive. Treatment with mist and racemic epinephrine usually relieves the stridor. The child should be observed until the effect of the racemic epinephrine is gone.

You should be familiar with the common emergencies in the newborn, eg, diaphragmatic hernia, tracheoesophageal fistula, and gastroschisis. The intitial treatment of these children in the delivery room as well as the anesthesia care should be reviewed. There are some anomalies with anesthetic implications, eg, the Pierre Robin syndrome, that should be reviewed.

Questions

DIRECTIONS (Questions 1 through 15): Each of the numbered items or incomplete statements in this section is followed by answers or by completions of the statement. Select the ONE lettered answer or completion that is BEST in each case.

1. The total dosage of lidocaine for a child should not exceed

   (A) 1 mg/kg
   (B) 3.5 mg/kg
   (C) 5 mg/kg
   (D) 7 mg/kg
   (E) 10 mg/kg

2. An infant under anesthesia loses body heat by all of the following routes EXCEPT

   (A) the metabolism of brown fat
   (B) breathing dry gases
   (C) conduction to cold surroundings
   (D) cold preparation solutions
   (E) exposure of abdominal contents

3. Urinary output during anesthesia in a child should be

   (A) 1 ml/kg/hour
   (B) 2 ml/kg/hour
   (C) 3 ml/kg/hour
   (D) 4 ml/kg/hour
   (E) 5 ml/kg/hour

4. The only early sign of malignant hyperthermia in an anesthetized infant is

   (A) rapid rise in body temperature
   (B) tachycardia
   (C) hot skin
   (D) arrhythmia
   (E) hot circle absorber

5. The blood volume of an infant with a normal hemoglobin is estimated to be

   (A) 30 ml/kg
   (B) 40 ml/kg
   (C) 50 ml/kg
   (D) 60 ml/kg
   (E) 80 ml/kg

6. The major factor associated with the closure of patent ductus arteriosus (PDA) in the newborn is

   (A) increased P_{CO_2}
   (B) decreased P_{CO_2}
   (C) increased P_{O_2}
   (D) decreased P_{O_2}
   (E) increased pulmonary artery pressure

7. The normal dead space in an infant is

   (A) 0.5 ml/kg of body weight
   (B) 1 ml/kg of body weight
   (C) 2 ml/kg of body weight
   (D) 3 ml/kg of body weight
   (E) 4 ml/kg of body weight

8. If a heated humidifier is used during anesthesia, the fluid management of a small child

   (A) will be unchanged
   (B) will require an increased amount of fluid
   (C) will require more sodium to be infused
   (D) must take into account that respiratory insensible loss is eliminated
   (E) will require more fluid to replace increased urinary losses

9. The most important factor in maintaining normothermia in the operating room is

   (A) body temperature at the beginning of the procedure
   (B) room temperature
   (C) use of a warming blanket
   (D) use of warm fluids
   (E) temperature of "prep" solutions

10. In the newborn infant, the spinal cord extends to the

(A) first lumbar vertebra
(B) second lumbar vertebra
(C) third lumbar vertebra
(D) fourth lumbar vertebra
(E) fifth lumbar vertebra

11. The surface area of a neonate relative to that of an adult is

(A) ¼
(B) ⅙
(C) ⅓
(D) ⅑
(E) 1/20

12. The number of saccules and primitive alveoli in a full-term infant as compared to an adult is

(A) the same
(B) 8%
(C) 25%
(D) 50%
(E) 75%

13. A child is admitted for general anesthesia for closure of a severe scalp laceration. He had eaten 2 hours before his accident. He should

(A) always have a rapid sequence induction with thiopental and succinylcholine
(B) have a nasogastric tube passed to remove gastric contents before induction
(C) not be operated on for 6 hours
(D) have vomiting induced
(E) be allowed to awaken with the endotracheal tube in place at the end of the procedure

14. If a child who is admitted with an incarcerated inguinal hernia has a mild upper respiratory tract infection

(A) the surgery should be cancelled
(B) the surgery should be allowed to proceed, but the child should not be intubated
(C) the child should be started on antibiotics, and the surgery should proceed
(D) the surgery should proceed with careful monitoring
(E) the patient should be operated on only under spinal anesthesia

15. Classic signs of congenital diaphragmatic hernia include all of the following EXCEPT

(A) decreased movement of the hemithorax
(B) rounded abdomen
(C) mediastinal shift
(D) bowel sounds in chest
(E) bowel pattern in chest by x-ray

DIRECTIONS (Questions 16 through 30): For each of the items in this section, ONE or MORE of the numbered options is correct. Choose the answer

A if only 1, 2, and 3 are correct,
B if only 1 and 3 are correct,
C if only 2 and 4 are correct,
D if only 4 is correct,
E if all are correct.

16. Pulmonary vascular resistance in newborns decreases because of

(1) closure of the ductus
(2) lung expansion
(3) decreased pH
(4) improved oxygenation

17. Retinopathy of prematurity

(1) may be a potential until the retina is completely vascularized at 44 weeks
(2) is directly related to the F_{IO_2}
(3) is related to the oxygen tension of the retinal artery blood
(4) occurs only after exposure to hyperoxemia for at least 24 hours

18. Drugs are handled differently by neonates because of differences in

(1) absorption
(2) total body water
(3) albumin levels
(4) metabolism

19. Less muscle relaxant is needed by a neonate because

(1) musculature is poorly developed
(2) muscle mass is less
(3) the myoneural junction is not well developed
(4) total body water is greater

20. The Mapleson D system

(1) is useful only for children over 20 kg
(2) can be used for spontaneous or controlled ventilation
(3) provides moist gas flows
(4) has a pop-off valve at the end of the expiratory tube

21. The administration of sodium bicarbonate to a newborn infant with an Apgar score of 2 at 2 minutes

(1) will increase the P_{O_2}
(2) is contraindicated
(3) may cause hepatic necrosis if given through a venous catheter whose tip is in the liver
(4) should be given intramuscularly

22. The work of breathing in a newborn infant

    (1) involves overcoming elastic forces
    (2) involves overcoming resistive forces
    (3) is least when the infant breathes at 35 times per minute
    (4) is less if the child is breathing very rapidly

23. The systolic blood pressure in infants

    (1) is less than that of adults
    (2) is of less importance than in an adult
    (3) is between 65 and 75 mm Hg at birth
    (4) is equal to adult pressure by age 2

24. The metabolic activity of a child

    (1) is lower than that of an adult
    (2) is highest in the first 2 years of life
    (3) is lowered by a febrile illness
    (4) rises with onset of puberty

25. The airway of the newborn, as compared to the adult, has

    (1) a more cephalad-placed larynx
    (2) an epiglottis that has the same shape in each
    (3) vocal cords slanted upward and backward
    (4) the most narrow area at the rima glottidis

26. A 4-year-old child develops postintubation laryngeal edema after a tonsillectomy. The treatment for this includes

    (1) inhalation of mist
    (2) steroids

    (3) racemic epinephrine
    (4) sedation

27. The child with epiglottitis typically

    (1) lies on the right side
    (2) has a sudden onset of symptoms
    (3) has a hacking cough
    (4) is febrile

28. The typical child with laryngotracheobronchitis has

    (1) a gradual onset of symptoms
    (2) a barking cough
    (3) a low-grade fever
    (4) a subglottic obstruction

29. Postintubation laryngeal edema in a child

    (1) is most common in the newborn period
    (2) can be decreased by the use of an appropriate lubricant
    (3) is noted particularly on exhalation
    (4) should be treated with oxygen and mist

30. The premature newborn infant who requires surgery

    (1) needs no anesthesia, since pain fibers are not developed
    (2) will not react to pain
    (3) should have an anesthetic course of oxygen and relaxant
    (4) should be evaluated for anesthesia using the same criteria as any patient

Answers and Explanations

1. **(D)** The dose of lidocaine in a child should not exceed a total dose of 7 mg/kg. This dose, as all doses, depends on the route and the speed of administration. If a dose of lidocaine is give intravenously, 7 mg/kg will be excessive. For infiltration of a laceration, the dose would be appropriate. *(178:230; 179:284)*

2. **(A)** The metabolism of brown fat is a heat-producing mechanism. All of the other options are common methods of losing heat in an operating room. The temperature must be monitored and methods initiated to prevent heat loss. *(177:19; 178:209)*

3. **(A)** Urinary output for a child should be 1 ml/kg/hour. This should be monitored if appropriate for the procedure. *(177:143; 178:212)*

4. **(B)** Tachycardia is an early sign of malignant hyperthermia. If one waits for the development of fever, hot skin, and hot absorber, the syndrome has already developed quite far. *(75:460; 177:frontispiece, 245)*

5. **(E)** The normal blood volume in an infant is 80 ml/kg. A premature infant has a higher volume per unit of weight. *(177:123; 178:553)*

6. **(C)** The major factor that causes closure of the PDA is the Po_2. Hypoxia in the early newborn period may delay closure. The level of Pco_2 is not involved, nor is pulmonary artery pressure. *(1:1731; 177:177)*

7. **(C)** The normal dead space in an infant is 2 ml/kg. This has always been one of the problems inherent in the equipment used for pediatrics. The dead space of the equipment exceeded the infant's dead space, making effective ventilation difficult. *(75:672; 178:59–60)*

8. **(D)** Heated humidifiers provide fluid to the child, and this must be accounted for in the fluid plan for the procedure. Normal plans for replacement include the insensible losses from the respiratory tract. This wil not occur with humidification. The fluid infusion should be reduced by the amount of insensible loss. For long-term ventilation, this also may be a problem. *(75:537; 178:144)*

9. **(B)** Most operating rooms are kept at a low temperature for the comfort of the staff. The infant loses heat by conduction to the cold table, by convection by the cold air, by evaporation, and by radiation. Once the child is covered, some of the heat loss decreases, but if a cavity is opened, more surface is available for heat loss. *(177:116; 178:208)*

10. **(C)** The spinal cord extends to the L-3 level in the newborn. When doing any spinal anesthesia, this must be kept in mind. In the adult, the spinal cord is at the level of the upper edge of L-2. *(75:1290; 177:258)*

11. **(D)** The surface is about 1/9 the surface area of an adult. *(178:12)*

12. **(B)** At birth, the infant has about 25 million primitive alveoli for air exchange. An adult has about 300 million. If a disease intervenes, complete development may not occur. *(1:2340; 177:9)*

13. **(E)** The child should have an induction that is most appropriate for his clinical condition. If there has been a large amount of blood lost, a rapid sequence induction with thiopental and succinylcholine may not be appropriate. Passing a nasogastric tube may not remove all of the stomach contents. The procedure should not be delayed to allow the stomach to empty. Once the injury has occurred, the stomach action probably stops, and the contents will still be there 6 hours later. The child should be allowed to awaken with the endotracheal tube in place. *(177:29; 178:574)*

14. **(D)** The child who has an incarcerated hernia is going to need surgery to reduce the hernia lest strangulation occur. An upper respiratory infection

is not the ideal situation, but since the procedure must be done, it should be done with careful attention to detail, including monitoring. If intubation is indicated, the child should be intubated. If the infection is deemed to be viral, antibiotics will not be of value. A spinal anesthetic may be used but is not the only solution to the problem. *(178:530; 180:349)*

15. **(B)** The child with a diaphragmatic abdomen classically has a scaphoid abdomen. There is decreased movement of the hemithorax and a mediastinal shift. The bowel sounds and bowel pattern on x-ray may be seen. *(177:50; 180:83)*

16. **(C)** Pulmonary vascular resistance decreases with lung expansion and improved oxygenation. A decrease in pH will increase pulmonary vascular resistance. The closure of the ductus does not affect vascular resistance. *(1:1730; 178:63)*

17. **(B)** There is controversy concerning the role of oxygen in retinopathy of prematurity. The retina is at risk until the vascularization is complete at about 44 weeks. It is not related to F_{IO_2} but is related to oxygen tension. It is also related to other factors, ie, oxygen tension is not the only factor. Retinopathy has been reported after very short exposures to oxygen. *(1:1157; 177:30)*

18. **(E)** Infants differ from adults in drug handling in absorption. The infant stomach has a higher pH, leading to increased absorption of some drugs. The total body is greater in the infant, making distribution different. The albumin levels are lower, leading to more unbound drug. The immaturity of the liver leads to decreased drug metabolism of some drugs. *(1:1763)*

19. **(A)** Lower doses of muscle relaxant are needed for the neonate because of poorly developed musculature, smaller muscle mass, and an immature myoneural junction. The greater total body water provides a dilutional effect. This would require larger doses. *(1:1776; 75:354,1286)*

20. **(C)** The Mapleson D system is most useful in the small child, under 10 kg. The flows are dry. The circuit can be used for spontaneous and controlled ventilation. The pop-off valve is placed near the end of the expiratory tube. *(1:1773; 177:275)*

21. **(B)** Administration of sodium bicarbonate to a newborn will increase the P_{O_2} if the pulmonary vascular resistance is decreased, allowing better ventilation. Care must be taken to avoid liver damage from injection into the liver. The drug must be given intravenously. *(1:1745)*

22. **(A)** The work of breathing involves overcoming both elastic and resistive forces. As the child breathes very fast, the work is increased, since turbulent flow is more prevalent. The optimal rate is 35 breaths per minute. *(178:59)*

23. **(B)** The systolic blood pressure in an infant is lower than that in an adult, but it is of equal importance. At birth, the systolic pressure is between 65 and 75 mm Hg and rises slowly. It remains relatively low until age 6, when it starts to increase to approach adult levels. *(177:11)*

24. **(C)** Metabolic activity rises with puberty but is highest in the first 2 years of life. The metabolic rate is higher in a child than in an adult. Febrile illnesses cause a rise in metabolic rate. *(178:21)*

25. **(B)** The infantile airway has a more cephalad-placed larynx and vocal cords that are slanted. The epiglottis is long and narrow. The most narrow portion of the infant airway is at the level of the cricoid cartilage. *(75:1258; 178:16)*

26. **(A)** Posttraumatic or postintubation croup is treated with mist inhalations, steroids, and racemic epinephrine. Steroids are not immediately effective, and some question their use at all, but they usually are given. Sedation of the child is based on the decision whether or not the child's anxiety may be contributing to the problem. Sedation should not be a routine order. *(177:265; 178:639; 180:437)*

27. **(C)** The child with epiglottitis typically is sitting up to allow better handling of the secretions. Since the child has pain on swallowing, drooling is common. The onset is sudden, and the child is febrile. *(177:180; 180:257)*

28. **(E)** The child with laryngotracheobronchitis (croup) has a gradual onset of symptoms, has a barking cough, a low grade, if any, fever, and a subglottic obstruction. *(177:164; 180:257)*

29. **(D)** Postintubation croup is uncommon in the newborn unless the tube is place for long periods of time. This may result in subglottic stenosis. Lubricants are of no help in reducing croup. Oxygen and mist are appropriate therapy. Croup is manifest on inspiration. *(177:265; 178:639; 180:436)*

30. **(D)** The newborn infant requires anesthesia and should receive anesthesia. Studies have demonstrated that the newborn reacts to pain. If the child has an unstable cardiovascular system and cannot tolerate anesthesia, resuscitation should proceed, and the anesthesia should be resumed after stability is restored. This does not differ from our treatment of adults. *(75:1263; 182:3)*

CHAPTER 11

Respiratory Therapy
Review

There is much overlap in the fields of anesthesiology and respiratory therapy, since both are greatly concerned with the respiratory system. Exposure to respiratory therapy equipment varies with the training programs and may be affected by the interest of the teaching staff and the time spent out of the operating room. Rotations through intensive care units bring us into contact with the equipment and give us a chance to become familiar with the various forms of therapy.

The field of respiratory therapy has come a long way from the time it was the oxygen therapy service in the hospital. Acuity of medical care has required an intensified approach to the respiratory care of the patient. The widespread use (and abuse) of intermittent positive pressure breathing (IPPB) in the postoperative patient has been supplanted by a systematic approach to the postoperative patient and giving care suited to the need.

This field has grown and, unfortunately, so has the long list of abbreviations. One must work to remain current with the constant developments in equipment and techniques.

The basic science of respiratory therapy is the same as that of anesthesiology. Anatomy and physiology of the respiratory system as well as pharmacologic applications are already known to you. The approach to the patient with an artificial airway is a part of our daily activity. We should all review the aseptic approach to the artificial airway. In the operating room, this is often done poorly. We cannot expect the personnel in the intensive care units to use aseptic technique when we have a more cavalier attitude in the operating room.

Ventilatory techniques useful in the long-term care of the patient are not used in the operating room. When we use a ventilator in the operating room, it is to control the ventilation. Techniques in use in the intensive care units will control the ventilation of some patients and supplement the respiration of others.

The various modes of ventilator maintenance therapy should be reviewed, including intermittent mandatory ventilation (IMV), synchronized intermittent mandatory ventilation (SIMV), and pressure support systems. Positive end-expiratory pressure (PEEP) ventilation, with its indications and contraindications, is an important mode of therapy today. In addition, the various forms of high-frequency ventilation are becoming more common. Studies of the effectiveness and uses of these techniques are still being carried out.

The applications of continuous positive airway pressure (CPAP) in the infant and adult should be reviewed. This technique has applications also in the patient being weaned from artificial ventilation.

One of the most common areas of overlap with the respiratory therapist is in the care of the postoperative patient in the recovery room and the postsurgical units. Methods to ensure patent airways and alveoli are very important to each of us. We must be aware of all of the maneuvers in use to prevent and treat alveolar collapse. The current use of incentive spirometry has improved the care of the postoperative patient.

Respiratory therapy is not without its own risks. Barotrauma and cross-infection are common occurrences. Since the patients who are receiving the therapy often are debilitated, these added complications may be an important factor in their recovery.

Questions

DIRECTIONS (Questions 1 through 15): Each of the numbered items or incomplete statements in this section is followed by answers or by completions of the statement. Select the <u>ONE</u> lettered answer or completion that is <u>BEST</u> in each case.

1. Which of the following is not a contraindication to the use of intermittent positive pressure breathing (IPPB)?

   (A) atelectasis
   (B) active tuberculosis
   (C) hemoptysis
   (D) shock
   (E) pneumothorax

2. Intermittent positive pressure breathing (IPPB) has the following physiologic effect

   (A) decrease in mean airway pressure
   (B) decrease in inspiratory mechanical bronchodilatation
   (C) decrease in the work of breathing
   (D) a preservation of the patient's inspiratory/expiratory (I:E) ratio
   (E) a decrease in tidal volume

3. The efficiency of respiratory therapy is primarily dependent on the

   (A) patient's condition
   (B) medication used
   (C) therapist
   (D) nurse at the bedside
   (E) machine being used

Questions 4 and 5
Please refer to the following figure:

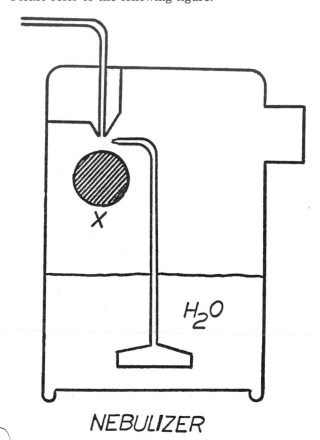

NEBULIZER

4. In the figure, the object marked with an X is

   (A) an atomizer
   (B) an injector
   (C) a heat element
   (D) a baffle
   (E) a screen

5. The purpose of the object depicted with an X is to

   (A) provide large droplets to be delivered
   (B) heat the incoming air

(C) provide small, uniform-sized droplets
(D) obstruct gas flow
(E) sterilize the gas flow

6. Aerosol therapy is useful in providing all of the following EXCEPT

(A) improved bronchial hygiene
(B) humidification
(C) a means to deliver medication
(D) decreased coughing
(E) expectoration promotion

7. If a drug is administered by inhalation, the blood level will most likely resemble that of the

(A) intravenous route
(B) subcutaneous route
(C) intramuscular route
(D) oral route
(E) rectal route

8. A partial rebreathing mask contains a small reservoir bag that

(A) requires an added oxygen flow
(B) leads to increased carbon dioxide
(C) leads to decreased carbon dioxide
(D) provides a high F_{IO_2} and conserves oxygen
(E) has no effect on blood gases

9. A technique most useful in treatment of bronchopleural fistula is

(A) spontaneous breathing with a mask
(B) assisted ventilation with positive pressure
(C) controlled ventilation with a mechanical ventilator
(D) positive end-expiratory pressure
(E) high-frequency jet ventilation

10. The usual inspiratory/expiratory (I:E) ratio during spontaneous breathing is

(A) 1:1
(B) 2:1
(C) 1:2
(D) 1:3
(E) 1:4

11. All of the following statements regarding suctioning of the airway in the patient with an artificial airway are true EXCEPT it

(A) should be done at least every hour
(B) may lead to bradycardia
(C) may lead to hypoxemia
(D) may cause trauma to the mucosa
(E) may lead to mucosal bleeding

12. Negative pressure during expiration

(A) decreases atelectasis
(B) decreases mean intrathoracic pressure
(C) decreases air trapping
(D) is useful in emphysema
(E) has no effect on small airways

13. The partial rebreathing oxygen mask

(A) is used to increase the patient's carbon dioxide
(B) is less efficient than an oxygen cannula
(C) can provide oxygen concentration over 60%
(D) can provide 100% oxygen
(E) provides over 60% oxygen regardless of mask fit

14. Absorption atelectasis

(A) is clinically unimportant
(B) occurs primarily with low-flow oxygen therapy
(C) occurs when high partial pressures of nitrogen are present
(D) occurs more with early airway closure
(E) is never seen when denitrogenation has been used

15. The pressure within a tracheal tube cuff that will interrupt mucosal blood flow is

(A) 5 mm Hg
(B) 10 mm Hg
(C) 15 mm Hg
(D) 20 mm Hg
(E) 30 mm Hg

DIRECTIONS (Questions 16 through 30): For each of the items in this section, ONE or MORE of the numbered options is correct. Choose the answer

A if only 1, 2, and 3 are correct,
B if only 1 and 3 are correct,
C if only 2 and 4 are correct,
D if only 4 is correct,
E if all are correct.

16. Racemic epinephrine administered by aerosol

(1) is a mixture of epinephrine and norepinephrine
(2) is a potent alpha and beta stimulant
(3) causes mucosal edema
(4) is a mild bronchodilator

17. When a drug is delivered by aerosol, it

(1) will not be effective
(2) may have a topical effect
(3) will only reach the larynx
(4) may have a systemic effect

SUMMARY OF DIRECTIONS

A	B	C	D	E
1, 2, 3 only	1, 3 only	2, 4 only	4 only	All are correct

18. Aerosol therapy may cause
    (1) lower airway obstruction
    (2) fluid overload
    (3) contamination of the airway
    (4) decreased bronchospasm

19. The pulmonary changes characteristic of the post-operative period include
    (1) decreased total lung capacity
    (2) decreased functional residual capacity
    (3) decreased residual volume
    (4) increased compliance

20. The use of blow bottles in the postoperative period
    (1) leads to decreased pleural pressure
    (2) causes alveolar opening
    (3) will decrease atelectasis
    (4) is an expiratory meaneuver

21. In order to avoid postoperative atelectasis
    (1) alveolar collapse must be avoided
    (2) closed alveoli must be opened
    (3) maneuvers to keep alveoli open must be repeated hourly
    (4) inhaled volume is most important

22. The mark "Z-79" on an endotracheal tube
    (1) refers to the size of the tube
    (2) refers to a committee of the American Standards Institute
    (3) refers to the manufacturer of the tube
    (4) identifies the tube as nontoxic

23. A patient being maintained on artificial ventilation becomes infected with *Serratia marcescens*. This may have come from a
    (1) contaminated nebulizer
    (2) caretaker's contaminated hands
    (3) contaminated drug vial
    (4) contaminated ventilator

24. Intermittent mandatory ventilation (IMV)
    (1) allows spontaneous ventilation
    (2) gives a prescribed number of ventilations per minute

    (3) ventilates the patient independent of his or her own breathing
    (4) is the same as assisted ventilation

25. Positive end-expiratory pressure (PEEP)
    (1) causes a decreased functional residual capacity
    (2) may cause decreased blood pressure
    (3) causes a decreased compliance
    (4) may cause barotrauma

26. The optimal PEEP level depends on the
    (1) degree of hypoxemia
    (2) type of lung disease
    (3) state of hydration
    (4) state of left ventricular function

27. The use of postural drainage is an effective method to augment lung clearance mechanisms. The prone position with the head down
    (1) will assist in drainage of the lower lobes
    (2) will inhibit drainage of apical segments
    (3) may be dangerous in the neurosurgical patient
    (4) may increase intracranial pressure

28. The mask shown in the illustration

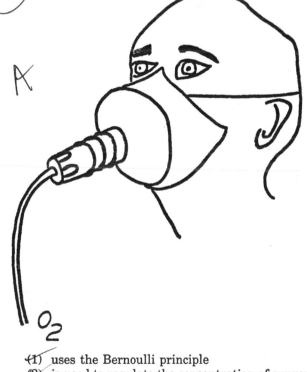

O₂

    (1) uses the Bernoulli principle
    (2) is used to regulate the concentration of oxygen
    (3) uses oxygen to entrain air
    (4) depends on the patient's respiration to determine oxygen concentration

29. Protocols for suctioning the patient with an artificial airway should include

   (1) preoxygenation
   (2) use of a catheter as close to the size of the airway as possible
   (3) application of suction for less than 15 seconds
   (4) bagging the patient with room air after suctioning is completed

30. In order to cough and deep-breathe adequately, a patient must

   (1) have a vital capacity of 20 ml/kg (or three times the tidal volume)
   (2) be alert and cooperative
   (3) have a functioning ciliary mechanism
   (4) be free of all narcotics

Answers and Explanations

1. **(A)** Atelectasis is not a contraindication to IPPB. It is one of the indications for its use. IPPB should not be employed in the patient with tuberculosis for fear of spreading the disease or in the patient with hemoptysis, shock, or pneumothorax lest those conditions be made worse. *(1:1131; 32:128)*

2. **(C)** IPPB will decrease the work of breathing. Mean airway pressure is increased. Bronchodilatation is increased. The tidal volume is increased, and the patient's I:E ratio is altered. *(1:1131; 32:124)*

3. **(C)** The purpose of IPPB is to increase the patient's tidal volume. Studies have shown that the factor most important in achieving that purpose is the therapist. The machine, the disease, the medication, and the nurse are all of secondary importance. *(32:127)*

4. **(D)** The object marked by the X is a baffle. This is an integral part of the nebulizer. The baffle is placed in the path of the air flow. The air, containing water particles, strikes the baffle. The water particles break up into small and large particles. The small particles are swept away with the gas flow, and the larger ones fall back into the water reservoir. *(1:2181; 32:101)*

5. **(C)** See answer to Question 4. *(1:2180; 32:101)*

6. **(D)** An increase in cough after mobilizing the secretions is one of the aims of aerosol therapy. This leads to improved bronchial hygiene. The aerosol may also be used to deliver medication. *(32:106)*

7. **(A)** Aerosol therapy is delivered into the lung with a large surface area. Uptake of medication is close to that of intravenous administration. For this reason, the blood level may rise rapidly. *(1:59; 32:113)*

8. **(D)** The partial rebreathing mask provides an increased F_{IO_2} and conserves oxygen. The oxygen flow can be decreased. Oxygen tension in the blood should be increased. There is no effect on carbon dioxide. *(1:2178; 32:184)*

9. **(E)** The patient with a bronchopleural fistula requires a method of ventilation that does not increase the flow across the fistula. Spontaneous ventilation with a mask is seldom sufficient, and methods employing positive pressure may not be able to accomplish ventilation because of loss of inspired air through the fistula. In these patients, the use of high-frequency ventilation may be lifesaving. *(32:447; 75:933)*

10. **(C)** The normal I:E time is 1:2. The longer expiratory time allows the airways to clear the inhaled gases. The patient with obstructive lung disease has prolonged expiratory times. We must be concerned with the ratio, since efficient ventilation requires that the times be adjusted to the individual patient. *(32:347)*

11. **(A)** Suctioning of the artificial airway is not a benign procedure. Even with the best technique there may be hypoxemia, with resultant bradycardia, and trauma to the airway. For this reason, suctioning should be done only when indicated. There should be some evidence of secretions that can be cleared. In addition, aseptic technique must be employed. *(1:2182; 32:252)*

12. **(B)** Negative pressure during exhalation decreases the mean intrathoracic pressure, allowing airways to collapse. This expiratory maneuver is no longer in use, since it has been shown to increase atelectasis and to close the small airways. The present treatment is to provide expiratory retard to keep the airways open. *(32:404; 34:120)*

13. **(C)** The partial rebreathing mask can provide an oxygen concentration over 60% but not 100%. The mask is more efficient than an oxygen cannula. The mask is not used to increase carbon dioxide. *(1:2178; 32:184)*

14. **(D)** Absorption atelectasis occurs with high oxygen concentrations. It is more important when the nitrogen concentration is low. If denitrogenation is

used, absorption atelectasis is more likely. Early airway closure increases the risk of absorption atelectasis. This is clinically important, since shunting can occur around the atelectatic units. *(1:1157; 32:339)*

15. **(E)** The pressure within the cuff that will interrupt mucosal flow is 30 mm Hg. The pressure at the venous end is 18 mm Hg. For this reason, the cuff pressure should be kept at about 15 mm Hg. This should prevent some of the tracheal damage. *(1:533; 32:273)*

16. **(D)** Racemic epinephrine is a mild bronchodilator. This drug is a 50/50 mixture of the levo- and dextro-isomers of epinephrine. Compared with epinephrine, the drug has little alpha and beta effects. It is a good mucosal decongestant. *(32:120)*

17. **(C)** A drug delivered by aerosol may have a topical and/or systemic effect. If the particles are small, they are transmitted to the distal bronchial tree and have an effect. *(32:113)*

18. **(A)** Aerosol therapy can cause obstruction of the lower airway due to swelling of the retained secretions that are present. The secretions swell, since they take up the water that is being used in the aerosol. Any aerosol can lead to fluid overload if the fluid delivered is not considered in the overall fluid plan. Contamination of respiratory therapy equipment is a constant threat. Aerosols may lead to bronchospasm because of irritation of the airways. *(32:108)*

19. **(A)** The postoperative period is marked by a decreased lung capacity, decreased functional residual capacity, and decreased residual volume. Respiratory therapy maneuvers in the postoperative period are aimed at increasing these volumes. The compliance is decreased. *(32:518, 75:1410, 207:1017)*

20. **(D)** The use of blow bottles in the postoperative period is an expiratory maneuver. It is an ineffective measure to increase the volumes, since the pressure closes the alveoli and will increase atelectasis. The effectiveness is in the deep breath that is needed to use the bottles. If the instructions are to finish the exercise by taking a final deep breath, it might be helpful. Inspiratory maneuvers are more effective. *(75:941; 207:1018)*

21. **(E)** All of the options are true. Alveolar collapse must be prevented and treated when it occurs. Inhaled volume is more important than pressure. If maneuvers are to be effective, they must be used hourly. Incentive spirometers that can be placed at the bedside are effective, since the patient can use

them without the presence of a therapist. *(32:150; 207; 1018)*

22. **(C)** The mark "Z-79" on an endotracheal tube refers to a committee of the American Standards Institute. The mark identifies the tube as nontoxic and in compliance with the standards set down. The initials "I.T." stand for implant tested and also show that the tube is nontoxic. *(32:239; 75:548)*

23. **(E)** *Serratia marcescens* was at one time considered a nonpathologic contaminant and was used to test distribution of air flows throughout buildings. It is now known to be a pathogen, and it is especially a problem with respiratory therapy equipment. Contaminated vials of drugs used for nebulizers have been common sites for growth, but hands and equipment also are common culture sites. *(2:578; 32:108 109)*

24. **(A)** IMV allows the patient to maintain his or her own breathing and receive a prescribed number of breaths per minute from the ventilator. It differs from assisted ventilation in that the breaths from the ventilator do not augment the patient's breaths. *(1:2164,2206; 32:384)*

25. **(C)** The use of PEEP may cause decreased blood pressure, especially in the hypovolemic patient. Since it causes increased intrathoracic pressure, one must be aware that barotrauma may occur. *(32:408; 75:1412)*

26. **(E)** The optimal PEEP level depends on the degree of hypoxemia. One need not go to high levels if the degree of hypoxemia is low. The type of lung disease also will affect the amount of PEEP used. The patient with emphysema and blebs in the lung will not benefit from PEEP and is more prone to barotrauma. Hydration and cardiac status are also important, since the patient with dehydration and poor contractility may not be able to withstand any increase in intrathoracic pressure. On the other hand, these patients may be helped by an increase in oxygenation. Careful titration is required. *(32:429; 75:1461)*

27. **(E)** Postural drainage is helpful in ridding the lungs of secretions, but other effects must be understood and considered. The patient with increased intracranial pressure may be injured by the head-down position needed to clear the lower lobes. *(32:137,138)*

28. **(A)** The Venturi mask uses oxygen flow to entrain air and regulate the oxygen concentration. This works on the Bernoulli principle. The patient's respiration is not a determinant. *(1:2178; 32:181)*

29. **(B)** Protocols for suctioning include preoxygenation and the use of a catheter smaller than the internal diameter of the tube. This allows air to pass down along the suction catheter and prevents the creation of a vacuum in the lungs when suction is applied. In addition, the suction should be applied for short periods (less than 15 seconds), and the patient should be bagged with 100% oxygen at the end of the procedure. *(1:2182; 32:251)*

30. **(A)** The ability to cough requires a good vital capacity, an alert and cooperative patient and a functioning ciliary mechanism. If any of these is missing, the cough will be less effective. Narcotics may reduce the pain of the cough, and the patient may be able to cooperate better. *(32:84,126)*

CHAPTER 12

Anesthesia Equipment
Review

The anesthesia machine and the ancillary equipment that are necessary for us to practice our profession have changed dramatically in the past decade. Machines that were fairly simple have become covered with new devices that measure flows, oxygen concentration, and pressures and scavenge our excess gases. Monitoring has grown from a blood pressure cuff and precordial stethoscope to a myriad of machines to record temperature, end-tidal carbon dioxide, oxygen saturation, and agents. Many of the devices have alarms that give a signal when a certain measure is out of the programmed acceptable range. The noise level is increasing. This has transformed some of our vigilance aids into distractions.

Equipment now has a very short life span before becoming obsolete. New machines are being designed and produced to make anesthesia safer for the patient and for the operating room environment. Even the textbooks on equipment become outdated very soon after they are published.

These facts make it harder to become familiar with anesthesia equipment. One should understand the physics of the components when that is appropriate and know the basic function of the anesthesia machine. The book *Understanding Anesthesia Equipment* by Dorsch and Dorsch (see reference 170) is an excellent text for study. The major textbooks of anesthesiology have brief sections, but they are not comprehensive. An anesthesiologist should be aware of the function of the equipment not only for the welfare of the patient but also for his or her own safety.

The use of compressed gases is an important part of our profession. It is a useful exercise to think through the movement of a gas, such as oxygen, from the tank outside your hospital to its delivery to the patient at the Y-piece. The entire piping system, the safety systems employed, and the problems associated with them should be reviewed. The diameter index safety system (DISS) and the pin index safety system should be a part of your knowledge. Methods to jerry-rig a system to circumvent these safety features have led to disaster on more than one occasion. The handling and storage of cylinders are important since we are the primary users of this supply of gases and are responsible for its storage and use.

The gas laws, covered in the section on respiration and physics, should be reviewed.

Regulators and devices to provide gases at usable pressures in our systems are important for the anesthesia machine. The fail-safe systems and the newer gas proportioner systems are of great value, and you should have a knowledge of their function.

The variety of vaporizers has decreased over the past decade. Although some of the older units are still in use, they are being replaced by newer models that are more efficient and safer. Features have been introduced to prevent the simultaneous delivery of two agents. The lockout methods vary with the machines. It is still possible to put the wrong agent in a vaporizer. Efforts to provide specific filling tubes for specific agents have not been well received. Overfilling has been eliminated by new design.

Flowmeters are manufactured as a unit. The float and the tubing are calibrated together. If one is lost or broken, the entire system must be replaced. Floats are designed to be read at the top of the float, except for the ball float, which is read at the middle of the ball. The float should always be floating freely and spinning in the tubing to demonstrate that it is not stuck. Dirty tubing can lead to a stuck float, leading to incorrect flow readings. The physics of the flowmeter tube and the gas flow through it should be reviewed.

The various gas delivery systems—circle, nonrebreathing, and closed—should be reviewed. The circle system is the one in most widespread use today in the adult patient. The varied arrangements of the components of the system and the functions of the components should be reviewed. The chemistry of soda lime or barium absorbents should be known.

The nonrebreathing system is in use mostly for the pediatric patient. Most use the Mapleson D modification of the system. Another modification, the Bain circuit, has gained wide usage. The flow requirements in the spontaneously breathing patient and the patient whose ventilation is being controlled should be reviewed.

The scavenger systems that are now a part of our machines have led to decreased trace gases in the operating room but have themselves introduced new problems.

Collapsed reservoir bags and increased system pressure have been reported. The problem of trace gases in general and the associated (causative?) diseases should be known. Methods to decrease the amount of trace gases should be reviewed not just for our protection but for the protection of all in the operating room suite.

The references detail the methods of cleaning the anesthesia equipment that has been in contact with the patient. With the current concern with the AIDS patient, this must become a part of our knowledge base.

Questions

DIRECTIONS (Questions 1 through 30): Each of the numbered items or incomplete statements in this section is followed by answers or by completions of the statement. Select the ONE lettered answer or completion that is BEST in each case.

1. The vapor pressure of a liquid is most dependent on

   (A) the atmospheric pressure
   (B) the specific heat of the container
   (C) the temperature
   (D) the conductivity of the container
   (E) the partial pressure of the gas

2. The most significant risk of a free-standing vaporizer is

   (A) using the wrong agent
   (B) tipping
   (C) foaming of the agent
   (D) leakage
   (E) overfilling

3. The Bain circuit is a modification of the

   (A) Mapleson A system
   (B) Mapleson B system
   (C) Mapleson C system
   (D) Mapleson D system
   (E) Mapleson E system

4. The lifetime of a canister filling of soda lime

   (A) depends on the method of filling
   (B) is independent of the volume of CO_2 exhaled
   (C) is independent of the location of the relief valve
   (D) is prolonged by low gas flows
   (E) is shortened by channeling

5. The hardness of soda lime

   (A) is assured by the addition of silica
   (B) is of little importance
   (C) is undesirable because as the granule disintegrates, it becomes more absorptive
   (D) causes channeling
   (E) imparts a uniform-sized granule

6. The advantages of using a Bain circuit include all of the following EXCEPT

   (A) rewarming of the fresh gas by the exhaled gas
   (B) good humidification
   (C) reduced weight of the system
   (D) concentric design
   (E) ease of scavenging waste gases

Questions 7 and 8
Please refer to the following figure:

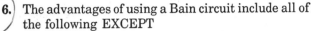

7. The system depicted in the figure is the

   (A) Georgia valve
   (B) Jackson-Rees system
   (C) T-piece
   (D) Bain circuit
   (E) Mapleson A system

8. The reported disadvantages of the circuit in the illustration include all of the following EXCEPT

   (A) inability to use spontaneous ventilation with the system
   (B) requirement for low flow
   (C) inability to scavenge waste gases
   (D) presence of overflow valve farther from the patient
   (E) kinking of inner delivery tube

9. In the closed system, the one measure that must be met is

   (A) the tidal volume
   (B) the minute volume
   (C) the respiratory rate
   (D) the oxygen consumption
   (E) the needed anesthesia

10. If either the Fluomatic or Fluotec Mark II vaporizer is tipped over

    (A) the wick will become saturated
    (B) the vaporizer must be returned to the factory
    (C) the concentration of the vapor will be higher than calculated
    (D) a low concentration will result
    (E) the vaporizer should be righted and put into use

11. The Tec-4 vaporizers are

    (A) temperature and pressure compensated
    (B) temperature compensated only
    (C) pressure compensated only
    (D) neither pressure nor temperature compensated
    (E) most accurate at 30°C

12. The Vapor 19.1 vaporizer is temperature compensated as a result of a(n)

    (A) bimetallic band
    (B) copper element
    (C) expansion element in the vaporizing chamber
    (D) sintered disc
    (E) heating element that keeps the vaporizer at a constant temperature

13. The pumping effect in reference to a vaporizer

    (A) leads to a decreased concentration of the agent
    (B) refers to a method of filling the vaporizer
    (C) refers to a method of cleaning the vaporizer
    (D) leads to a decreased flow through the vaporizer
    (E) is more pronounced at low flow rates

14. If halothane is being used, the flow through the kettle is 100 ml, the room temperature is 20°C, and the flow of gases is 2 L of oxygen and 2 L of nitrous oxide, the concentration of halothane is

    (A) 0.5%
    (B) 1%
    (C) 1.25%
    (D) 2%
    (E) 3%

15. All of the following flowmeter indicators are read at the top EXCEPT the

    (A) nonrotating float
    (B) plumb bob float
    (C) skirted float
    (D) ball float
    (E) H float

16. Disadvantages of heated humidifiers include all of the following EXCEPT

    (A) tracheal burn due to increased heat
    (B) fluid overload of the patient
    (C) decreased airway resistance

    (D) bulkiness
    (E) water accumulation in the delivery hoses

17. All of the following are rules for safe use of cylinders EXCEPT that

    (A) cylinders should be stored in airtight rooms
    (B) cylinders should not be stored near flammable materials
    (C) flammable gases and gases that support combustion should be stored separately
    (D) cylinders should not be stored by a source of heat or flame
    (E) empty and full cylinders should be stored separately

18. Wood's metal is

    (A) an alloy used in fusible plugs of cylinders
    (B) used in flowmeters
    (C) used in vaporizers
    (D) used in circle systems to conduct heat
    (E) used to facilitate CO_2 absorption

19. The anesthesia system depicted in the illustration is a

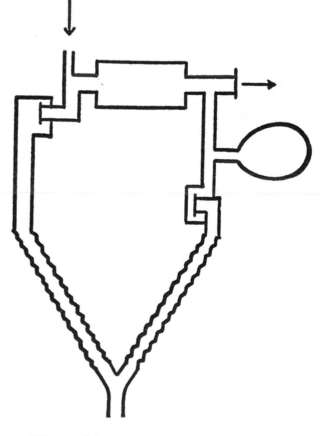

    (A) to-and-fro system
    (B) Magill system
    (C) circle system
    (D) nonrebreathing system
    (E) T-piece

20. The purpose of cracking an oxygen cylinder is to

(A) remove gaseous impurities
(B) establish that there is gas in the tank
(C) establish that the gas in the tank is oxygen
(D) remove dust or other flammable substances from the yoke
(E) check the cylinder valve

21. The pin index system prevents

(A) the connection of the wrong gas to the cylinder manifold
(B) the delivery of the wrong gas from the wall
(C) the delivery of a hypoxic mixture from the flow-meter
(D) starting a case with empty tanks
(E) improper pipe fittings from the source of gas to the wall

22. In the illustration, the oxygen flowmeter should be at position

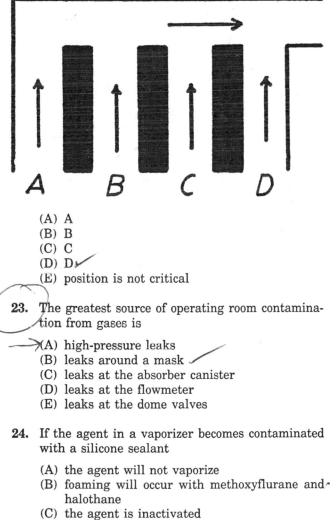

(A) A
(B) B
(C) C
(D) D
(E) position is not critical

23. The greatest source of operating room contamination from gases is

(A) high-pressure leaks
(B) leaks around a mask
(C) leaks at the absorber canister
(D) leaks at the flowmeter
(E) leaks at the dome valves

24. If the agent in a vaporizer becomes contaminated with a silicone sealant

(A) the agent will not vaporize
(B) foaming will occur with methoxyflurane and halothane
(C) the agent is inactivated
(D) no adverse effect will occur
(E) discoloration will occur

25. Overfilling of a vaporizer

(A) will cause the vaporizer not to function
(B) will yield a concentration of halothane lower than that dialed
(C) is eliminated in modern vaporizers
(D) is not a problem with a copper kettle
(E) will decrease oxygen delivery

26. The patient in the posttonsillectomy position

(A) lies on his or her back
(B) has the down-side leg kept straight
(C) has the down-side arm flexed
(D) has the up-side arm straight
(E) is kept prone

27. In the kidney position, proper technique includes

(A) arms at side
(B) kidney rest under the lower rib cage
(C) lower leg flexed
(D) upper leg flexed
(E) head kept flat on the table

28. The position best tolerated by the surgical patient is the

(A) lithotomy position
(B) prone position
(C) horizontal supine position
(D) Trendelenburg position
(E) Fowler position

29. A factor NOT involved in the stretch mechanism responsible for brachial plexus injury is the

(A) pectoralis minor tendon attachment to the coracoid process
(B) clavicle
(C) first rib
(D) subclavian artery
(E) head of the humerus

30. The nervous structures most likely involved in improper positioning are nerves of the

(A) cervical plexus
(B) brachial plexus
(C) lumbar plexus
(D) sciatic system
(E) autonomic system

DIRECTIONS (Questions 31 through 60): For each of
the items in this section, ONE or MORE of the numbered options is correct. Choose the answer

A if only 1, 2, and 3 are correct,
B if only 1 and 3 are correct,
C if only 2 and 4 are correct,
D if only 4 is correct,
E if all are correct.

31. The Cole tube

(1) has a lower resistance when compared to a tube
of similar size
(2) is the tube of choice for nasotracheal intubation
(3) carries less likelihood of endobronchial intubation
(4) should be inserted to the maximum distance
possible to get a good fit

32. When using a Macintosh blade for laryngoscopy,
the

(1) epiglottis is lifted directly
(2) laryngoscope is held in the right hand
(3) blade enters the mouth on the left side
(4) tip is advanced to the space between the base of
the tongue and the epiglottis

33. The Macintosh laryngoscope blade

(1) has a straight spatula
(2) has no flange
(3) has a pointed tip
(4) is manufactured in various sizes

34. Nasopharyngeal airways are contraindicated in the
patient with

(1) nasal polyps
(2) sepsis of the nasopharynx
(3) a very low platelet count
(4) the jaw wired shut

35. The use of a mask to administer anesthesia may be
complicated by

(1) contact dermatitis
(2) trigeminal nerve injury
(3) an increased incidence of nausea and vomiting
(4) conjunctival edema

36. A regulator used on a compressible gas cylinder

(1) reduces the pressure of the gas as it rises from
the cylinder
(2) is an instrument of measure
(3) permits the expansion of the compressed gas to
a lower pressure
(4) measures the pressure of the gas in pounds per
square inch(psi)

37. Cylinders for compressed gases

(1) are marked only with letters designating the
gas contained
(2) are designated by a letter referring to the size
(3) are made of aluminum
(4) have a letter designation, and the gas capacity
increases as one advances in the alphabet

38. Safe practices recommended by the Compressed
Gas Association include

(1) do not handle cylinders or apparatus with oily
hands
(2) to detect leaks, an open flame may be used
(3) fully open the cylinder valve when the cylinder
is in use
(4) leave the wrapper on the cylinder when it is in
use

39. The oxygen analyzer

(1) is a good disconnect alarm
(2) should be placed on the exhalation side of the
circuit
(3) is unaffected by humidity
(4) should be placed on the fresh gas side of the
circuit

40. When a gas stream passes through a vaporizing
chamber, the

(1) most energetic molecules are swept out
(2) molecules with the most surface force are swept
out
(3) mean energy of the liquid falls
(4) temperature of the liquid increases

41. The reaction of carbon dioxide and soda lime produces

(1) $CaCO_3$
(2) Na_2CO_3
(3) H_2O
(4) HCl

42. Soda lime granules

(1) are manufactured to be smooth and round
(2) are of a size 4 to 8 mesh
(3) of a small size give a lower resistance
(4) of a small size give better absorption function

43. The function of the reservoir bag is to

(1) accumulate gas during expiration
(2) provide a means for assisting or controlling
respiration
(3) serve as a monitor of ventilation
(4) serve as a pressure buffer because of its compliance

44. The vapor pressure of a liquid

   (1) is a function of its temperature
   (2) decreases with an increase in temperature
   (3) is not affected by the total barometric pressure above the liquid
   (4) increases with a decrease in temperature

45. If using a multiple-agent vaporizer, confusion will be avoided if

   (1) one always checks the agent present by smell
   (2) one always labels the vaporizer
   (3) drainage of one agent is followed immediately by filling with another
   (4) one always discards the agent if the identity of the agent is in question

46. The standard measurement(s) for anesthesia and ventilator fittings is (are)

   (1) 12 mm
   (2) 15 mm
   (3) 18 mm
   (4) 22 mm

47. In a nonrebreathing system

   (1) inspired gas tensions may be held constant
   (2) humidification is optimal
   (3) change of flow produces rapid changes in inspired concentrations
   (4) one adds oxygen in amounts just to satisfy metabolic requirements

48. The advantage(s) of the semiclosed system is (are)

   (1) decreased resistance to ventilation
   (2) fast change of concentration
   (3) moisture collection in the system
   (4) constancy of inspired concentration

49. The fail-safe system installed on anesthesia machines

   (1) prevents delivery of a hypoxic mixture
   (2) prevents flow unless the oxygen flowmeter is on
   (3) requires that oxygen tanks be full
   (4) works on a pressure principle

50. The float in a flowmeter

   (1) may stick at a high level if the tube is dirty
   (2) is made to remain static during flow
   (3) may give an inaccurate reading if back pressure builds up
   (4) may be replaced with another if it is lost

51. The Fluotec-4 vaporizer

   (1) is an in-circuit vaporizer
   (2) is temperature compensated
   (3) is calibrated for halothane and enflurane
   (4) diverts only a portion of the flow into the vaporizing chamber

52. The ideal anesthesia system would have

   (1) accuracy and precision
   (2) low dead space
   (3) low resistance
   (4) conservation of moisture

53. Sterilization of medical equipment with gamma radiation

   (1) can be done on prepackaged equipment
   (2) is not associated with a rise in temperature
   (3) requires no airing period
   (4) does not cause toxic effects on polyvinylchloride plastics

54. The diameter index safety system (DISS)

   (1) prevents attachment of gas-administering equipment to the wrong type of gas
   (2) prevents incorrect yoke–tank connections
   (3) is based on matching specific bores and diameters
   (4) is not used on suction hoses

55. In order to calculate the concentration of an agent when using a kettle vaporizer, you must know the

   (1) temperature
   (2) temperature—vapor pressure curve
   (3) volume of inflow gas
   (4) total flow

56. The nerve(s) most likely to be injured in the lithotomy position is (are) the

   (1) obturator nerve
   (2) femoral nerve
   (3) saphenous nerve
   (4) peroneal nerve

57. In the supine position, the patient's weight is borne by the

   (1) occiput
   (2) sacrum
   (3) scapulae
   (4) heels

58. In the prone position, points that must be protected from pressure and compression include

   (1) eyes
   (2) male genitalia
   (3) breasts
   (4) toes

SUMMARY OF DIRECTIONS				
A	**B**	**C**	**D**	**E**
1, 2, 3 only	1, 3 only	2, 4 only	4 only	All are correct

59. Nerve injuries occurring during anesthesia are
    (1) more frequent with long nerves
    (2) always due to poor positioning
    (3) more frequent with superficial nerves
    (4) less common in the patient with ischemic disease

60. Symptoms referable to positioning may involve the
    (1) circulatory system
    (2) respiratory system
    (3) nervous system
    (4) neuromuscular system

41/60

Answers and Explanations

1. **(C)** The vapor pressure of a liquid is most dependent on the temperature. It is independent of the atmospheric pressure. The heat conductivity of the container may affect the temperature, but it does not directly affect the vapor pressure. The specific heat of the container and the partial pressure of the gas are not determinants. *(75:104,526; 170:77)*

2. **(B)** The most troublesome problem with free-standing vaporizers is the danger of tipping, which can lead to very high concentrations of the agent. Use of the wrong agent, foaming, leaking, and overfilling are problems seen with all vaporizers and are not specific for free-standing vaporizers. *(75:522; 170:129)*

3. **(D)** The Bain circuit is a modification of the Mapleson D system. This system has a fresh gas inlet at the patient end, a piece of corrugated tubing that connects the inflow to the relief valve. The relief valve is adjacent to the reservoir bag. *(1:139; 75:532; 170:187)*

4. **(E)** Channeling of the airflow shortens the life of soda lime by allowing passage of the exhaled gas along channels of low resistance. This expends the soda lime along the channels, and carbon dioxide will flow through the system without being absorbed. The method of filling does not affect the length of soda lime usefulness. The relief valve position does have an effect. The valve should be placed to vent the air that has the highest concentration of carbon dioxide. The higher the gas flow, the longer the soda lime will last. *(170:218)*

5. **(A)** The hardness of soda lime is due to the addition of silica. The hardness decreases the amount of dust that is present. The dust can cause channeling and increased resistance and can be carried throughout the system. *(1:124; 75:534; 170:214)*

6. **(D)** The concentric design of the Bain circuit has led to some of the more serious problems. The inner tube may be disconnected or kink, leading to disruption of fresh gas flow. The other options are advantages of this system. *(1:140; 170:190)*

7. **(D)** The circuit shown is a Bain circuit, which is a modification of the Mapleson D system. *(1:140; 75:533; 170:187)*

8. **(E)** See answer to Question 6. *(1:140; 75:532; 170:190)*

9. **(D)** In any anesthesia system, the one factor that must be provided for is oxygen. All other considerations are secondary. *(170:309)*

10. **(C)** If a vaporizer tips over, liquid agent may find its way into the tubing. This will cause an increased concentration of anesthetic agent in the system. If tipping occurs, it is not necessary to return the vaporizer to the factory, but it must be righted and allowed to air out. It should not be put into immediate use. *(75:522; 170:129,309)*

11. **(B)** The Tec-4 series of vaporizers are temperature compensated. A steady back pressure will reduce the output of the vaporizer; therefore, they are not pressure compensated. *(75:519; 170:101)*

12. **(C)** The Vapor 19.1 vaporizer accomplishes temperature compensation by virtue of an expansion element that extends into the vaporizing chamber. Older vaporizers used the bimetallic band. No heating elements are involved. *(75:521; 170:115)*

13. **(E)** The pumping effect refers to the increase in anesthetic concentration from a vaporizer during assisted or controlled ventilation. This effect is more pronounced at low flow rates. *(75:518; 170:88)*

14. **(C)** The kettle vaporizer is not in widespread use today because of many problems inherent in its use. The formula to determine the concentration is detailed in the references. It would be helpful to understand the formula, not for use with the kettle but to understand vaporizers in general. *(1:129; 170:83)*

15. (D) The ball float is read at the midpoint of the ball. If one reads the flow at the bottom of a float designed to be read at the top, there is a considerable difference in flows. This may not be important in all machines or in all cases, but the effect is magnified at low flow rates. *(170:56)*

16. (C) Humidification causes increased airway resistance. The heated humidifier has many advantages, but the disadvantages can be troublesome. Water overload must be prevented. The system must be monitored for increased temperature that will be transmitted to the patient. Most humidifiers are bulky and not easy to use. Water accumulation in the hoses can present a problem. *(1:135; 170:171)*

17. (A) Cylinders should be stored in well-ventilated areas. Storage in areas near open flames or areas near flammable materials is discouraged. Empty and full containers should be stored separately to avoid confusion. Gases that are combustible and those that support combustion should be stored separately. *(170:10)*

18. (A) Wood's metal is an alloy that is employed in the fusible plug of a cylinder. This plug is designed to melt at a temperature of 200°F. If the cylinder is exposed to high heat, the plug will melt and the contents will be discharged before an explosion can occur. *(170:8)*

19. (C) The system in the picture is a circle system. This system has an absorber that contains soda lime or a similar absorbent, a fresh gas inlet, valves to direct flow, a relief valve, pressure gauge, breathing tubes, reservoir bag, and Y-piece. An oxygen analyzer is also a part of the system. *(1:142; 170:211)*

20. (D) Cracking a cylinder refers to the release of a small amount of gas from the cylinder before placing it on the yoke. Its purpose is to remove dust or other flammable material from the opening. *(170:13)*

21. (A) The pin index safety system is one of the safety systems built into the compressed gas system to prevent delivery of the wrong gas. This system is effective at the gas machine. On the other side of the wall, pipes may be transposed without our knowledge. This accentuates the importance of the oxygen analyzer. *(75:18; 170:10)*

22. (D) Placement of the oxygen in the position nearest to the common gas outlet will avoid delivery of a hypoxic mixture should a crack occur in the flowmeter tubing. If a leak occurs in this position, all components of the gas will leak out the crack in the tubing. *(75:513; 170:58)*

23. (A) The greatest source of operating room contamination with trace gases is from high-pressure leaks. These leaks, at wall outlets and machine connections, can contaminate the area even when the machine is not in use. *(1:152)*

24. (B) Foaming of halothane (and methoxyflurane) may occur if even small amounts of silicone sealants find their way into the vaporizing chamber. These materials should be avoided in the maintenance of vaporizers. The agent will continue to vaporize, but the foaming may cause liquid agent to be propelled out of the vaporizer, leading to high concentrations of the agent. *(170:312)*

25. (C) Overfilling of the vaporizer is mainly a problem of the past. Modern vaporizers are designed to avoid this hazard. When overfilling of a vaporizer occurs, the hazard of high concentrations is present due to delivery of liquid agent. *(75:522; 170:309)*

26. (B) The patient in the posttonsillectomy position lies on the side with the face downward. The downside leg is kept straight, the upper leg is flexed, and a pillow is placed between the legs. The down-side arm is extended slightly behind the torso, and the up-side arm is flexed with the hand near the head. *(16:12,158)*

27. (C) In the kidney position, the lower leg is flexed to give some stability to the position. The upper leg is kept straight. The arms are placed in a neutral position. The head is supported. If a kidney rest is used, it should be on the dependent iliac crest. *(16:249; 75:654)*

28. (C) The horizontal supine position is the one best tolerated, but even that one has its problems. Merely because the patient does not have to be moved should not cause one to be complacent with positioning. Pressure points should be padded, the superficial nerves protected, and the eyes protected. *(75:645)*

29. (D) The subclavian artery is not involved in brachial plexus injuries. The other options are important. One should check to determine if there is any tension in the position. The arm should be as free of tension as possible. This should be checked frequently during the procedure. *(1:403; 75:651)*

30. (B) The brachial plexus has been determined to be the most frequent source of nerve injuries. The second most frequent is the saphenous nerve. Although these may be reflections of the numbers of procedures in which these are at risk, all nerves should be protected. *(16:303)*

31. **(B)** The Cole tube is a tube with a small diameter at the distal end but a larger proximal end. The supposed advantage is that the tube cannot be placed in an endobronchial position. The resistance is lower, since the diameter is larger for part of the tube. There is no guarantee that endobronchial intubation will not occur. The tube should be advanced to a distance judged to be correct for the patient, not to the maximum distance. *(170:357)*

32. **(D)** The Macintosh blade is used by placing it in the space between the base of the tongue and the epiglottis. The laryngoscope is held in the left hand, and the blade enters the mouth on the right. *(1:529; 170:348)*

33. **(D)** The Macintosh blade is manufactured in various sizes. It has a flat tip, a curved spatula, and a flange. *(75:547; 170:339)*

34. **(A)** Any instrumentation of the nose should be done after taking a history to ascertain the absence of a condition likely to precipitate problems. Nasal polyps that may bleed or be sheared off, a low platelet count, and sepsis of the nasal areas are contraindications to the use of a nasopharyngeal airway. A wired jaw, in itself, is not a contraindication to a nasopharyngeal airway. *(170:333)*

35. **(E)** Application of a mask can lead to complications, especially if the application is used for prolonged periods. Contact dermatitis may occur with short exposures. *(170:330)*

36. **(B)** A regulator is a device to allow the compressed gas in a cylinder to be delivered at a usable pressure. It is not a device of measurement. *(170:43)*

37. **(C)** The cylinder markings indicate the serial number, the service pressure, the type of metal, the manufacturer, the type of manufacture, and the retest date. The cylinders are designated by letter, the larger cylinders having a letter higher in the alphabet. The cylinders are made of steel. *(170:5)*

38. **(B)** Cylinders should be unwrapped when in use. Flames should not be used to detect the presence of a gas. The cylinder valve should always be fully open when in use. Oily hands can lead to slippage, dropping the cylinder, and damage to the cylinder or rupture of it. This may lead to its being propelled as a missile. *(170:11)*

39. **(D)** The oxygen analyzer should be placed on the fresh gas side of the system. It is not a good disconnect alarm, since the time lag is too great. Analyzers may be affected by humidity by becoming nonfunctional. *(170:155)*

40. **(B)** When a gas stream passes through a vaporizer, the most energetic molecules, the ones above the liquid, are swept out. As vaporization occurs, the energy level falls, and the temperature decreases. Molecules with the most surface activity stay in the liquid. *(75:516; 170:80)*

41. **(B)** The reaction of carbon dioxide and soda lime yields calcium carbonate, sodium carbonate and water. No hydrochloric acid is formed. *(1:124; 75:534; 170:214)*

42. **(C)** Soda lime granules are in the size of 4 to 8 mesh. Smaller granules give a larger absorptive surface for the number of granules but cause more resistance. The irregular shape is better to give more absorptive area. *(1:124; 75:534; 170:214)*

43. **(E)** The reservoir bag on the machine has the function, besides being a reservoir, of a monitor, a ventilation assist device, and a pressure buffer. The reservoir of gases must be present to accommodate the needs of the inspiratory flow rate. *(170:144)*

44. **(B)** The vapor pressure is primarily a function of the temperature. It is not affected by the atmospheric pressure above the liquid. The vapor pressure decreases with temperature drops and increases with increased temperature. *(75:104,516; 170:77)*

45. **(C)** It is difficult to check the agent present in a vaporizer by smell because some vapors have such strong odors that they mask the presence of other agents. When changing from one agent to another, it is important to allow the vaporizer to be completely drained and completely evaporated before adding another agent to it. This question is not pertinent in the modern anesthesia machine. Our vaporizers are not used interchangeably. However, it is still possible to fill the vaporizer with the wrong agent, and one must know the proper steps to take to correct the mistake. *(1:128; 75:516; 170:127)*

46. **(C)** Standard fittings on the modern anesthesia machine are 15 mm and 22 mm. *(170:144)*

47. **(B)** In a nonrebreathing system, the anesthesia concentrations can be held constant. Changes can be made rapidly also, since there is no reservoir that must be equilibrated. Humidification is not good because no rebreathing occurs and the gases are discharged. Oxygen is always provided in amounts sufficient to provide a wide latitude of consumption. *(1:137; 170:207)*

48. **(D)** The advantage of a circle system is the constancy of inspired concentration. This is also a disadvantage if a fast change in concentration is needed.

There is more moisture in the system, which, if collected on the one-way valves, can be a problem. There is an increased resistance in the system. *(1:141; 170:232)*

49. **(D)** The fail-safe system is another safety system built into the machine. It is important to understand that this system is strictly pressure-related. As long as there is oxygen pressure in the machine, it is possible to deliver a hypoxic mixture to the patient. In contrast, newer machines have oxygen flow protectors, requiring either a certain flow of oxygen or that a certain proportion of the total flow be oxygen. These protect the patient from hypoxic mixtures. It is important to understand the system being employed. *(170:51)*

50. **(B)** The float may stick if the tubing is dirty. If back pressure can build up in the system, the reading may be inaccurate. The float should rotate to show that oxygen is flowing. If one component of the flowmeter set is broken or lost, the entire set must be replaced. *(75:512; 170:164)*

51. **(C)** The Fluotec-4 is an out-of-system vaporizer, is temperature compensated, and is calibrated only for halothane. These vaporizers divert only a measured amount of the inflow gas into the vaporizing chamber. *(75:517; 170:101)*

52. **(E)** The ideal system would have all of the characteristics listed. No such system is available today. *(1:135)*

53. **(E)** All of these options are correct. If polyvinylchloride materials are sterilized by gamma radiation and later sterilized with ethylene oxide, toxic products may be produced. *(32:214; 170:418)*

54. **(B)** The DISS prevents attachment of gas administration equipment to the wrong gas. The system is based on matching specific bores and diameters, which are assigned to the specific gases. This is not the protective system for cylinder–yoke attachments. That is the pin index safety system. Suction hoses are not included in the DISS. *(170:24)*

55. **(E)** In order to calculate the concentration of an agent delivered from a kettle vaporizer, one must know the agent, the temperature, the vapor pressure curve, the volume of the inflow gas, and the total flow. *(1:129,131; 170:83)*

56. **(E)** In the lithotomy position, all of the nerves listed may be injured. The peroneal nerve usually is injured by pressure against the stirrups, the other nerves by compression due to flexion of the legs on the trunk. *(1:405; 16:48)*

57. **(E)** In the supine position, the weight of the body is borne by the occiput, the scapulae, the sacrum, and the heels. These areas must be supported during procedures. During long procedures or in the very thin patient with little natural padding, additional padding should be provided. *(16:33; 75:647)*

58. **(E)** The prone position provides many opportunities for positioning problems. The pressure points must be carefully checked and padded as necessary. *(16:211; 75:659)*

59. **(B)** The nerves that are most subject to injury are those that are superficial and run a long course. The ulnar nerve is an example. The patient with ischemic disease, eg, arteriosclerosis or diabetes mellitus, is more subject to injury. One must also remember that not all postoperative nerve injuries are due to positioning. Some may be due to injections or direct damage to the nerve. *(1:403; 16:306)*

60. **(E)** Symptoms produced by positioning may involve the circulatory system, eg, hypotension, the nervous system, eg, nerve damage, the respiratory system, eg, restriction of ventilation, and the neuromuscular system, eg, pain from muscle damage due to the position. *(16:83)*

CHAPTER 13

Disease States
Review

It would be impossible in a short review to discuss the entire list of diseases that an anesthesiologist must deal with. Many of the specific diseases are dealt with in the specific organ system; others are included in questions in this chapter.

The major journals have a section in each issue for case presentations. These discuss the anesthetic management of various disease states. It would be helpful to review several volumes of the journals to study approaches to various disease entities.

Specific areas dealt with in this section are pain management, endocrine disease, urologic problems, blood administration, air embolism, and a host of unusual diseases.

Questions

DIRECTIONS (Questions 1 through 109): Each of the numbered items or incomplete statements in this section is followed by answers or by completions of the statement. Select the ONE lettered answer or completion that is BEST in each case.

1. An example of a central pain state is

    (A) postoperative incision pain
    (B) gallbladder pain
    (C) phantom limb pain
    (D) bone fracture pain
    (E) headache

2. Occipital neuralgia involves

    (A) the greater occipital nerve
    (B) the cervical plexus
    (C) a pain distribution confined to the occipital area
    (D) the scapular nerve
    (E) trophic lesions of the skull

3. Coccygodynia

    (A) is common in males
    (B) is best treated by coccygectomy
    (C) responds to local application of counterirritants
    (D) always responds to caudal anesthesia
    (E) is a difficult syndrome to treat, and success is limited

4. Signs of causalgia include

    (A) hypoesthesia
    (B) coldness or hyperthermia
    (C) pain that is of short duration
    (D) pliable nails
    (E) osteopetrosis

5. The effectiveness of a neurolytic agent is dependent on all of the following EXCEPT

    (A) location of the injection
    (B) concentration
    (C) histology of the nerve
    (D) volume
    (E) needle size

6. In the pain theory proposed by Wall and Melzack, the interneurons proposed as the mediators of pain are in the

    (A) lateral horn
    (B) corticospinal tract
    (C) substantia gelatinosa
    (D) cerebral cortex
    (E) thalamus

7. If a patient undergoing thoracotomy receives intercostal blocks with bupivacaine, his postoperative period will

    (A) be little different from controls
    (B) show marked improvement in respiratory function over controls
    (C) show little difference in vital capacity but marked pain relief
    (D) be marked by hyperventilation
    (E) be marked by increased incidence of atelectasis

8. If a patient has prerenal failure, the urine will

    (A) be dilute
    (B) be concentrated
    (C) have a specific gravity of 1.010
    (D) be excreted in large amounts
    (E) have a reddish tinge due to presence of red blood cells

9. In order to provide an adequate sensory level for prostate resection, the sensory level must be

    (A) T-4
    (B) T-6
    (C) T-8
    (D) T-10
    (E) T-12

10. A patient is undergoing transurethral resection under general anesthesia. The urologist is heard to complain to the circulating nurse that the irriga-

tion device is not working properly. The anesthesiologist notices loss of relaxation and irregular respirations. You should immediately think of

(A) massive hemoptysis
(B) electrolyte disturbance
(C) a perforation
(D) increased blood loss
(E) pulmonary embolus

11. A 75-year-old man undergoes prostate resection under general anesthesia. After 30 minutes of resection, the blood pressure, previously 130/78, is recorded as 154/92. The most likely cause of this is

(A) bladder distention
(B) absorption of irrigating fluid
(C) hypercarbia
(D) hypoxemia
(E) an allergic reaction

12. A muscle relaxant that should be avoided for renal transplantation is

(A) curare
(B) metocurine
(C) gallamine
(D) succinylcholine
(E) pancuronium

13. In the patient with liver disease

(A) the albumin level will be elevated, making thiopental more effective
(B) osmolarity will be high
(C) pancuronium is more effective
(D) gamma globulin will be low
(E) less thiopental is required

14. The optimal anesthetic regimen for a patient with liver disease

(A) will avoid thiopental
(B) will avoid nondepolarizing relaxants
(C) is a balanced technique
(D) will avoid halogenated hydrocarbons
(E) will depend on the cause of the liver disease and the patient's status

15. The patient with active liver disease

(A) is not affected by surgical procedures
(B) is an acceptable candidate for general anesthesia for elective surgery if the liver disease is mild
(C) is a candidate for elective surgery only if it is mandatory and only when the patient is in optimum condition
(D) should have a thiopental induction
(E) should never have a general anesthetic

16. A patient with recent onset of jaundice is scheduled for surgery for a semiurgent procedure. Your approach should be to

(A) delay the procedure until a definitive diagnosis is established if that is possible
(B) proceed under regional anesthesia
(C) proceed using nitrous oxide and a narcotic
(D) refuse to give the anesthesia
(E) proceed using isoflurane

17. The patient with jaundice

(A) should receive blood over 5 days old if transfusion is necessary
(B) should have glucose infusions withheld in the postoperative period
(C) has elevated liver glycogen
(D) should always have a nasogastric tube inserted during general anesthesia
(E) should have prothrombin time performed preoperatively

18. A patient underwent a thyroidectomy at 0800, and at 2200 he complained to the nurse of difficulty in breathing. She took his blood pressure, which was moderately elevated above previous determinations, but she also noticed that his wrist flexed when the blood pressure cuff remained inflated. The cause of the stridor is probably

(A) vocal cord paralysis
(B) partial cord paralysis
(C) laryngeal edema
(D) cervical hematoma
(E) hypocalcemia

19. A patient with untreated hypothyroidism (myxedema) is admitted for emergency abdominal surgery. A finding consistent with the myxedematous state is

(A) fine, soft hair
(B) moist skin
(C) bradycardia
(D) heat intolerance
(E) pitting edema of the eyelids

20. Fluid and blood replacement in the patient with myxedema

(A) should be guided by blood pressure
(B) should be guided by electrocardiographic voltage
(C) does not differ from that in normal patients
(D) must be guided by as many hemodynamic monitors as possible
(E) should be accompanied by full digitalization

21. A patient with a recent onset of clinical hyperthyroidism is admitted for repair of a tendon laceration. He has been off propylthiouracil for 4 days. At
this time

    (A) the patient should be essentially euthyroid
    (B) should be considered as a high-risk hyper-
thyroid patient
    (C) the drug has reached a dosage level where hy-
pothyroidism may result
    (D) the patient would have bradycardia
    (E) the patient should have general anesthesia if
at all possible

22. The heart disease usually associated with hyperthyroidism is

    (A) a shocklike state brought about early in the
disease
    (B) due to valvular dysfunction
    (C) due to intracardiac shunts
    (D) due to production of low peripheral resistance
    (E) a function of the hypertension and increased
peripheral resistance

23. A patient is anesthetized for the implantation of a
knee prosthesis. She has been on cortisone for rheumatoid arthritis for 6 months. During the procedure, there is a sudden drop in blood pressure.
The first step to be taken is

    (A) administer prednisolone, 300 mg IV
    (B) establish the cause of the hypotension
    (C) cancel the procedure
    (D) administer a vasopressor
    (E) turn off all anesthesia

24. The time required for a patient to develop adrenal
suppression from cortisone treatment is

    (A) 2 weeks
    (B) 4 weeks
    (C) 8 weeks
    (D) 12 weeks
    (E) unknown

25. The patient with a diagnosis of pheochromocytoma

    (A) requires immediate surgery
    (B) should be treated for 7 to 12 days with alpha
blockers
    (C) can be anesthetized regardless of the level of
blood pressure readings
    (D) is usually hypervolemic
    (E) should have a Swan-Ganz catheter in place pre-
operatively

26. The most important goal in the treatment of the
diabetic patient undergoing anesthesia is to

    (A) keep blood sugar in the normal range
    (B) prevent glycosuria

    (C) prevent hypoglycemia
    (D) prevent ketoacidosis
    (E) prevent acetonuria

27. Insulin shock in the awake patient

    (A) is identical to that in the anesthetized patient
    (B) is characterized by bradycardia
    (C) is characterized by hypertension
    (D) may be manifested by convulsions
    (E) is characterized by a marked parasympathetic
response

28. A male diabetic patient is anesthetized for the incision and drainage of a large abscess. His usual dose
of Lente insulin is given in the morning, and the
procedure lasts only 15 minutes. After surgery you
would expect his insulin requirement to

    (A) decrease
    (B) be unaffected
    (C) increase greatly; therefore, he should have fre-
quent injections empirically
    (D) remain high for 72 hours
    (E) be roughly double his preoperative require-
ment

29. Hyperosmolar coma

    (A) usually occurs in young people
    (B) occurs at osmolar levels of 150 to 175 mOsm/L
    (C) occurs in the absence of ketonemia
    (D) is usually accompanied by oliguria
    (E) requires treatment with large doses of insulin

30. The circulatory effect of droperidol is

    (A) short-lived
    (B) 6 to 12 hours
    (C) 12 to 18 hours
    (D) 18 to 24 hours
    (E) over 24 hours

31. During cardiopulmonary perfusion, patients

    (A) need a large dose of muscle relaxants
    (B) require very little muscle relaxation
    (C) should have PCO_2 maintained at about 45 torr
    (D) should have their lungs hyperinflated
    (E) should have continued ventilation

32. The patient who has complete heart block should
have pacer wires inserted under

    (A) general anesthesia
    (B) local anesthesia
    (C) local anesthesia unless he or she becomes un-
comfortable, in which case general anesthesia
should be initiated
    (D) nitrous oxide analgesia
    (E) local anesthesia with thiopental used as needed
for sedation

33. Before induction of anesthesia for a patient with a pacemaker in place, pacer function must be assured by

(A) palpation of the pulse
(B) monitoring the electrocardiogram
(C) taking a history
(D) starting an isoproterenol drip
(E) administering epinephrine subcutaneously

34. Causes of complete heart block include all of the following EXCEPT

(A) ischemic heart disease
(B) Lenegre's disease
(C) rheumatic heart disease
(D) ventricular aneurysm
(E) cardiomyopathy

35. If a patient with a pacemaker in place requires surgery that entails the use of cautery

(A) the indifferent plate of the electrocautery unit should be as close to the power pack as possible
(B) electrocardiographic monitoring is necessary only if the patient is being paced
(C) electrocardiographic monitoring will give the best information
(D) little danger is present if the pacer is a demand unit
(E) constant palpation of the pulse or listening to an esophageal stethoscope is necessary

36. The patient with a pacemaker in place may develop competing rhythms when a normal sinus rhythm is present and the unit has been converted to the asynchronous mode. If the pacing stimuli fall on the T wave of the previously conducted beats

(A) ventricular fibrillation will follow
(B) there is little danger, since the energy output is so low with the current pulse generators
(C) ventricular fibrillation is less likely if hypoxemia is present
(D) ventricular fibrillation is less likely with catecholamine release
(E) ventricular fibrillation is less likely with myocardial infarction

37. Intraaortic balloon counterpulsation is a circulatory assist device that

(A) is used for patients with aortic aneurysms
(B) is used for patients with aortic insufficiency
(C) causes an intraaortic balloon to be inflated during systole
(D) increases coronary blood flow
(E) increases impedance to the opening of the left ventricle

38. The clamping of the thoracic aorta in aneurysm repair is followed by

(A) immediate hypotension
(B) immediate hypertension
(C) cardiac standstill
(D) no change
(E) loss of blood pressure in the right arm

39. Clamping of the distal aorta will be followed by

(A) increased cardiac output
(B) decreased arterial blood pressure
(C) decreased systemic vascular resistance
(D) increased stroke volume
(E) stable heart rate

$$CO = HR \times SV$$
$$SV = \frac{CO}{HR}$$

40. A complication of aortic surgery is paraplegia that is due to

(A) pressure on the spinal cord during surgery
(B) long periods of hypotension
(C) hypothermia associated with the surgery
(D) spinal cord ischemia
(E) loss of cerebrospinal fluid

41. Hypovolemia may occur during abdominal aneurysm procedures as a result of all of the following EXCEPT

(A) blood loss
(B) inadequate fluid replacement
(C) use of vasopressors
(D) loss of fluid into the bowel
(E) expansion of the vascular bed during occlusion

42. The normal flow rate for an adult on total bypass is

(A) 15 ml/kg/minute
(B) 35 ml/kg/minute
(C) 55 ml/kg/minute
(D) 85 ml/kg/minute
(E) 115 ml/kg/minute

43. The flow during total bypass

(A) is independent of temperature
(B) is nonpulsatile
(C) provides a pulsatile pressure
(D) is a pulsatile flow
(E) mimics normal flow in all respects

44. Problems with oxygenators include all of the following EXCEPT

(A) denaturation of proteins
(B) platelet destruction
(C) hypercapnia
(D) sterility hazards
(E) coagulation defects

45. When a patient is on total bypass

    (A) arterial pressure should be maintained at about 50 torr
    (B) blood is pumped from the venae cavae and drains by gravity into the aorta for circulation
    (C) a sump is placed in the left ventricle to drain the coronary sinus blood
    (D) venous pressure elevation is of no consequence
    (E) venous return to the pump is always started before arterial infusion

46. Anesthesia for carotid artery surgery

    (A) causes a decreased oxygen consumption
    (B) involves the use of hypotension
    (C) carries no danger of cerebral infarction
    (D) should always be preceded by tests to show if clamping can be tolerated
    (E) requires general anesthesia

47. Anesthesia for carotid endarterectomy is best achieved by all of the following EXCEPT

    (A) hypercapnia
    (B) normal or slightly increased arterial oxygen tension
    (C) normal or slightly increased arterial pressure
    (D) systemic heparinization
    (E) normothermia

48. During carotid artery surgery, the stump pressure is

    (A) dependent on collateral circulation
    (B) decreased by hypocapnia
    (C) increased by hypercapnia
    (D) decreased by hypertension
    (E) a measure of the pressure proximal to the surgically occluded carotid artery

49. Of the many factors affecting intracerebral blood flow, which of the following is a correct description?

    (A) vasomotor paralysis: vasoconstriction of vessels in or near ischemic areas
    (B) autoregulation: ability of vessels to respond in a manner consistent with maintaining homeostasis
    (C) luxury perfusion: metabolic requirements in excess of blood flow
    (D) intracerebral steal: decrease of blood flow in normal areas with increased flow to ischemic areas
    (E) inverse steal: diversion of flow to normal areas from ischemic areas

50. A factor of great importance in the mortality associated with fractured hip is

    (A) time from injury to admission
    (B) number of blood transfusions
    (C) type of anesthesia
    (D) duration of anesthesia
    (E) age of the patient

Questions 51 and 52

A 67-year-old male was anesthetized for a total hip replacement. After induction with thiopental, anesthesia was maintained with isoflurane, nitrous oxide, and oxygen. Immediately after the implant was placed in the femur, cardiac arrest occurred.

51. The cardiac arrest may be due to all of the following EXCEPT

    (A) hypotension
    (B) hypoxemia
    (C) hypovolemia
    (D) hypervolemia
    (E) fat embolization

52. The cement substance, methylmethacrylate

    (A) is a liquid hydrocarbon
    (B) generates considerable heat while setting
    (C) is associated with hypertension
    (D) is always mixed preoperatively
    (E) is used only for hip fractures

53. Clinical manifestations of fat emboli include all of the following EXCEPT

    (A) petechiae
    (B) hypoxemia
    (C) confusion
    (D) bradycardia
    (E) cyanosis

54. The average amount of blood lost during surgery for hip fracture is

    (A) 300 ml
    (B) 500 ml
    (C) 800 ml
    (D) 1300 ml
    (E) 2000 ml

55. When ventilating the patient with a head injury, all of the following statements are true EXCEPT

    (A) the patient should be kept supine
    (B) the P_{CO_2} should be kept at 25 to 30 torr
    (C) PEEP should be used if needed
    (D) hypoxia and hypercarbia should be avoided
    (E) the patient should be prevented from bucking

56. Mannitol may lead to subdural hematoma by

    (A) causing cerebral edema
    (B) affecting clotting mechanisms
    (C) leading to cortical vein disruption
    (D) causing hypertension
    (E) leakage through the vein wall

57. The best agent to decrease cerebral oxygen requirement is

(A) a muscle relaxant
(B) a glucose solution
(C) an anticonvulsant, eg, phenytoin
(D) a barbiturate
(E) oxygen by mask

58. The normal level of intracranial pressure is

(A) 1 to 10 torr
(B) 10 to 30 torr
(C) 40 to 60 torr
(D) 60 to 80 torr
(E) 80 to 100 torr

59. The Glasgow Coma Score is based on

(A) response to eye opening, verbal response, and motor response
(B) assessment of knee jerk
(C) assessment of pupil size
(D) assessment of respiration
(E) assessment of EEG

60. Focal ischemia may be treated with all of the following drugs EXCEPT

(A) thiopental
(B) naloxone
(C) isoflurane
(D) nimodipine
(E) halothane

61. The intracerebral steal

(A) is a term used to describe focal flow decrease caused by cerebral vasodilatation
(B) is a phenomenon caused by alkalosis
(C) is a condition caused only by brain tumors
(D) always occurs during anesthesia
(E) is always helpful to ischemic tissue

62. In the $Paco_2$ range of 20 to 60 torr, the cerebral blood flow increases for each 10 torr

(A) 1 to 2 ml/100 g/minute
(B) 2 to 4 ml/100 g/minute
(C) 4 to 6 ml/100 g/minute
(D) 6 to 8 ml/100 g/minute
(E) 8 to 10 ml/100 g/minute

63. The use of succinylcholine to facilitate tracheal intubation in patients with increased intracranial pressure is associated with

(A) increased levels of intracranial pressure
(B) no change in intracranial pressure
(C) incomplete relaxation
(D) conditions more satisfactory than those with the use of pancuronium
(E) high levels of potassium

64. The incidence of air embolism during surgery in the sitting position is

(A) 25 to 30%
(B) 5 to 15%
(C) 20 to 25%
(D) 30 to 40%
(E) less than 2%

65. The major intracranial buffer against increased intracranial pressure is the

(A) dural sinus
(B) cerebrospinal fluid
(C) white matter
(D) gray matter
(E) glial cells

66. In the artificially ventilated neurosurgical patient, PEEP

(A) should be used routinely
(B) should be used on selected patients, and the patient's head should always be down
(C) has no effect on intracranial pressure
(D) should be withheld in all cases
(E) should be titrated against O_2 requirements and neurologic status

Questions 67 and 68

The graph shows the relationship between intracranial pressure and volume.

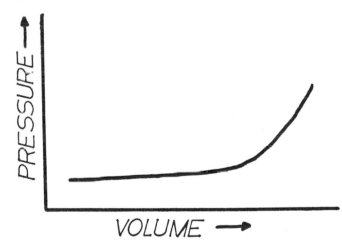

67. On the relatively flat part of the curve

(A) there is a slow pressure increase with increased volume
(B) there is a slow pressure increase showing poor compensatory effect
(C) pressure increases are compensated for by increased blood flow
(D) there is a large pressure increase
(E) compensatory mechanisms are not functional

68. Intracranial pressure measurements similar to those shown in the graph are obtained from a

(A) needle in the caudal canal
(B) spinal epidural needle
(C) transducer in the extradural space
(D) carotid artery transducer
(E) jugular bulb transducer

69. The most profound chemical stimulus for cerebral autoregulation is

(A) metabolic alkalosis
(B) hypothermia
(C) hyperthermia
(D) carbon dioxide
(E) acidosis

70. The oxygen reserves of the brain are

(A) infinite
(B) capable of maintaining function for 25 minutes
(C) greater under anesthesia
(D) very low
(E) carried primarily in the cerebral hemispheres

71. Treatment of the neurosurgical patient with mannitol may be followed by all of the following EXCEPT

(A) initial hypervolemia
(B) decreased urine volume
(C) hypovolemia
(D) decreased venous pressure
(E) a fall in arterial pressure

72. Nitrous oxide should be avoided in patients with

(A) brain tumor
(B) cerebral hemorrhage
(C) head injury
(D) recent air encephalography
(E) meningioma

73. In neurosurgical patients, the fluid 5% dextrose in water

(A) is the fluid of choice
(B) may cause excessive diuresis
(C) may lead to cerebral edema
(D) does not provide sufficient calories
(E) leads to water retention

74. Signs of air embolism include all of the following EXCEPT

(A) arrhythmia
(B) hypertension
(C) heart murmur
(D) bubbles at the operative site
(E) decreased end-expired carbon dioxide

75. As the neurosurgeon manipulates tissue in the posterior fossa, there is a sudden arrhythmia. You should

(A) lower the head
(B) administer lidocaine
(C) inform the neurosurgeon
(D) turn off all anesthesia
(E) turn off the nitrous oxide

76. During a neurosurgical procedure, the P_{CO_2} should be maintained at

(A) 25 to 35 torr
(B) 20 to 30 torr
(C) 15 to 20 torr
(D) 35 to 40 torr
(E) 40 to 45 torr

77. Loss of cerebral autoregulation

(A) will cause the cerebral blood pressure to fall with systemic hypertension
(B) always affects the entire brain at the same time
(C) may be focal
(D) only affects the lower end of the blood pressure range
(E) has no clinical significance

78. Cerebrospinal fluid pressure may be increased by

(A) cough
(B) long expiratory time
(C) short expiratory time
(D) low expiratory resistance
(E) negative expiratory phase

79. In a patient who receives 4 units of warmed blood in 1 hour

(A) electrocardiographic changes are expected
(B) serum calcium will fall to very low levels
(C) signs of tetany will be seen even with normal calcium values
(D) calcium chloride, 10 g/hour, should be administered
(E) no treatment is necessary

80. Acidosis may accompany the rapid transfusion of blood to control hemorrhage, and

(A) the blood should always be warmed to 120°F
(B) the blood should be warmed to 38°C
(C) each unit has an acid load of 18 mEq/unit
(D) sodium bicarbonate should be administered at a rate of 44 mEq/2 units
(E) the acidosis should be treated with lactate

81. The treatment of suspected transfusion reaction includes all of the following EXCEPT

(A) stopping the transfusion
(B) infusion of 20% mannitol, 100 g
(C) treating hypotension
(D) giving fluids at a rate sufficient only to keep intravenous lines open
(E) alkalinizing the urine

82. The blood component with the least risk of hepatitis is

(A) fibrinogen
(B) fresh frozen plasma
(C) packed red cells
(D) frozen washed red cells
(E) albumin/plasma protein fraction

83. The shelf life of blood stored in citrate phosphate dextrose (CPD) solution is

(A) 1 week
(B) 2 weeks
(C) 3 weeks
(D) 4 weeks
(E) 5 weeks

84. The shelf life of blood stored in citrate phosphate dextrose-adenine (CPD-adenine) solution is

(A) 2 weeks
(B) 3 weeks
(C) 4 weeks
(D) 5 weeks
(E) 6 weeks

85. Fresh frozen plasma is useful for the treatment of

(A) factor VIII deficiency
(B) platelet deficiency
(C) factor II deficiency
(D) multiple coagulation factor deficiency
(E) factor VII deficiency

86. The minimum number of platelets needed for surgical hemostasis is

(A) $40,000/mm^3$
(B) $50,000/mm^3$
(C) $100,000/mm^3$
(D) $200,000/mm^3$
(E) $300,000/mm^3$

87. The average unit of packed red cells, processed by centrifugation, has a hematocrit of

(A) 40%
(B) 50%
(C) 60%
(D) 70%
(E) 90%

88. Preparation for surgery of the patient with sickle cell disease should include all of the following EXCEPT

(A) transfuse to a hemoglobin level of 10 g
(B) treat infection
(C) maintain good hydration
(D) provide good pulmonary care
(E) avoid stasis of blood flow

89. A child is admitted with acute appendicitis. He is known to have phenylketonuria. His preanesthetic medication should consist of

(A) atropine only
(B) heavy doses of narcotic
(C) barbiturates only
(D) diazepam only
(E) a narcotic, a barbiturate, and scopolamine

90. Children with phenylketonuria are prone to all of the following EXCEPT

(A) convulsions
(B) hypoglycemia
(C) sensitivity to narcotics
(D) coarse skin
(E) sensitivity to anesthetics

91. A woman is admitted with an alleged mental disorder, red urine, and abdominal pain. A diagnosis of acute intermittent porphyria is made. Drugs that may be used for sedation include all of the following EXCEPT

(A) chlorpromazine
(B) promazine
(C) morphine
(D) pentobarbital
(E) meperidine

92. If a patient has methemoglobinemia, a drug to be avoided is

(A) thiopental
(B) meperidine
(C) prilocaine
(D) halothane
(E) morphine

93. The infant with hypothyroidism presents many difficulties for the anesthesiologist, including

(A) hyperthermia
(B) hypoventilation
(C) resistance to narcotics
(D) small mouth and tongue
(E) hyperkinetic heart

94. A 40-year-old male is admitted for open reduction of a fractured femur. The patient has Huntington's disease. A drug that should be avoided is

    (A) morphine
    (B) isoflurane
    (C) nitrous oxide
    (D) fluphenazine (Prolixin)
    (E) thiopental

95. In the surgical correction of torticollis in an adult, complications may occur

    (A) if preanesthetic medication is given
    (B) on induction
    (C) on intubation
    (D) during maintenance of anesthesia
    (E) postoperatively as a result of airway difficulty

Questions 96 and 97

A 55-year-old woman is admitted for surgical procedures on the digit of both hands. She has rheumatoid arthritis.

96. Important factors that should be checked before induction of anesthesia include all of the following EXCEPT

    (A) mobility of neck
    (B) liver enzyme levels
    (C) reaction to previous anesthetics
    (D) chest x-ray
    (E) electrocardiogram

97. The patient has limited mobility of the neck and has full dentition. The anesthetic of choice is

    (A) local
    (B) regional
    (C) general under mask
    (D) general with intubation
    (E) general with awake intubation

98. A patient is to be operated on for tumor of the small bowel. In your questioning, you elicit a history of flushing, diarrhea, and joint pain. There is a history compatible with heart failure. A likely diagnosis is

    (A) Zollinger-Ellison syndrome
    (B) carcinoid syndrome
    (C) pheochromocytoma
    (D) Peutz-Jeghers syndrome
    (E) adrenal tumor with metastasis

99. A 16-year-old patient with Down's syndrome is admitted for dental extractions. In the preoperative preparation

    (A) atropine should be avoided
    (B) narcotics should be avoided
    (C) neck mobility should be documented

    (D) heavy sedation is required
    (E) anticonvulsants should be withheld

100. A patient with esophageal obstruction is to have a general anesthetic for esophagoscopy. He has had a barium swallow the day before. One of the greatest dangers of the planned procedure is

    (A) bleeding
    (B) hypotension
    (C) difficult intubation
    (D) aspiration
    (E) arrhythmia

101. Hurler's syndrome (gargoylism) is a disturbance of mucopolysaccharide metabolism. Anesthesia is complicated by all of the following EXCEPT

    (A) dwarfism
    (B) macroglossia
    (C) hypertelorism
    (D) hepatosplenomegaly
    (E) short neck

102. If a patient has been a chronic user of amphetamines in high doses, hypotension occurring during anesthesia should be treated with

    (A) ephedrine
    (B) metaraminol
    (C) norepinephrine
    (D) dopamine
    (E) dobutamine

Questions 103 and 104

Wernicke's encephalopathy (beriberi) is a nutritional disease seen with thiamine deficiency. It is rarely seen in isolated form but may accompany alcoholism. Patients show neurologic and cardiovascular changes.

103. The cardiovascular disease is characterized by

    (A) high output failure
    (B) low output failure
    (C) rapid response to digitalis
    (D) high peripheral resistance
    (E) aneurysm formation

104. In the management of patients with beriberi heart disease, the anesthetic of choice is

    (A) regional
    (B) nitrous oxide
    (C) halothane
    (D) isoflurane
    (E) balanced anesthesia

105. The anesthetic relatively contraindicated in patients with multiple sclerosis is

(A) spinal
(B) halothane
(C) isoflurane
(D) nitrous oxide
(E) narcotic

Questions 106 and 107

Scleroderma is a disease characterized by widespread sclerosis that affects almost all body organs.

106. Problems that may be encountered include all of the following EXCEPT

(A) small mouth
(B) arterial dilatation
(C) pulmonary edema
(D) contractures
(E) pericarditis

107. The pulmonary disease of scleroderma is characterized by all of the following EXCEPT

(A) increased compliance
(B) diffuse fibrosis
(C) decreased vital capacity
(D) hypoxemia
(E) increased V_D/V_T ratio

108. In the patient who has a bullous-type skin disorder, it is important to rule out, before anesthesia

(A) renal disease
(B) heart disease
(C) porphyria
(D) pulmonary disease
(E) neurologic disease

109. A patient with Sipple's syndrome (multiple endocrine adenomatosis) is scheduled for a thyroidectomy. Soon after induction, hypertension of 210/130 is recorded. A likely cause for this is

(A) light anesthesia
(B) pheochromocytoma
(C) inadvertent injection of a pressor agent
(D) hypercarbia
(E) allergic response to anesthesia

DIRECTIONS (Questions 110 through 216): For each of the items in this section, ONE or MORE of the numbered options is correct. Choose the answer

A if only 1, 2, and 3 are correct,
B if only 1 and 3 are correct,
C if only 2 and 4 are correct,
D if only 4 is correct,
E if all are correct.

110. Percutaneous cordotomy

(1) may be performed under local anesthesia
(2) is usually done bilaterally
(3) is as effective as open cordotomy
(4) is useful only in relatively healthy patients

111. In treating pain of somatic origin, the following is (are) true

(1) the target is usually the dorsal root ganglion
(2) alcohol injections into the peripheral nerve may produce a neuritis
(3) treatment leading to loss of bowel or bladder function should be used only in those with terminal disease
(4) absence of sensation by the patient may be worse than the pain

112. A patient with obstructive lung disease develops a causalgia syndrome involving the right arm after a nerve injury. Treatment of the syndrome may involve

(1) stellate ganglion block
(2) physical therapy
(3) application of moist heat
(4) axillary block

113. The placebo effect occurs

(1) only in patients who are emotionally unstable
(2) with normal individuals
(3) only in those who are faking pain
(4) with pharmacologically active substances

114. The factor(s) most important in the drug therapy of chronic pain is (are)

(1) drug
(2) vehicle of the drug
(3) timing of administration
(4) patient

115. Diagnostic blocks may be used in the treatment of chronic pain. Such blocks

(1) elicit the type of pain being suffered
(2) use 6% phenol as the agent
(3) include differential spinal blocks
(4) seek a permanent interruption of the pathways

116. Of the two principal neurolytic agents, alcohol and phenol

(1) alcohol has the greater tendency to produce neuritis
(2) alcohol is used in 6% concentration
(3) alcohol has the more rapid onset of action
(4) phenol is used in a 50% concentration

SUMMARY OF DIRECTIONS				
A	B	C	D	E
1, 2, 3 only	1, 3 only	2, 4 only	4 only	All are correct

117. Pain theories being proposed currently postulate a

    (1) straight stimulus-to-nervous-system path
    (2) system involving large fibers only
    (3) system with inhibition exerted by small fibers
    (4) system involving excitatory and inhibitory input with resulting sensation

118. Anesthetic agents and adjuncts acceptable for renal transplantation include

    (1) halothane
    (2) gallamine
    (3) thiopental
    (4) enflurane

119. In a patient undergoing a prostatic resection under spinal anesthesia, fluid absorption in large amounts is heralded by

    (1) a rise in systolic and diastolic blood pressure
    (2) bradycardia
    (3) mental change
    (4) pain

120. The patient who absorbs fluid during transurethral surgery is in danger of pulmonary edema as a result of

    (1) increased intravascular pressure
    (2) position on the operating table
    (3) decreased osmotic pressure
    (4) increased sodium concentration

121. During transurethral resection of the prostate, fluid uptake through venous sinuses may lead to

    (1) increased circulating fluid volume
    (2) hemolysis of red cells
    (3) hemodilution of electrolytes
    (4) increased serum sodium concentration

122. The irrigating fluids for prostatic resection should be

    (1) nonhemolytic
    (2) close to water in composition
    (3) isoosmolar
    (4) electrolyte solutions

123. Mechanisms by which blood glucose can increase during surgery include

    (1) intravenous intake
    (2) secretion from the liver secondary to a decreased insulin secretion
    (3) secretion from the liver secondary to an increased catecholamine output
    (4) uptake of glucose into tissue

124. Insulin should be administered to a diabetic patient during surgery

    (1) by adding it to the container of intravenous fluids
    (2) only when monitoring urine and blood for sugar
    (3) in the usual daily dosage
    (4) only if glucose is being infused

125. The juvenile-type diabetic is noted for

    (1) heavy habitus
    (2) good response to oral hypoglycemics
    (3) blood sugar in the range of 50 to 100 mg/dl
    (4) lack of insulin activity in the blood

126. Oral hypoglycemic drugs are noted for which of the following durations of activity?

    (1) tolbutamide: 6 hours
    (2) chlorpropamide: 33 hours
    (3) acetohexamide: 20 hours
    (4) tolazamide: 3 hours

127. A major operation is attended with a stress response that helps achieve homeostasis. This response may not occur in the

    (1) neonate
    (2) chronically ill
    (3) very old
    (4) patient with adrenal hyperplasia

128. Hormones secreted by the adrenal cortex include

    (1) mineralocorticoids
    (2) glucocorticoids
    (3) sex hormones
    (4) norepinephrine

129. The patient with myxedema may have

    (1) heart failure
    (2) cardiomegaly
    (3) pleural effusion
    (4) tachycardia

130. A patient with a thyroid tumor develops hypertension during the procedure. This may be due to

    (1) light anesthesia
    (2) pheochromocytoma
    (3) hypercarbia
    (4) myxedema

131. Glucocorticoids are

    (1) produced in the adrenal cortex under influence of ACTH

(2) active in carbohydrate metabolism
(3) active in protein metabolism
(4) synonymous with aldosterone

132. In diabetes insipidus

(1) the serum sodium is high
(2) the osmolality of the serum is high
(3) the urine is dilute
(4) thirst need not be present

133. The patient with hyperthyroidism

(1) has an increased MAC
(2) should not have medication the day of surgery
(3) should be heavily sedated
(4) may require propranolol intravenously

134. Anticholinergic agents are omitted from premedication in the patient with hyperthyroidism because they

(1) interfere with interpretation of pulse rate
(2) interfere with pupillary constriction
(3) interfere with sweating mechanisms
(4) slow gastric emptying

135. Many of the clinical manifestations of hyperthyroidism are related to compensatory changes that counteract the increased heat production. These include

(1) sweating
(2) vasoconstriction
(3) tachycardia
(4) shivering

136. The patient with hyperaldosteronism usually has

(1) excess secretion of hormone from the adrenal medulla
(2) hypertension
(3) acidosis
(4) hypokalemia

137. If a patient has elevated blood pressure in the postoperative period, one must think of

(1) hypercapnia
(2) increased sympathetic activity
(3) pain
(4) error in the diagnosis of hypertension

138. Anesthetic agents must be used with caution in patients with cardiac tamponade to avoid cardiac depression, and

(1) compensatory mechanisms must be preserved
(2) the heart should be kept full
(3) the heart rate should be kept high
(4) peripheral vasculature should be kept constricted

139. The patient with uremic pericardial effusion and tamponade

(1) requires high venous filling pressure
(2) has a high incidence of arrhythmias
(3) does not tolerate increased intrathoracic pressure
(4) should be hypoventilated to stimulate the sympathetic outflow

140. The transplanted heart has

(1) two sinoatrial nodes
(2) intact adrenergic receptors
(3) normal atrial-ventricular conduction
(4) a normal response to digitalis

141. In a patient who has had a heart transplant, you would expect heart rate changes with

(1) atropine
(2) pancuronium
(3) neostigmine
(4) propranolol

142. The high level of success achieved with cardiac surgery today is due to better

(1) perfusion technique
(2) surgical technique
(3) patient preparation
(4) anesthesia

143. A good anesthetic for cardiac surgery should

(1) cause a minimum of cardiovascular depression
(2) cause an increase in heart rate
(3) control the reflexes produced by painful stimuli
(4) cause an increase in blood pressure

144. The addition of nitrous oxide to an anesthetic for cardiac surgery

(1) causes increased ischemia
(2) causes sympathetic activation
(3) causes decreased myocardial contractility
(4) decreases pulmonary vascular resistance

145. The vasodilator properties of droperidol are due to

(1) sympathetic stimulation
(2) a vagolytic effect
(3) a beta-adrenergic effect
(4) alpha-adrenergic blockade

146. The administration of fentanyl in large doses (100μg/kg) to patients with valvular heart disease results in

(1) bradycardia
(2) decreased cardiac output
(3) stable blood pressure
(4) more profound changes than seen with morphine

SUMMARY OF DIRECTIONS				
A	**B**	**C**	**D**	**E**
1, 2, 3 only	1, 3 only	2, 4 only	4 only	All are correct

147. In the anesthetic management of patients with coronary artery disease and those with severe valvular disease, the primary aim is to

    (1) minimize myocardial oxygen consumption
    (2) maintain a fast heart rate
    (3) maintain coronary blood flow
    (4) maintain light anesthesia

148. In the presence of heart disease, fast sinus tachycardia

    (1) is desirable
    (2) may cause hypotension
    (3) decreases the energy requirements of the heart
    (4) may cause pulmonary edema

149. A patient with aortic insufficiency enters the operating room with a blood pressure of 160/40. After induction with thiopental, anesthesia is maintained on halothane and oxygen, and curare, 6 mg, is administered. This is accompanied by a fall in pressure to 80/20 and bradycardia. This is accompanied by

    (1) vasoconstriction
    (2) decreased cardiac output
    (3) decreased left atrial pressure
    (4) decreased coronary filling pressure

150. The primary determinant(s) of myocardial oxygen supply is (are)

    (1) the oxygen-carrying capacity of the blood
    (2) FIO_2
    (3) coronary blood flow
    (4) age

151. The major complication(s) attributed to ketamine when used for coronary artery surgery is (are)

    (1) hypertension
    (2) hallucinations
    (3) tachycardia
    (4) hypoxia

152. Many drugs have been used during induction of anesthesia for coronary artery procedures. Of those commonly used

    (1) diazepam maintains stable hemodynamics
    (2) droperidol may blunt the autonomic response to intubation
    (3) ketamine may increase myocardial oxygen consumption
    (4) thiopental increases myocardial contractility

153. When used for anesthesia of a patient for coronary surgery, fentanyl has the advantage over morphine of

    (1) increasing the heart rate
    (2) earlier emergence
    (3) increased oxygen supply to the heart
    (4) a shorter period of required ventilation

154. Many patients admitted for coronary artery surgery are taking propranolol. The following are facts to be considered in the decision to continue the medication

    (1) the plasma half-life of propranolol is 3 to 6 hours
    (2) there are no side effects from prompt discontinuation
    (3) the beta-blocking effect is related to plasma concentration
    (4) the drug can be stopped without difficulty if supplemental oxygen is being administered

155. Hemodilution performed before bypass may cause

    (1) bradycardia
    (2) decreased cardiac output
    (3) decreased myocardial oxygen consumption
    (4) an improved tissue flow

156. If the lungs are allowed to collapse during cardiopulmonary bypass

    (1) shunt will not change from preoperative values
    (2) more atelectasis will be present
    (3) compliance will not change from preoperative values
    (4) lung rupture is more likely to occur in the recovery period

157. The continuance of ventilation during bypass

    (1) leads to hypercarbia
    (2) leads to better ventilation
    (3) decreases time on a ventilator during recovery
    (4) leads to surfactant depletion

Questions 158 and 159

A 15-year-old girl had a spinal fusion with Harrington rod instrumentation. On emergence, the patient was unable to move her left lower extremity.

158. The cause(s) of this may be

    (1) overcorrection of the scoliotic curve
    (2) cord compression due to hematoma
    (3) surgical damage to the cord
    (4) electrolyte imbalance

159. In the patient, the proper course to follow when the loss of function is discovered is to

(1) extubate the trachea, start blood
(2) observe for 24 hours
(3) establish baseline neurologic function and observe
(4) reexplore immediately

160. The blood loss in operations for total hip replacements correlates with

(1) type of anesthesia
(2) type of disease present
(3) intraoperative blood pressure
(4) whether the procedure is the first or second procedure of the day

161. The morbidity and mortality of patients undergoing corrective surgery for hip fractures

(1) are significantly lower with spinal anesthesia
(2) depend on the agent used
(3) are significantly higher with general anesthesia
(4) are essentially the same for spinal and general anesthesia

162. Fat emboli in the lungs may be found after

(1) external cardiac massage
(2) soft tissue injury
(3) burns
(4) bone injury

163. In the patient with an acute stroke, there is evidence that barbiturate anesthesia

(1) is harmful
(2) is helpful in focal ischemia
(3) is less protective than halothane
(4) is not protective in global ischemia

164. Mannitol given to a head-injured patient

(1) may lead to hyperosmolar coma
(2) removes water from the normal brain tissue
(3) may lead to cerebral edema if the blood–brain barrier is impaired
(4) is effective in doses of 0.25 g/kg

165. Dexamethasone, given to the neurosurgical patient

(1) will reduce the edema due to brain tumor
(2) has an effect because of its osmolar property
(3) is less effective in control of edema secondary to injury
(4) is effective only in preventing Addison's disease

166. The normal brain

(1) has a constant metabolic rate
(2) has autoregulation of flow over the blood pressure range of 50 to 150 torr
(3) has a constant blood flow
(4) requires fructose for energy

167. Induction of anesthesia with nitrous oxide, 66%, and oxygen

(1) leads to increased intracranial pressure
(2) leads to cerebrovascular dilatation
(3) may cause decompensation of intracranial relationships
(4) is not associated with any difficulty

168. Attention must be given to levels of intracranial pressure on induction. Increased intracranial pressure may lead to

(1) internal herniation
(2) localized areas of brain ischemia
(3) lowering of cerebral perfusion pressure
(4) brain retraction

169. Air embolism may be a fatal complication, depending on

(1) the amount of air present
(2) the site of entry
(3) the rate of entry
(4) whether a Swan-Ganz catheter is in place

170. The G-suit is employed during neurosurgical procedures done in the sitting position to

(1) stop bleeding
(2) prevent hypotension
(3) decrease intracranial pressure
(4) treat hypotension

171. Factors of importance in regulation of intracranial pressure include the

(1) cerebrospinal fluid
(2) intracranial tissue
(3) blood
(4) dura

172. Anesthetic agents that increase intracranial pressure in the neurosurgical patient include

(1) fentanyl
(2) halothane
(3) thiopental
(4) nitrous oxide

173. Treatment of cerebral edema includes

(1) osmotic agents
(2) loop diuretics
(3) steroids
(4) surgical decompression

SUMMARY OF DIRECTIONS				
A	B	C	D	E
1, 2, 3 only	1, 3 only	2, 4 only	4 only	All are correct

174. Halothane, used in the neurosurgical patient

    (1) adds to cerebrovascular tone
    (2) is a vasodilator
    (3) decreases cerebral blood flow
    (4) should be used with controlled ventilation to produce hypocapnia

175. When hypothermia is used in the neurosurgical patient

    (1) cerebral metabolism is decreased
    (2) cerebral vascular resistance increases
    (3) cerebral vasculature remains responsive to carbon dioxide
    (4) more glucose is needed for metabolism

176. The blood–brain barrier is

    (1) relatively impermeable to morphine
    (2) readily permeable to glucose
    (3) readily permeable to carbon dioxide
    (4) readily permeable to bicarbonate

177. Mannitol is preferred over urea as an osmotic agent in cerebral edema because mannitol

    (1) has a longer duration
    (2) has less rebound effect
    (3) has a higher molecular weight
    (4) causes permanent effects

178. Hyperventilation may lead to

    (1) cerebral vasodilatation
    (2) tetany
    (3) shift of the oxyhemoglobin dissociation curve to the right
    (4) decreased cardiac output

179. If the patient is to be operated on in the sitting position

    (1) the legs should be wrapped with elastic bandages
    (2) the legs should be kept at a level below the heart
    (3) the head should be firmly fixed
    (4) the patient should be positioned as quickly as possible to avoid loss of monitors

180. Premedication with depressant drugs should be minimized in

    (1) infants
    (2) patients with increased intracranial pressure
    (3) comatose patients
    (4) very anxious patients

181. The use of induced hypotension in neurosurgery

    (1) usually is needed for short intervals
    (2) is best provided with phenoxybenzamine
    (3) causes increased physiologic dead space
    (4) is relatively contraindicated

182. Air embolism

    (1) is most common in the sitting position
    (2) occurs most often with occipital craniectomy
    (3) occurs through the diploic veins and venous sinuses
    (4) requires a relatively negative pressure

183. Treatment of air embolism requires

    (1) the head-up position
    (2) removal of intracardiac air
    (3) hypotension
    (4) elevation of venous pressure in the head

184. Causes of arrhythmia associated with neurosurgical procedures include

    (1) orbital decompression
    (2) carotid ligation
    (3) tonsillar herniation
    (4) trigeminal nerve surgery

185. During a cerebral aneurysm procedure, sodium nitroprusside was infused. You can expect

    (1) short duration of action
    (2) bradycardia
    (3) acidemia
    (4) nitric acid toxicity

186. The Doppler ultrasonic flowmeter for detection of air embolus

    (1) can ideally detect 0.5 ml of air
    (2) functions at 15 Hz
    (3) should be placed over the right side of the heart
    (4) will not detect carbon dioxide

Questions 187 and 188

A comatose patient with a history of severe headaches has an intracranial pressure monitor in place. Oxygen and nitrous oxide administered to the patient lead to an increased intracranial pressure.

187. The increased intracranial pressure may be blocked by administration of

    (1) halothane

(2) diazepam
(3) ketamine
(4) thiopental

188. The effect of agents or drugs to modify a response of increased intracranial pressure

(1) varies with the individual
(2) is constant
(3) depends on the summation of influences on cerebrovascular tone
(4) is independent of ventilation effects

189. Reactions to transfusions are

(1) immediate
(2) fatal in most cases
(3) always of a hemolytic nature
(4) to be anticipated and must be monitored for carefully

190. The incidence of hepatitis after blood transfusion

(1) is usually due to non-A, non-B hepatitis
(2) is 1/100 units transfused
(3) is lower if blood donation is limited to volunteers
(4) is higher after transfusion of red cells

191. Von Willebrand's disease

(1) is a congenital bleeding disorder
(2) involves only females
(3) involves bleeding primarily from mucous membranes
(4) is caused by factor VII deficiency

192. Vitamin K-dependent coagulation factors are

(1) II
(2) VII
(3) IX
(4) X

193. During blood storage, there is an increased concentration of

(1) potassium
(2) dextrose
(3) ammonia
(4) bicarbonate

194. Hemolysis of blood may be caused by

(1) overheating
(2) infusion under pressure
(3) cardiopulmonary bypass
(4) cooling to 4°C

195. Surgical procedures or conditions known to predispose to a bleeding diasthesis include

(1) abruptio placentae
(2) prostate surgery
(3) portacaval shunt
(4) small bowel resection

196. The advantage(s) of citrate phosphate dextrose (CPD) over acid citrate dextrose (ACD) storage is (are)

(1) one-half as rapid loss of 2,3-DPG in CPD
(2) lower pH with CPD
(3) longer red cell survival with CPD
(4) higher plasma potassium with CPD

197. Sickling of the red cell is more likely with

(1) low oxygen tension
(2) low temperature
(3) low pH state of the blood
(4) low hematocrit

198. Hypoglycemia occurring during an anesthetic

(1) can be prevented in all cases by infusion of glucose
(2) is readily detected
(3) can be diagnosed accurately only by blood glucose determination
(4) cannot be detected if a glucose solution is running

199. Wilson's disease is an inborn error of copper metabolism. Anesthetic implications include

(1) possible hepatic involvement
(2) drug metabolism
(3) possible prolongation of neuromuscular blockade
(4) renal tubular disease

200. Patients with gout who are to undergo anesthesia should

(1) have generous intravenous fluids
(2) be deprived of lactate solutions
(3) not receive enflurane
(4) receive no premedication

201. Marfan's syndrome (arachnodactyly) is not always diagnosed before a disastrous event. Many of these patients have another illness. Anesthetic considerations include

(1) avoidance of hypertension to avoid dissection
(2) aortic stenosis
(3) difficult intubations
(4) short stature, making airway management difficult

SUMMARY OF DIRECTIONS				
A	B	C	D	* E
1, 2, 3 only	1, 3 only	2, 4 only	4 only	All are correct

202. An obstetric patient is admitted for delivery. She has methemoglobinemia. Total hemoglobin level is given as 14 g/dl. It is important to know

(1) the level of the methemoglobin
(2) the cause of her methemoglobinemia
(3) if methylene blue has been used successfully in treatment
(4) her family history

203. Patients with pneumoconioses, eg, asbestosis and silicosis, often require surgery of other organs. In the preoperative assessment, one must recognize that

(1) the lung volumes will be increased
(2) the x-ray abnormality may not reflect the functional changes
(3) normal diaphragmatic movement is retained until the very late stages
(4) fibrosis usually is present

204. If anesthesia is required for a patient who chronically smokes marijuana, you would expect

(1) withdrawal symptoms
(2) bronchitis
(3) hepatic dysfunction
(4) tachycardia

205. In giving anesthesia to a patient with syringomyelia

(1) coughing on the endotracheal tube should be prevented
(2) depolarizing muscle relaxants should be avoided
(3) there may be increased sensitivity to nondepolarizing relaxants
(4) ventilation/perfusion (V/Q) ratios may be disturbed

Questions 206 and 207

A 14-year-old boy is brought to the hospital for treatment of facial fractures suffered from a fall after he had been sniffing glue.

206. Physiologic derangements seen with inhalation of these fumes include

(1) hepatic disorders
(2) anemia
(3) renal disorders
(4) white blood count depression

207. If anesthesia is needed, the following should not be used

(1) isoflurane
(2) halothane
(3) narcotics
(4) enflurane

208. Patients who are acutely poisoned with cocaine exhibit

(1) depression
(2) hypertension
(3) sympathetic blockade
(4) tachycardia

209. If patients with multiple myeloma require general anesthesia, it is important to have preoperative documentation of

(1) serum calcium
(2) renal studies
(3) bone involvement
(4) serum chloride

210. A patient who has a bullous type of skin disorder requires an anesthetic technique that avoids

(1) the use of tape
(2) intubation
(3) friction
(4) deep anesthesia

211. In the patient with amyotrophic lateral sclerosis, anesthetic techniques should include

(1) avoidance of succinylcholine
(2) avoidance of respiratory depressants
(3) minimal use of relaxants
(4) avoidance of halothane

212. Autonomic hyperreflexia

(1) occurs with a lesion above T-5
(2) is initiated only by bladder distention
(3) is accompanied by severe hypertension
(4) is accompanied by tachycardia *brady*

213. In the anesthesia of a patient with myotonic dystrophy, it is important to consider that

(1) halothane may cause shivering postoperatively and precipitate a myotonic response
(2) myotonia can be relieved by nondepolarizing relaxants
(3) myotonia can be precipitated by succinylcholine
(4) neostigmine prevents myotonia

214. The Pierre Robin syndrome presents anesthetic difficulty because of the prevalence of

(1) heart problems
(2) lung problems
(3) renal problems
(4) intubation problems

215. Patients with polycystic kidneys also have a higher incidence of

(1) lung cysts
(2) liver cysts
(3) thyroid cysts
(4) cerebral aneurysms

216. A patient with neurofibromatosis may present anesthetic difficulties due to

(1) the possibility of tumor occurring in the larynx
(2) lung disease
(3) the possibility of pheochromocytoma
(4) heart disease

Answers and Explanations

1. **(C)** Phantom limb pain is an example of central pain. Another example is postherpetic neuralgia. The other options are examples of somatic pain. Central pain is usually amenable to the same treatment as somatic pain. *(1:2078,2083; 159:11)*

2. **(A)** Occipital neuralgia involves the greater occipital nerve and leads to a chronic headache that may extend to the shoulder or forward to the area around the eye. It may be due to compression of the occipital nerve within the skull. The scapular nerve is not involved nor is the cervical plexus. *(75:795; 120:21)*

3. **(E)** Coccygodynia is difficult to treat. Coccygectomy is not successful in most cases. In some patients, repeated caudal injections may lead to some relief. The syndrome is more prevalent in women. *(120:21)*

4. **(B)** The signs of causalgia are hyperesthesia, extremities that may be cold or warm, pain that is long-lasting, and trophic changes. These may include brittle nails and osteoporosis. *(1:2089; 75:1442; 120:19)*

5. **(E)** The size of the needle used to deposit the neurolytic agent is not important. What is important are the location of the injection (proximity to the nerve), the concentration of the neurolytic agent, the volume of the agent, and the histology of the nerve. Smaller nerves are easier to block than larger nerves. *(1:2097; 75:1447; 121:161–162)*

6. **(C)** The pain theory of Wall and Melzack proposed mediators in the substantia gelatinosa. This theory has been expanded and is not the currently held theory. However, it was their article that stimulated further research into pain mechanisms. *(8:311; 123:685)*

7. **(B)** There is some controversy concerning the usefulness of intraoperative blocks. Some reports did not demonstrate any difference in postoperative ventilation. Most current authors have found that the postoperative course is easier and shorter if blocks are done at the time of the thoracotomy. Most use bupivacaine. There is still a danger of a total spinal block and of administration of a toxic dose of the local anesthetic drug. *(1:1426; 75:940)*

8. **(B)** When trying to diagnose the cause of renal failure, one should obtain a urine specimen before treatment is begun. The urine will be concentrated in the patient with prerenal failure and will have a higher specific gravity. The urine need not be blood tinged. Oliguria is present *(1:2237; 75:1095)*

9. **(D)** Adequate anesthesia for a prostatic resection involves a level to at least T-10. *(75:1112)*

10. **(C)** Perforation is a possibility with transurethral resection. An electrolyte disturbance is possible, and the patient may have had a pulmonary embolus, but the most likely problem in the situation cited is a perforation. *(1:1659; 75:1111)*

11. **(B)** The timing of the problem is consistent with fluid absorption. An allergic reaction usually is heralded by a fall in pressure. Bladder distention may occur but is usually not a problem. One must not assume that hypoxemia and hypercarbia are not the problem but must rule them out as possibilities. *(75:1110; 125:621; 127:1)*

12. **(C)** Gallamine requires kidney function for excretion. Curare, pancuronium, and metocurine require renal excretion to some degree. Succinylcholine may increase serum potassium levels. *(1:1656; 75:1094)*

13. **(E)** Decreased protein levels decrease thiopental binding and allow more free thiopental. There may be lower metabolism also. Both of these effects may be offset by a higher blood volume in which the thiopental is distributed, making the dose less effec-

tive. Serum osmolarity is low, and gamma globulin is higher in liver disease. Pancuronium has a larger volume of distribution and is less effective for a given dose. *(75:1154)*

14. **(E)** There is no ideal technique. Halothane is not contraindicated, nor are the other halogenated agents. One must titrate the effects of the agents against the patient response. *(75:1155)*

15. **(C)** The patient with active liver disease should not be a surgical candidate unless there is a good reason. Most techniques lead to a decreased hepatic blood flow and will put the patient at risk. In addition, the patient with hepatitis places the operating room team at risk. A general anesthetic is appropriate if it is appropriate for the procedure. Thiopental may be used. *(1:1665; 75:1154)*

16. **(A)** See preceding answer. The patient is at risk for further deterioration. In some cases, the only way to determine the cause is to do an abdominal exploration. The risk should be discussed before anesthesia. *(1:1675)*

17. **(E)** Determination of clotting ability is necessary before induction. Fresh blood should be used to get the clotting factors needed. Glucose should be provided. Liver glycogen is decreased. The use of a nasogastric tube may lead to bleeding if the patient has esophageal varices. *(1:1675; 75:1142)*

18. **(E)** Stridor occurring 14 hours after thyroidectomy and accompanied with signs of tetany is most likely due to hypocalcemia. This patient has an airway problem, and that should be given priority in management. All of the options may be correct. The patient should be observed and intubated if necessary to protect the airway. *(75:1189; 133:214)*

19. **(C)** Patients with myxedema have coarse hair and dry skin. Heat intolerance is not present, but cold intolerance is. The edema is nonpitting. The patients do have bradycardia. *(75:1189; 133:224)*

20. **(D)** These patients should be well monitored. Digitalization may lead to myocardial infarction. The electrocardiogram and blood pressure are not sufficient alone to monitor the fluid status. *(75:1190; 133:224)*

21. **(B)** The mean time for onset of action for propylthiouracil is 8 days, and it takes about 6 weeks before the euthyroid state is reached. The patient would still have a tachycardia. If a regional anesthetic is possible, it would be more easily managed. *(1:273; 75:1188; 134:588)*

22. **(D)** The heart disease associated with hyperthyroidism is usually of a high output failure variety. It is due to low peripheral resistance. *(134:586)*

23. **(B)** A likely cause of hypotension is surgical stress in a patient who has been on cortisone. However, there are many other causes, and one must rule them out before assuming that the steroid problem is responsible. *(75:1200; 108:3)*

24. **(E)** There are many estimates of time to development of adrenal suppression, but the definite time is not known. For this reason, many will cover anyone who has been on steroids within the previous 6 months. *(75:1200; 108:3)*

25. **(B)** The patient with pheochromocytoma should be well prepared preoperatively. This may take 2 weeks. Such patients are usually hypovolemic. The level of monitoring varies with the patient. A pulmonary artery catheter may be needed, but it is not mandatory in all cases. *(1:269; 75:1202)*

26. **(C)** The most important goal is to prevent hypoglycemia. One can monitor glucose levels and try to keep them in a normal range, but this should not be done at the risk of hypoglycemia. Many regimens are proposed to handle the sugar and insulin, but the one thing that is necessary is to avoid hypoglycemia. *(1:258; 75:1202; 135:3)*

27. **(D)** Insulin shock may be manifest as a convulsion. Tachycardia is usually present, and the skin is cold and clammy. There is a sympathetic discharge. *(75:1206)*

28. **(E)** After surgery, the insulin requirement will be increased for a short time. For the first 72 hours after surgery, there should be close monitoring of the sugar. *(95:362; 162:18)*

29. **(C)** Hyperosmolar coma occurs in the absence of ketosis. The osmolar levels are over 300 (normal is about 285). The condition is seen more often in the elderly. Polyuria is seen. Treatment is with rehydration and small doses of insulin. *(75:1206)*

30. **(A)** The circulatory effects of droperidol are short-lived. The effect of potentiation of narcotics is much longer lasting. *(15:352)*

31. **(B)** During bypass, little muscle relaxation is needed. The lungs can be left deflated. The carbon dioxide is usually kept in the normal range. *(75:998)*

32. **(B)** A patient with complete heart block should have pacer wires placed under local anesthesia to avoid the depressant effects of anesthesia on the

heart. If, for some reason, local anesthesia is not possible, sedation or general anesthesia may be used, avoiding agents that depress the heart. *(1:1488; 75:424)*

33. **(B)** If a pacemaker is in place, the electrocardiogram should be checked to ascertain the function of the pacer. It is also necessary to know the type of pacemaker, the rate, and how to modify the rate if necessary. *(1:293; 19:97)*

34. **(D)** Ventricular aneurysms usually are not associated with heart block. The other options frequently are accompanied by heart block. *(136:128)*

35. **(E)** Constant monitoring of the heart beat by palpation or listening is necessary. The indifferent plate should be placed away from the power pack. If the pacer is in demand mode, it may sense the cautery current as depolarization and shut off. Since the electrocardiogram usually is distorted by the cautery, palpation will give an appraisal of the heart beat. *(1:293; 136:129)*

36. **(B)** With modern pacemaker units, the energy output is so low that there is little danger of fibrillation. However, ventricular fibrillation is more common in the patient with a high catecholamine titer, myocardial infarction, and hypoxemia. *(136:129)*

37. **(D)** The intraaortic balloon pump is deflated during systole. It is rapidly inflated during diastole, thereby increasing coronary blood flow. It decreases impedance to the left ventricle. It is contraindicated in the patient with aortic insufficiency. *(19:48; 75:1002)*

38. **(B)** Clamping of the thoracic aorta leads to an immediate increase in blood pressure. Assuming the heart can withstand the markedly increased afterload, there should not be standstill or hypotension. Blood pressure readings are lost in the left arm, but the pulse in the right arm should be present, depending on the placement of the clamp relative to the take-off of the vessels to the arms. *(75:1030)*

39. **(E)** Clamping of the distal aorta leads to an increased vascular resistance and decreased stroke volume, cardiac output, and blood pressure. The heart rate usually is stable. *(19:314)*

40. **(D)** A complication of aortic surgery is spinal cord ischemia due to the compromise of the radicular arteries. These arteries are not constant, and the large artery to the spine, the artery of Adamkiewitz, may be compromised, leading to ischemia. Pressure on the cord can lead to ischemia. Hypothermia may be protective. Loss of cerebrospinal fluid is not a factor. Long periods of hypotension may lead to ischemia. *(19:315; 75:1035)*

41. **(E)** The expansion of the vascular bed that occurs is following the release of the clamps. It is due to a reactive vasodilatation. The other factors, blood loss, inadequate fluid replacement, vasopressors, and extravasation of fluid, are all important. *(19:315; 75:1034)*

42. **(C)** The flow rate on total bypass can be varied to achieve the perfusion pressure that is desired. This must be varied with the state of resistance. *(75:998)*

43. **(B)** The flow during bypass is nonpulsatile in both flow and pressure. This has been studied to determine if a more physiologic pattern would be beneficial. *(19:372)*

44. **(C)** Oxygenator problems include denaturation of proteins, platelet destruction, sterility hazards, and coagulation defects. Hypocapnia is another problem. *(75:990)*

45. **(A)** When the patient is on bypass, the pressure should be kept at about 50 torr. Lower pressures can be tolerated, and there is not agreement on any specific perfusion pressure. The blood drains from the venae cavae into the pump and is pumped back into the aorta. The sump in the left ventricle drains blood that accumulates from the thebesian veins and from aortic regurgitation. *(19:377,383)*

46. **(D)** Tests should be done to determine if the artery can be clamped. Anesthesia causes decreased oxygen consumption. Hypotension is not a part of carotid surgery. Cerebral infarction is a possibility. General anesthesia is not mandatory, and many have advocated local anesthesia. Shunting procedures are used in many cases to provide flow during clamping. *(1:1624; 19:318)*

47. **(A)** Hypercapnia is not necessary for carotid artery surgery. The vasodilatation has not proven to be helpful. Oxygen tension and blood pressure are kept at levels that are normal or slightly above normal. Normothermia is used, as is systemic heparinization. *(1:1624; 19:321)*

48. **(A)** Stump pressure is dependent on collateral circulation. It is a measure of the pressure distal to the occlusion and the pressure that is perfusing the brain. It is not decreased by hypertension. The effects of hypocapnia and hypercapnia are not uniform. *(1:1624; 19:318)*

49. **(B)** The definition of autoregulation is correct. Vasomotor paralysis involves a vasodilatation. Luxury perfusion is perfusion in excess of requirement. Intracerebral steal involves blood flow away from ischemic areas. Inverse steal involves diversion of

flow from normal areas to ischemic areas. *(1:1256; 75:819; 137:374)*

50. **(E)** All of the factors have some bearing on the outcome of the patient for hip fracture surgery, but the age of the patient is the one determinant that is most important. *(75:1175)*

51. **(D)** Hypervolemia does not contribute to the problem at the time of implant placement. Hypotension may follow a period of hypovolemia that is aggravated by peripheral dilatation. Fat emboli may contribute. *(75:1176)*

52. **(B)** Methylmethacrylate is an acrylic cement. It does generate heat when setting. It is mixed at the time of usage. Placement may lead to hypotension. It is a glue used for many types of fractures. *(75:1176)*

53. **(D)** Fat emboli may be seen with fractures. The emboli are associated with petechiae, hypoxemia, and confusion. Cyanosis may be apparent. There is usually a tachycardia. *(2:528; 75:1172)*

54. **(D)** The average amount of blood lost during a procedure for hip fracture is 1300 ml. *(75:1173; 146:1005)*

55. **(A)** The patient with a head injury should have meticulous care from a ventilatory standpoint. He or she should be kept with the head elevated, the P_{CO_2} controlled in the range of 25 to 30, and PEEP used judiciously as needed. Increases in pressure should be avoided, and, of course, hypoxia and hypercarbia should be avoided. *(160:155)*

56. **(C)** Mannitol may lead to vein disruption, leading to hematoma. This may be more of a problem in the elderly. Mannitol may also lead to cerebral edema but that does not lead to hematoma. This drug may leak through vein walls and may cause hypervolemia, but these factors do not contribute to the development of hematomas. *(1:1571)*

57. **(D)** The best agent for decreasing cerebral oxygen requirement is a barbiturate. A muscle relaxant may contribute if the patient is fighting while being ventilated. Oxygen may be helpful to avoid hypoxia. Glucose and phenytoin may be adjuncts. *(1:805; 75:852)*

58. **(A)** The usual cerebrospinal fluid pressure is 1 to 10 torr or about 13 to 20 cm H_2O pressure. *(1:2253; 75:852)*

59. **(A)** The Glasgow Coma Score is based on the ability to open the eyes, the verbal response, and the motor response. Responses to knee jerk, pupil size, respiration, and EEG are assessed in a general neurologic workup but are not part of the Glasgow Coma Score. *(1:236; 75:1367)*

60. **(E)** Focal brain ischemia is not treated with halothane, since that will cause brain vasodilatation. Thiopental has been used effectively. The calcium channel blocker, nimodipine, has been used. Naloxone and isoflurane have been used successfully. *(1:1632; 75:870)*

61. **(A)** Intracerebral steal describes a change in flow in ischemic tissue due to vasodilatation. It is present with tumors and with ischemia due to stroke. It may occur during anesthesia depending upon how ventilation is handled. The phenomenon is not helpful to compromised tissue. *(2:751; 75:821,870)*

62. **(E)** Cerebral blood flow increases greatly with increases in Pa_{CO_2}. For this reason it is important to have good airway control at all times when dealing with patients with increased intracranial pressure. *(1:1257; 75:850)*

63. **(A)** The intracranial pressure may increase with succinylcholine administration. This effect can be attenuated with prior use of a nondepolarizer. The important factor is to continue ventilation to avoid build-up of CO_2. Serum potassium will not rise above the usual 0.5 to 1.0 mEq/L. *(1:1257; 75:837)*

64. **(C)** The incidence of air embolism depends on the method used to search for it. With the Doppler, the rate has been quoted up to 25%. This must be compared with the 12% incidence in a flat position with an infratentorial exploration. *(1:1580; 75:860)*

65. **(B)** The major buffer against increases in intracranial pressure is the cerebrospinal fluid. The dural sinuses, which contain blood, are also a buffer. The other options are tissues that do not act as buffers. *(1:1564; 75:852)*

66. **(E)** PEEP has a place in the ventilation of the neurosurgical patient, but it should not be used on a routine basis. The level of PEEP should be titrated to the need and effect. The intracranial pressure must be watched to ascertain that the PEEP is not causing harm. The head should be elevated. *(75:837)*

67. **(A)** On the flat part of the compliance curve, there is a slow rise in pressure for increases in volume. In this area of the curve, there is good compensation. As one moves to the right, there is a sudden increase in pressure with little change in volume. *(1:1566; 75:835)*

68. **(C)** The tracings are obtained with transducers in the extradural space. Small increments of volume

are added, and the pressure changes are noted. *(1:1566; 75:835)*

69. **(D)** The most profound stimulus for cerebral auto-regulation is carbon dioxide. Changes in electrolytes and acid-base balance may have an effect, but the predominant effect is from CO_2. *(1:1257; 75:850)*

70. **(D)** The oxygen reserves are very low. The reserves are not changed under anesthesia, but oxygen use is decreased. Since oxygen reserves are so low, the brain is subject to hypoxia with any bout of ischemia. *(1:1250; 75:819)*

71. **(B)** Urinary volume will increase with mannitol administration. The patient may become hypervolemic at first but may become hypovolemic after diuresis. The venous pressure and arterial pressure may fall. *(1:1571; 153:71–72)*

72. **(D)** Nitrous oxide may cause increased intracranial pressure. Therefore, its use must be considered carefully in the patient with head injury, hemorrhage, and tumor. The biggest problem is in the patient with recent air studies, since the nitrous oxide may diffuse into the air-containing spaces. *(1:639; 153:78)*

73. **(C)** Dextrose solutions may diffuse into the brain and cause or aggravate cerebral edema. The dextrose can lead to diuresis if the glucose level is excessive. The fluid does not lead to fluid retention. *(75:870; 153:80)*

74. **(B)** Air embolism is associated with arrhythmia, heart murmur (when there is a large amount of air), bubbles at the operative site, and decreased end-tidal CO_2. Hypotension usually is seen. *(1:1583; 75:860; 153:84)*

75. **(C)** Any traction in the posterior fossa may lead to arrhythmias. The surgeon should be informed immediately. If the arrhythmia persists, lidocaine may be indicated. It is not necessary initially to change the anesthetic or lower the head. *(75:859; 153:85)*

76. **(A)** There is general consensus that the P_{CO_2} should be kept at 25 to 35 torr. If the CO_2 tension is lowered below 20 torr, the effect is self-defeating. *(2:753; 154:2)*

77. **(C)** Loss of autoregulation may be focal and only affect part of the brain. For this reason, changes in P_{CO_2} may cause diversion of blood from the areas that are ischemic to areas that are still regulated. Loss of autoregulation may have great significance, but it is difficult to know how to manipulate the CO_2 to get the best effect. *(1:1276; 154:2)*

78. **(A)** Cerebrospinal fluid pressure is increased with coughing. This causes a transmitted pressure to the cranial vault. Bucking on an endotracheal tube has the same effect. Any maneuver that decreases intrathoracic pressure will decrease intracranial pressure. *(1:2255; 75:835)*

79. **(E)** If blood is warmed as it is given, there should be no ill effects, and no treatment is necessary. The serum calcium will not fall, and there will be no signs of tetany. *(1:1345)*

80. **(B)** Blood should be warmed to 100°F (38°C). Hemolysis may occur if the blood is overheated. There is no need for bicarbonate administration unless there is a documented acidosis. If an acidosis occurs, it should be treated with bicarbonate, not lactate. *(1:1339,1347)*

81. **(D)** If transfusion reaction occurs, fluids should be given in large amounts to keep the kidneys open. Mannitol is given for the same reason. The rest of the options are true. *(1:1351)*

82. **(E)** The least risk of hepatitis is present with albumin/plasma protein fraction that has been treated to kill the virus. All of the other units carry about the same risk per unit, 1 in 100 units transfused. *(75:719)*

83. **(C)** The shelf life of blood stored in CPD is 3 weeks. The red cell survival is about 28 days, but government approval is for only 3 weeks. *(1:1334; 161:6)*

84. **(D)** CPD-adenine has a shelf life of 5 weeks. This added time has helped the patient who wants to give his or her own blood before a surgical procedure. *(1:1335; 161:40)*

85. **(D)** Fresh frozen plasma is recommended for the treatment of multiple coagulation factor deficiency. It should not be used for a volume expander or for undocumented replacement of coagulation factors. *(161:19)*

86. **(B)** The minimum number of platelets needed for coagulation is controversial. The two references cite two different numbers, 50,000 and 100,000. The recent "Transfusion Alert" (ref. 164) cites the figure of 50,000 as being acceptable for surgery. *(1:1358; 161:14; 164:1)*

87. **(D)** Most units of red cells have a hematocrit of 70%. Some blood banks can centrifuge the blood to a hematocrit of 90%. *(1:1356; 161:9)*

88. **(E)** The patient with sickle cell disease need not be transfused to a specific hemoglobin level. To push the patient may cause heart failure. Many centers

are now giving exchange transfusions to lower the percentage of sickle cells present. The preparation should strive for good hydration, good pulmonary care, and during the procedure, avoidance of hypothermia and stasis. *(1:320; 75:450)*

89. **(A)** The child should be given atropine only, since the other drugs all are sedatives, and the child with phenylketonuria has an unpredictable response to sedatives. *(167:216; 176:35)*

90. **(D)** Phenylketonuria is not associated with coarse skin. The other options are all true. The child has a tendency to convulsions and hypoglycemia. As already noted, they may be very sensitive to sedative medications. *(75:479; 167:216; 176:35)*

91. **(D)** The patient with acute intermittent porphyria should not receive barbiturates. All of the other drugs can be used without difficulty. *(75:470; 167:217; 176:28)*

92. **(C)** Prilocaine can lead to methemoglobinemia. Few other therapeutic agents will cause this. *(75:391; 176:595)*

93. **(B)** Hypoventilation is a problem for the anesthesiologist in treating the baby with myxedema. Hypothermia is also present in many cases. The children are sensitive to narcotics. The mouth is of normal size, and the tongue may appear large. The heart is not hyperkinetic as in hyperthyroidism. *(176:318)*

94. **(E)** There is a report in the literature of an abnormal response to thiopental with delayed awakening, generalized tonic spasm, and tight jaws. *(75:446; 176:487)*

95. **(E)** Adult patients who have torticollis may develop postoperative airway difficulties, since they frequently have an underlying disease contributing to the symptoms. They should be watched carefully in the recovery room. Intubation is usually of no difficulty. *(176:487)*

96. **(B)** Liver enzymes are not a prerequisite unless there is some other factor that may lead to liver damage. The neck mobility, the chest x-ray, and the electrocardiogram should be checked. One should always check to determine if there were any previous anesthesia experiences. *(75:452; 176:487)*

97. **(B)** A conduction-type anesthetic should be employed if possible to avoid the problems of intubation and airway maintenance. If the procedure requires a general anesthetic, an intubation under topical anesthesia may be advisable. *(167:441)*

98. **(B)** The symptoms are compatible with carcinoid syndrome. The Zollinger-Ellison syndrome is associated with hypersecretion of stomach acid. Pheochromocytoma is associated with hypertension and a catecholamine-secreting tumor. Peutz-Jeghers syndrome is associated with multiple polyps of the gastrointestinal tract. *(1:317; 75:1129; 176:438)*

99. **(C)** About 13 to 18% of patients with Down's syndrome have an atlanto-axial subluxation. A sensitivity to atropine was thought to be present in these children, but that was later disproved. The children can receive sedatives and narcotics if needed. Anticonvulsants should be given as usual. *(1:308; 176:70; 183:89)*

100. **(D)** Aspiration is possible, since the esophagus may contain the barium from the examination as well as other intake. The esophagus should be suctioned before induction. *(176:387)*

101. **(C)** Hurler's syndrome is associated with all of the options listed. Hypertelorism may be present, but it should not be a factor complicating the anesthetic. *(176:387)*

102. **(C)** Amphetamines cause a depletion of catecholamine stores. If hypotension occurs, it should be treated with a direct-acting drug, eg, norepinephrine. The other drugs act by liberating another substance. *(15:264; 176:729)*

103. **(A)** Beriberi heart disease is not seen often. It should be thought of in the patient with alcoholism. The heart disease is a high output failure. *(176:694)*

104. **(E)** There is no method of providing anesthesia that is better than any other. Perhaps a balanced plan with fentanyl or one of the derivatives will provide a safer course that can be titrated. *(176:459)*

105. **(A)** Since multiple sclerosis is a disease that has natural cycles, it is better to avoid an anesthetic that may be identified as the cause of one of the down cycles. The reference cites problems that have been identified with spinal anesthesia. *(75:444; 176:495)*

106. **(B)** Scleroderma is associated with many problems. Arterial dilatation is not one of the associated problems. The arterial problem is usually arterial constriction. Raynaud's phenomenon frequently is seen. *(75:453)*

107. **(A)** The pulmonary problem in scleroderma is a restrictive disease. The chest wall as well as the lung itself contributes to the restriction. There is fibrosis and a decreased vital capacity leading to decreased arterial saturation. The V_D/V_T ratio increases. *(176:24)*

108. (C) There are many bullous-type skin disorders. One of these is associated with porphyria. Since porphyria may cause anesthetic problems with thiobarbiturates, it is important to know the diagnosis before induction. *(75:454,476; 167:210; 176:28)*

109. (B) The patient with Sipple's syndrome who develops hypertension must be suspected of having pheochromocytoma. Light anesthesia and hypercarbia should be quickly ruled out. Allergic reactions are not usually associated with hypertension. The inadvertent injection of a pressor agent may occur but should be easy to rule out. *(75:120; 167:218)*

110. (B) Percutaneous cordotomy has been found to be as effective as open cordotomy. It is best in the patient with terminal pain. It is usually done unilaterally and can be done under local anesthesia. *(1:2105)*

111. (E) In treating chronic pain, one must remember that the pain may not be as bad as the loss of bowel and urinary control and the absence of sensation. The possibility must be discussed with patients before undertaking pain relief methods. *(121:165)*

112. (E) All of the options listed are important for the patient with causalgia. In the patient with obstructive lung disease, one may want to avoid the stellate ganglion approach, since there is a possibility of pneumothorax, which could be life-threatening. *(124:259)*

113. (C) The placebo effect is present in all therapeutic situations. It is not seen only in those who are unstable or who are faking symptoms but is seen in normal patients. *(125:17)*

114. (B) There are many factors in the treatment of chronic pain, but the most important for a given patient are the drug and the timing of its administration. The vehicle is not usually of importance. *(1:2082; 75:1433)*

115. (B) In many cases of chronic pain one can do a diagnostic block to establish the type of pain present. This may involve a short-acting local anesthetic or a differential spinal. It is not done with a neurolytic agent, such as phenol, which is permanent. *(1:2087; 120:19)*

116. (B) Alcohol has a faster onset of action but a greater tendency to produce neuritis. It is used in absolute concentration. Phenol is used in concentrations of 10%. *(1:1086; 75:1447)*

117. (D) Current pain theories involve the small and large nerves and a path through the dorsal root.

Both inhibitory and excitatory nerves are involved. *(15:634; 75:1431; 123:685)*

118. (B) Halothane and thiopental should cause no problem to the kidney. Gallamine may not be excreted in a timely fashion. Enflurane may lead to fluoride ion increases on metabolism and should be avoided on theoretical grounds. *(1:1656; 75:1094)*

119. (A) There is no pain with the absorption of fluid. The blood pressure rises, and the heart rate falls. There may be mental changes. The severity of these changes depends on the amount of fluid absorbed. *(75:1110; 125:621; 127:1)*

120. (B) The syndrome of fluid absorption may lead to pulmonary edema due to increased intravascular pressure and to decreased osmotic pressure. The serum sodium will fall. The position on the table is not a factor. *(75:1110; 125:621; 127:1)*

121. (A) The serum sodium is decreased. There is an increase of circulating fluid, and the electrolytes are diluted. Hemolysis of red cells may occur. *(75:1110; 125:621; 127:1)*

122. (B) The irrigating fluids should be nonhemolytic and isoosmolar. (Glycine is hypoosmolar. Cytal is isoosmolar.) The composition should not be close to water, since water is hypoosmotic. Electrolyte solutions interfere with the cautery. *(1:1658; 75:1109)*

123. (A) Blood sugar rises during surgery by many mechanisms, including administration of intravenous fluids, secretion from the liver due to catecholamines, and insulin suppression. Uptake into the tissues leads to a decrease in blood sugar. *(8:374; 75:1207)*

124. (C) Administration of insulin should be carefully monitored during surgery. Blood sugar should be followed closely. The intravenous line containing the insulin should not be the primary line but should be piggy-backed into another line. There is also concern that some of the insulin will be adsorbed to the intravenous tubing. The dosage should be titrated to needs. *(1:258; 75:1208)*

125. (D) The juvenile-type diabetic is usually brittle, with blood sugars in the higher ranges. These patients are usually thin. They have poor response to oral hypoglycemics. They do lack insulin in the blood. *(1:257; 8:377)*

126. (A) The first three options are correct. Tolazamide has an activity of 10 to 18 hours. *(1:420)*

127. (A) We depend upon the stress response for homeostasis in many cases. In the neonate, the chronically

ill, and the very old this response may not be present. This is important from two perspectives. First, the response may not be present, and cardiovascular stability will vanish. Second, we may administer drugs that will take away the stress response with the same result. *(2:991)*

128. **(A)** Mineralocorticoids, glucocorticoids, and sex hormones are secreted by the cortex. Norepinephrine is secreted by the medulla. *(1:263; 75:1194)*

129. **(A)** The patient with myxedema may have heart failure, cardiomegaly, and pleural effusion. Bradycardia is usually present. *(75:1189)*

130. **(A)** Hypertension may be caused by many factors. In this case, the first three options are correct. Myxedema is not associated with hypertension. Pheochromocytoma is possible if the tumor is part of the multiple endocrine adenoma syndrome. *(1:275; 75:1201)*

131. **(A)** Glucocorticoids are produced under stimulation by ACTH and are active in carbohydrate and protein metabolism. Aldosterone is a mineralocorticoid. *(1:263; 8:386; 75:1194)*

132. **(E)** In diabetes insipidus, the serum sodium is high and the serum osmolality is high. The urine is dilute. In spite of polyuria, thirst need not be present. *(75:740; 95:101)*

133. **(D)** The patient with hyperthyroidism does not have an increased MAC. Medication should be continued into the perioperative period. With modern techniques and preparation, heavy sedation and sneaking the patient are not necessary. Propranolol may be needed. *(1:273)*

134. **(B)** Anticholinergics interfere with interpretation of the pulse rate and with the sweating mechanisms. Pupillary activity and gastric emptying are not concerns in these patients. *(1:273; 134:590)*

135. **(B)** Sweating and tachycardia are compensatory mechanisms to rid the body of the increased heat being produced in the patient with hyperthyroidism. Vasoconstriction is not seen, but vasodilatation is. Shivering is not a heat-losing mechanism. *(134:586)*

136. **(C)** The patient with hyperaldosteronism has hypertension and hypokalemia. The excess secretion comes from the adrenal cortex. Alkalosis is present. *(8:385; 75:1197)*

137. **(E)** All of the options are possible and must be evaluated before treatment. It is important to take

the blood pressure yourself with the proper sized cuff. Hypercarbia must be ruled out. *(75:1402)*

138. **(E)** In caring for the patient with tamponade, the heart is kept full, the heart rate fast, the periphery constricted, and the compensatory mechanisms intact. This patient is living on compensatory mechanisms. *(1:1487; 19:297)*

139. **(A)** The patient with tamponade has a higher incidence of arrhythmias. These would be aggravated by hypoventilation. Increases in thoracic pressure will have an adverse effect on venous filling. *(1:1487; 19:297)*

140. **(A)** Surgery for the patient with a transplanted heart will be rare and in most cases will be done in centers where the transplant was performed. The transplanted heart is essentially denervated. Drugs that usually work directly have more effect. *(138:67; 163:26)*

141. **(D)** See preceding answer. *(138:67; 163:26)*

142. **(E)** Many factors have gone into the improvement of statistics for cardiac surgery. Improvements in anesthesia is one of these. *(131:331)*

143. **(B)** The anesthesia for cardiac surgery should avoid stress caused by painful stimuli and cause a minimum of cardiovascular depression. Heart rate should not be elevated, and the blood pressure should not be allowed to increase. *(75:982; 131:331)*

144. **(A)** Nitrous oxide does not decrease pulmonary vascular resistance. It does increase myocardial ischemia. Sympathetic stimulation is increased. When used with halothane, there is decreased myocardial contractility. *(75:990; 139:2)*

145. **(D)** Droperidol is an alpha-blocker. There are no sympathetic stimulating, vagolytic effects or beta-agonist effects. *(1:385; 15:352)*

146. **(B)** Administration of fentanyl will result in bradycardia, but the blood pressure is stable. The cardiac output will decrease to a mild degree. Morphine changes are more pronounced. *(1:754; 75:996)*

147. **(B)** The anesthetic goal in patients with coronary heart disease is to minimize the oxygen requirement and to maintain coronary flow. A fast heart rate increases oxygen consumption, as does light anesthesia. *(75:982)*

148. **(C)** In the presence of heart disease, tachycardia is undesirable, since it increases the energy requirements of the heart. This may lead to hypotension and pulmonary edema. *(1:1192; 15:182)*

149. (C) In the case described, the fall in pressure would be accompanied with vasodilatation, decreased cardiac output, increased left atrial pressure, and decreased coronary filling pressure. *(19:246)*

150. (A) The primary determinants of myocardial oxygen supply are blood flow and the oxygen-carrying capacity of the blood. Age is not a primary determinant. F_{IO_2} affects oxygen supply by increasing the amount of dissolved oxygen in the blood. *(75:173)*

151. (B) The major problems with ketamine are the production of hypertension and tachycardia, both of which will increase oxygen demand. The hallucinations are not a problem unless they lead to increased oxygen demand. Oxygen lack is not seen with ketamine. *(75:136)*

152. (A) Thiopental does not increase myocardial contractility. Diazepam usually maintains cardiovascular stability. Droperidol blunts the autonomic response to intubation. Ketamine, as noted in the preceding answer, will increase oxygen consumption. *(141:23)*

153. (C) Fentanyl will lead to earlier emergence and earlier extubation. The heart rate will be lower with fentanyl. The oxygen supply to the heart will not be increased. *(75:996; 141:23)*

154. (B) The effect of propranolol is related to the plasma concentration. The half-life is only 3 to 6 hours. Therefore, the drug should not be discontinued, since the withdrawal may lead to difficulty. The drug should be maintained throughout the perioperative period. *(75:181,597; 141:23)*

155. (D) Hemodilution may lead to improved tissue flow. It does not lead to bradycardia or to decreased cardiac output or decreased myocardial oxygen consumption. *(141:26)*

156. (B) The ideal method of maintaining the lungs during cardiopulmonary bypass to decrease postoperative complications is controversial. Stanley showed that the complications are fewer if the lungs are allowed to collapse during bypass. *(19:346; 145:394)*

157. (D) Continued ventilation during bypass may lead to depletion of surfactant. There is no evidence that it leads to better ventilation or that it improves the postoperative recovery time. It does not lead to hypercarbia. *(19:346; 145:394)*

158. (A) The deficit described may be the result of the first three options. An electrolyte imbalance is not a factor. *(147:527)*

159. (D) If the patient has a deficit that cannot be explained, the back should be reexplored to determine if there is a hematoma present. The patient should be left intubated, pending a decision. There is no advantage of waiting. If there is a cord compromise, it should be removed as early as possible. *(147:527)*

160. (A) The blood loss in total hip replacements has been correlated with the type of anesthesia (less with general), type of disease (more with degenerative and with a second procedure), and with intraoperative blood pressure. Whether the procedure is the first or second has no bearing. In some institutions, many procedures are done on the same day. There is no correlation of the blood loss with placement in the schedule. *(75:1176; 151:641)*

161. (D) There is controversy regarding the relative merits of each type of anesthesia. Studies are available for each viewpoint. If one looks at the mortality data at 1 month postoperatively, there is little difference. *(75:1175; 152:614)*

162. (E) Most of us think of fat emboli in the context of the bone fracture. Emboli have been described from sternotomy, liver fracture, and soft tissue injuries as well. *(2:528; 75:1172)*

163. (C) In global ischemia, there is no electrical activity. Since barbiturates protect by decreasing electrical activity, they have little effect in this situation. Thiopental is more protective than halothane. *(1:1632; 75:869)*

164. (E) Mannitol may lead to hyperosmolar coma if given in large doses. The drug has its effect by removing water from the normal tissues. If the blood–brain barrier is impaired, mannitol may pass into the cells and cause cerebral edema. The drug is effective in doses as low as 0.25 mg/kg. *(160:155)*

165. (B) Dexamethasone is effective in the treatment of the edema of patients with brain tumors. It is not effective in the patient with brain injury. The effect is by membrane stabilization. *(1:1572,2259; 75:1457)*

166. (A) The normal brain has a metabolic rate and blood flow that are relatively constant. The range of autoregulation is 50 to 150 torr. The energy requirements do not demand fructose as the source. *(2:753; 75:819)*

167. (A) Induction of anesthesia with nitrous oxide as a component will lead to increased intracranial pressure. In the patient with an already increased pressure, decompensation may occur. *(1:1264; 75:852)*

168. (A) If increased intracranial pressure occurs on induction, there may be areas of focal ischemia, her-

niation, and decreased perfusion pressure. Brain retraction will not occur. *(75:849,856)*

169. **(B)** Factors of importance in air embolism are amount and rate of entry. The site of entry is not important. A pulmonary artery catheter may be useful for the monitoring aspects, but the port is too small to be very helpful in the withdrawal of air. *(75:861)*

170. **(C)** The G-suit has be recommended to prevent hypotension and to treat hypotension. It has not been universally accepted and has had questionable effectiveness. *(2:768; 52:143)*

171. **(A)** Factors of importance in regulating the intracranial pressure are the cerebrospinal fluid, the intracranial tissue, and the blood flow. The dura is not a regulating mechanism. *(75:852; 112:1)*

172. **(C)** Fentanyl and thiopental do not increase intracranial pressure. Halothane and nitrous oxide do increase the pressure. *(1:1264; 75:820)*

173. **(E)** Treatment of cerebral edema includes all of the options: osmotic diuretics, chemical diuretics, steroids, and surgical decompression. *(1:1570; 2:771)*

174. **(C)** Halothane, used in the neurosurgical patient, should be combined with controlled ventilation to decrease intracranial pressure. It is a vasodilator. *(1:1267; 75:851)*

175. **(A)** When hypothermia is used, less glucose is needed. The cerebral metabolism decreases, resistance increases and the patient remains responsive to CO_2. *(2:536; 75:867)*

176. **(A)** The blood–brain barrier is readily permeable to drugs that have an affinity for the membrane lipid. Morphine, glucose, and carbon dioxide pass through. Bicarbonate does not. *(1:1259; 75:264,867)*

177. **(A)** Mannitol is preferred because of its longer duration, the smaller rebound effect, and the fact that it has a larger molecule. There are no permanent effects. *(15:428; 153:7)*

178. **(C)** Hyperventilation may lead to tetany and decreased cardiac output. The cerebral vasculature is constricted, and the oxyhemoglobin curve is shifted to the left. *(1:1159; 75:1374; 153:73)*

179. **(B)** Positioning the patient in the sitting position requires planning. The legs should be at a level above the heart, and the legs should be wrapped. The head must be firmly fixed in a head rest. Positioning should be done slowly to avoid hypotension. *(1:1579; 75:663; 153:70)*

180. **(A)** Premedication is used in small doses if at all in the very young, the patient with increased intracranial pressure, and comatose patients. The anxious patient should be made sedate if possible. *(75:486; 90:3)*

181. **(B)** The use of induced hypotension usually is needed for very short times during a neurosurgical procedure. It is best given with a short-acting drug, such as sodium nitroprusside. The use of hypotension may lead to increases in dead space. Hypotension is not contraindicated in the neurosurgical patient. Cottrell makes the point that hypotension is indicated today more than in the past. *(106:4,5; 153:81–82)*

182. **(E)** All of the options are true concerning air embolism. In order for air to reach the heart, there must be a relatively negative pressure. That does not require a great elevation of the head. *(75:664,860; 153:84)*

183. **(C)** Treatment of air embolism requires removal of the air in the heart. This can be accomplished by aspiration or by compression forcing the air into the pulmonary artery. Small amounts may be pushed into the artery. Large amounts should be aspirated. The venous pressure in the head should be elevated to prevent the aspiration of air. The position should be head-down. *(1:1586; 75:861; 153:84–85)*

184. **(E)** Any one of these procedures may be associated with arrhythmias. *(153:184–185)*

185. **(B)** Sodium nitroprusside is of short duration. It may cause an acidemia. It usually is associated with a tachycardia. The toxicity is cyanide toxicity. *(75:218; 106:3)*

186. **(B)** The Doppler flowmeter can detect air in quantities as little as 0.5 ml. The transducer is placed over the right side of the heart. The Doppler functions at 2.0 Hz. The transducer will detect CO_2, and some inject a small amount of CO_2 to check the function of the transducer. *(1:1583; 75:860)*

187. **(C)** Diazepam and thiopental may block the rises in intracranial pressure. Halothane and ketamine will lead to increases. *(1:1270; 75:852)*

188. **(B)** Drug effects on intracranial pressure are not constant but will vary among individuals. They depend on ventilation effects. The total effect on vascular tone will determine the effect on pressure. *(1:1270; 75:852)*

189. **(D)** Reactions to transfusions are to be expected. Most are not fatal. Many do not occur immediately. The reaction may be hemolytic, but it may be an allergic reaction. *(1:1350; 161:69,74)*

190. (A) Hepatitis may follow transfusion of blood products. The most common type is non-A, non-B. The incidence is lower if the donor pool is volunteers. Transfusion of red cells does not carry a higher risk. Current data list the risk as 1/100 units transfused. *(1:1384; 75:719; 164:2)*

191. (B) Von Willebrand's disease is a bleeding disorder that is congenital. It involves bleeding primarily from the mucous membranes. The defect is in factor VIII. The defect has an autosomal dominant transmission in most cases. It is not seen only in females. *(1:2389; 75:714)*

192. (E) Vitamin K-dependent factors are II, VII, IX and X. *(1:1209; 161:64)*

193. (B) During blood storage, there is an increasing concentration of potassium and ammonia. Dextrose and bicarbonate levels decrease. *(1:1335; 161:7)*

194. (A) Hemolysis of blood may be caused by overheating to over 100°F, infusion under pressure, and cardiopulmonary bypass. In the last, blood cells are destroyed in the oxygenator and in the suction devices that are needed. Cooling blood does not cause hemolysis. *(161:53)*

195. (A) Small bowel resection does not have any increased incidence of bleeding. The other options are all associated with bleeding. *(1:1718; 75:716)*

196. (B) CPD blood has better storage characteristics. There is longer survival and less loss of 2,3-DPG. The pH is higher with CPD, and the potassium does not rise as much (a reflection of the lower cell breakdown). *(1:1335; 161:7)*

197. (A) Sickling of susceptible red cells is more likely with low oxygen tension, low temperature, and low pH. A low hematocrit does not cause sickling but may help flow and thereby reduce sickling. *(1:320; 75:450)*

198. (B) Hypoglycemia in the anesthetized patient may be difficult to detect. In the patient who is known to have hypoglycemia, blood sugars should be determined. A glucose infusion will avoid hypoglycemia. Blood sugars can be determined even with an infusion running, but one should avoid drawing blood from the same extremity in which the infusion is running. *(75:1206; 176:8,9)*

199. (A) Wilson's disease is a metabolic derangement of copper metabolism. Hepatic involvement may affect drug metabolism. The action of neuromuscular blocking agents may be prolonged if the liver disease is severe. The kidneys are not involved. *(167:221; 176:44)*

200. (A) Patients with gout should be given generous amounts of fluids to ensure good urinary output. Lactate solutions have an uricemic effect and should be avoided. On theoretical grounds, enflurane should be avoided because of possible fluoride toxicity. *(176:45)*

201. (B) Marfan's syndrome is associated with aortic changes, making dissection more common. Hypertension should be avoided. The high-arched palate may make intubation more difficult. Aortic stenosis is not seen, but aortic insufficiency is common. The patients are tall with long extremities. *(167:215)*

202. (E) In a patient with methemoglobinemia, one must ascertain the cause. The disease may be inherited, or it may have been caused by drugs, eg, primaquine or nitrites. The level should be determined. It is helpful to know the past therapeutic experience. Most of these patients are cyanotic but have no dyspnea. The family history may reveal the cause. *(75:391; 176:250)*

203. (C) Pneumoconioses are associated with fibrosis. Since a restrictive component is present, the diaphragm may move very little. The x-ray may look much worse than the functional state. *(176:248)*

204. (C) The chronic use of marijuana leads to bronchitis and tachycardia. There is not a withdrawal syndrome to marijuana alone. The liver is not involved unless other drugs are involved. *(75:411; 176:737)*

205. (E) The pressure in the cranium is transmitted to the syrinx; therefore, any bucking or coughing should be avoided. Many of these patients have scoliosis, and the associated V/Q abnormalities may affect ventilation under anesthesia. If the disease has progressed, there may be muscle wasting, making the use of succinylcholine hazardous. In addition, there may be increased sensitivity to nondepolarizing relaxants. *(75:351; 176:493)*

206. (B) Patients who have a history of glue sniffing are prone to liver and renal disorders. There is no hematologic involvement. *(176:710)*

207. (C) Choice of anesthesia in a patient with a history of renal and hepatic toxins would make one avoid halothane and enflurane. A regional technique may be desirable. The patient and family must be told of the increased risk of anesthesia, since we cannot always predict hepatic blood flow. *(176:170)*

208. (C) Patients acutely toxic with cocaine are hypertensive and have tachycardia. This is due to the action of cocaine in preventing reuptake of norepinephrine. If the cocaine use is chronic, the patient may be more moody and violent. *(75:412; 176:729)*

209. **(A)** The patient with multiple myeloma has hypercalcemia. Bone pain is common, and the patient is subject to easy bone fractures. Renal failure may occur due to the deposition of the abnormal protein in the tubules. Serum chloride levels usually are not deranged. *(75:454; 176:344)*

210. **(B)** Patients with skin bullae present difficult anesthesia management problems. Tracheal intubation should be used if needed. The tube should be secured with wide cord or umbilical tape to avoid the use of adhesive tape. To do the procedure under mask requires pressure on the face, and that may cause skin deterioration. Any friction may lead to loss of skin. *(176:563)*

211. **(A)** The patient with amytrophic lateral sclerosis is chronically weak and has muscle wasting. Succinylcholine should be avoided. Muscle relaxants, if required, should be used in low doses. Respiratory depressants are avoided. If the patient has any respiratory compromise postoperatively, artificial ventilation is in order. *(75:351,447; 167:108)*

212. **(B)** Autonomic hyperreflexia occurs with spinal lesions above T-5. Any stimulation, eg, urinary catheter stimulation, will lead to hypertension accompanied by sweating and bradycardia. The anesthesiologist must be prepared to treat the hypertension immediately. *(75:1171; 176:650)*

213. **(B)** The patient with myotonic dystrophy presents many anesthetic problems. Succinylcholine may cause myotonia. Myotonic episodes are not reversed by nondepolarizers. Neostigmine may aggravate myotonia. Shivering in the recovery room may lead to myotonia. The approach to the procedure involves a careful history to determine which factors may make the particular patient worse. At the end of the procedure, artificial ventilation is preferable to reversal of muscle relaxants. *(75:351,441; 167:215; 176:535)*

214. **(D)** The Pierre Robin syndrome presents problems due to the recessed chin, making intubation very difficult. Tracheostomy may be necessary to avoid airway obstruction. There usually are no associated renal, cardiac, or lung problems. *(75:1741; 167:216)*

215. **(E)** Polycystic kidney disease is associated with cysts in other organs, including the lung, liver, and thyroid. Cerebral aneurysms are also more common. *(167:216)*

216. **(B)** The patient with neurofibromatosis presents problems on intubation due to the possible presence of tumors in the larynx. The fibromas may be present anywhere. There is an increased incidence of pheochromocytoma. Heart disease and lung disease are not increased in incidence. *(75:479; 167:220)*

CHAPTER 14

General Considerations
Review

Questions in this chapter deal with general aspects of anesthesiology and some aspects that do not fall specifically into another category. Areas covered are massive obesity, outpatient surgery, ophthalmic surgery, history of anesthesiology, medicolegal aspects of anesthesiology, and acupuncture.

There are many aspects that have not been discussed that should be reviewed before the examination, including endoscopy, lithotripsy, anesthesia for the patient with burns, radiology, and the cost of medical care.

The practice of anesthesiology today is not limited to the operating room. There is a constant input from hospital committees, third party carriers, and the government in relation to our practice. One cannot sit back and just practice medicine any more. One must remain current with the various interventions that affect us.

In addition to the extraneous data that we must be aware of, there is a constant need to remain up to date with the scientific aspects of our profession. New techniques are being developed, and new methods of delivering care are being used. Note the change in outpatient surgery. In the early 1970s there were few outpatient procedures; today 70% of some practices involve patients who are first seen on the day of surgery. This has drastically changed our practice. Other changes that we do not anticipate are ahead of us, and we must be prepared to meet them.

Questions

1. The statistical term for the spread of individual values is

   (A) mean
   (B) median
   (C) variance
   (D) standard deviation
   (E) standard error of the mean

2. Patients who undergo outpatient surgery with halothane should not drive or operate machinery for at least

   (A) 30 minutes
   (B) 1 hour
   (C) 3 hours
   (D) 7 hours
   (E) 16 hours

3. The preanesthetic use of atropine in patients with glaucoma

   (A) is contraindicated
   (B) is more dangerous in the patient with open-angle glaucoma
   (C) should not precipitate glaucoma
   (D) may cause miosis
   (E) will decrease the intraocular pressure significantly

4. A 5-year-old patient is admitted with an open eye secondary to severe globe laceration. He had eaten 1 hour before his accident. General anesthesia is required for the repair. The intubation should be accomplished

   (A) by an awake intubation
   (B) after injection of 100 mg of succinylcholine
   (C) after D-tubocurarine followed by succinylcholine

   (D) after vecuronium administration
   (E) after deep halothane by inhalation induction

5. The best method for prevention of the oculocardiac reflex is

   (A) preoperative atropine
   (B) a retrobulbar block
   (C) intravenous atropine during the procedure
   (D) administration of vecuronium
   (E) administration of neostigmine

6. The efferent limb of the oculocardiac reflex is the

   (A) ciliary nerve
   (B) trigeminal nerve
   (C) vagus nerve
   (D) facial nerve
   (E) ophthalmic nerve

7. The motto on the seal of the American Society of Anesthesiologists is

   (A) Safety
   (B) Vigilance
   (C) Excellence in Medicine
   (D) Ever Forward
   (E) Concern

8. The first person to hold a position as a chairman of a department of anesthesiology in an American university was

   (A) Magill
   (B) Guedel
   (C) Waters
   (D) Bert
   (E) Morton

9. The man who first administered ether in a public trial was

   (A) Wells
   (B) Long

(C) Morton
(D) Warren
(E) Abbott

10. The English physician who popularized chloroform was

(A) Magill
(B) Snow
(C) Richardson
(D) Simpson
(E) Jackson

11. Morbid obesity is associated with

(A) decreased cardiac output
(B) hypertension
(C) decreased pulmonary artery pressure
(D) decreased blood volume
(E) decreased cardiac workload

12. Technical difficulties in treating patients with morbid obesity include all of the following EXCEPT

(A) low blood pressure readings
(B) difficult venous access
(C) difficult intubation
(D) difficult airway maintenance with mask
(E) difficulty with nerve blocks

13. In obtaining informed consent, an anesthesiologist should

(A) have the surgeon explain the anesthesia procedures to the patient
(B) tell the patient only the common problems
(C) not paint too gloomy a picture lest the patient be frightened
(D) disclose the potential for death or serious harm
(E) answer only specific questions

14. The principal cause of lawsuits is

(A) negligence
(B) cardiac arrest
(C) failure to establish rapport with patients
(D) damaged teeth
(E) postoperative sore throats

DIRECTIONS (Questions 15 through 28): For each of the items in this section, ONE or MORE of the numbered options is correct. Choose the answer

A if only 1, 2, and 3 are correct,
B if only 1 and 3 are correct,
C if only 2 and 4 are correct,
D if only 4 is correct,
E if all are correct.

15. General anesthesia for electroconvulsion therapy

(1) should be performed without muscle relaxants

(2) requires an oral airway for the protection of the patient
(3) should not be preceded with oxygenation
(4) should be induced with a short-acting barbiturate

16. General anesthesia is indicated for computed tomography (CT) scanning when the patient

(1) is very young
(2) is restless
(3) has involuntary movements
(4) is febrile

17. Statistics useful in interpreting continuous numerical data include

(1) the mean
(2) variance
(3) standard deviation
(4) Student's *t*-test

18. The doctrine of *res ipsa loquitur* is applicable where the

(1) accident is of a kind that usually does not happen without negligence
(2) apparent cause of the accident is within the control of the defendant
(3) plaintiff could not have contributed to the accident
(4) defendant wants to settle out of court

19. If it is discovered at the end of a procedure that a tooth is missing, the anesthesiologist should

(1) awaken the patient as usual
(2) check the oropharynx and nasopharynx
(3) ask the family about the tooth when the patient is in the recovery room
(4) get x-rays of the head, chest, and abdomen

20. A child who undergoes outpatient anesthesia should

(1) not be intubated
(2) be watched for at least 1 hour postoperatively
(3) be kept NPO for at least 6 hours after surgery
(4) be admitted if croup develops

21. After outpatient surgery with halothane

(1) there is less psychomotor impairment than after anesthesia with diazepam
(2) the patient may return home alone after a 2-hour wait
(3) the patient should not ingest alcohol for 24 hours
(4) there is more psychomotor impairment than after anesthesia with methohexital

SUMMARY OF DIRECTIONS				
A	**B**	**C**	**D**	**E**
1, 2, 3 only	1, 3 only	2, 4 only	4 only	All are correct

22. Eyedrops that cause anesthesia difficulties include

(1) atropine
(2) phenylephrine
(3) echothiophate iodide
(4) antibiotics

23. Drugs affecting intraocular pressure include

(1) acetazolamide
(2) succinylcholine
(3) mannitol
(4) atropine

24. The oculocardiac reflex is associated with

(1) blood pressure changes
(2) bradycardia
(3) traction
(4) cardiac arrhythmias

25. A digital computer

(1) input is the information entered for processing
(2) memory stores the input

(3) functions using the binary system
(4) uses Boolean logic

26. The hazards known to be present in operating rooms for personnel include an increase in

(1) the incidence of spontaneous abortions
(2) the number of congenital abnormalities in the children of exposed males and females
(3) liver disease
(4) female cancer

27. Which of the following advantages are claimed for acupuncture?

(1) complete safety, since the physiology of the patient is not disturbed
(2) a tonic or regulatory effect on the body
(3) no residual effects
(4) an anti-inflammatory effect

28. Which of the following disadvantages are cited in the use of acupuncture?

(1) lack of complete analgesia
(2) no muscle relaxation
(3) traction of viscera provokes pain
(4) dyspnea during intrathoracic procedures

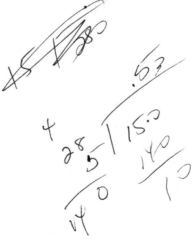

Answers and Explanations

1. **(D)** The statistical term for the spread of individual values is the standard deviation. The mean is the average of the data, and the standard error of the mean is a precision factor. Variance is the difference of each value from the mean. *(1:193; 75:53; 185:749)*

2. **(E)** Most of us tell the patients not to drive or operate machinery until the next day, but there are data suggesting that 2 days may be more appropriate. *(1:1909)*

3. **(C)** In the dosage needed for premedication, atropine should not cause problems in the patient with glaucoma. The theoretical problem is in the patient with closed-angle glaucoma. Atropine can cause mydriasis. Atropine does lower intraocular pressure due to its smooth muscle relaxation, but it is not significant. If given in large doses and there is a problem precipitated, the pressure will increase. *(1:389; 75:1053)*

4. **(C)** There is no consensus in answering this question. Succinylcholine alone is not good. An awake intubation is not good. If starting an intravenous line will cause such anxiety in a child that the intraocular pressure increases due to his thrashing around, that is unacceptable. In a given situation, I have used a gas induction with cricoid pressure successfully. The intravenous line was started after the child was asleep, and then vecuronium was given. Cricoid pressure was maintained until the airway was secure. I have also started an intravenous line with no difficulty with the child and then used vecuronium. If one chooses to use succinylcholine, the fasciculations must be blocked. It is important to explain the problem to the parents before the procedure. Let them know that there is a serious problem. *(1:1851; 75:1059; 179:242; 180:36)*

5. **(C)** One can find various answers in the literature. Atropine is espoused, but there are those who believe that the administration of atropine may lead to an increased incidence of arrhythmias and that prevention is not warranted. It is important to in-

form the surgeon as soon as bradycardia is seen. The reflex does fatigue early and usually is not persistent. *(1:1845; 75:1055)*

6. **(C)** The oculocardiac reflex is a trigeminovagal reflex, with the efferent nerve being the vagus. *(1:1845; 75:1055)*

7. **(B)** This motto is seen on the cover of every issue of *Anesthesiology*. It is just as important today when we have many monitors as it was when the ASA was founded. *(75:1055)*

8. **(C)** Ralph M. Waters was appointed chairman at the University of Wisconsin. Magill was responsible for the development of many anesthesia techniques in London. Bert was an early physiologist who worked on the physiology of narcosis. Morton was the first to demonstrate the use of ether in a public trial. *(1:14)*

9. **(C)** See preceding answer. Wells was a dentist who pioneered the use of nitrous oxide. Long was one of the first to use ether. There is a statue in his honor in Washington, DC. Warren was the surgeon who operated on the patient whom Morton put to sleep with ether. *(1:7; 75:6)*

10. **(D)** Simpson introduced anesthesia into childbirth. Chloroform was the method he espoused. Snow was also instrumental in the use of chloroform. *(75:7)*

11. **(B)** Hypertension is seen in 5 to 10% of patients with morbid obesity. The cardiac output is increased, as is the pulmonary artery pressure. Blood volume is increased, and the cardiac workload is increased. *(1:261; 75:1118)*

12. **(A)** Blood pressure readings usually are high due to the difficulty in obtaining a suitable cuff. Venous and arterial access is difficult. Intubation may be difficult. It may be impossible to get a suitable mask fit. Nerve blocks are difficult because of the problem in finding landmarks. *(75:1121)*

13. **(D)** In the preanesthetic discussion, one must be honest with the patient. The common problems must be discussed, and the possibility of death or serious problems should be explained. It is not necessary to be exhaustive in the discussion of problems, but problems that are a potential to the particular procedure or the particular patient should be discussed. *(1:30; 75:36)*

14. **(C)** The most important reason for the development of a suit is the lack of rapport. The most common problem that leads to some payment is damage to teeth. *(131:49)*

15. **(C)** Electroshock therapy requires an oral airway for patient protection. The anesthesia can be induced with a thiobarbiturate. Muscle relaxants are important to prevent injury to the patient. Preoxygenation is helpful in preventing desaturation when the seizure is induced, since it will increase oxygen consumption. *(2:790)*

16. **(A)** Most CT scans can be done without anesthesia. There are situations in which the patient cannot or will not hold still to get a good study. In those situations, anesthesia is helpful. In our hospital, even the very young are done with sedation. Little general anesthesia is employed. Fever is not an indication for general anesthesia. *(179:235; 187:425)*

17. **(E)** All of the options are useful in interpreting continuous numerical data. *(1:192,197; 75:54,59; 185:749)*

18. **(A)** The doctrine of *res ipsa loquitur* (the thing speaks for itself), is invoked if the accident usually does not happen without negligence, the plaintiff was not a factor, and the defendant usually has control of whatever caused the accident. Settling out of court is not a factor. *(75:36)*

19. **(C)** If it is discovered that a tooth is missing, immediate steps should be taken to ascertain the location. First, make sure that it was there when the case started. Examine the oropharynx and nasopharynx. This can be done visually and by x-ray. If the tooth is in the trachea, a bronchoscopy should be performed immediately. *(186:121)*

20. **(C)** An outpatient child can be intubated if the procedure calls for intubation. The child should be given fluids as soon as there is a desire expressed. If croup develops, the child should be observed for a period of time after treatment to make sure there are not going to be progressive symptoms. Admission may be necessary. *(177:32)*

21. **(B)** After halothane anesthesia for outpatients, there is less psychomotor impairment than after diazepam. Alcohol should not be ingested for at least 24 hours. Patients should not return home alone but should be driven. There is less psychomotor impairment after halothane than after methohexital. *(75:1357)*

22. **(A)** Eyedrops that can cause systemic difficulties are atropine, which may cause tachycardia, phenylephrine, which may lead to hypertension, and echothiophate iodide, which can lead to prolonged succinylcholine activity. Antibiotic drops, in the absence of allergy, should not be a problem. *(1:1846; 75:1056)*

23. **(E)** All of the options may cause changes in intraocular pressure. Acetazolamide lowers pressure in glaucoma. Mannitol will lead to decreased intraocular pressure. One must be sure that the patient has good renal function. Atropine may increase the pressure in patients with glaucoma, or it may decrease the pressure by relaxing smooth muscle. *(1:1842; 75:1053)*

24. **(E)** The oculocardiac reflex is associated with blood pressure changes if the heart rate drops to low levels. Traction on the muscle is not the only cause. Pressure on the eye and retrobulbar blocks has caused the reflex. Cardiac arrhythmias other than bradycardia also are seen. In some reports, other arrhythmias are seen more frequently after atropine has been given to prevent the reflex. *(1:1844; 75:1055)*

25. **(E)** Computers are now a part of our equipment, and it is important that we become familiar with the computers insofar as possible. *(1:165)*

26. **(E)** Studies have shown that there is an association between fetal anomalies and employment in an operating room. These anomalies occur in the offspring of both male and female employees. The studies have had some flaws, and some conclusions have been drawn that are not warranted, but it is important for us to make the operating room as safe as possible for all who work there. *(1:151; 75:70)*

27. **(E)** *(188:1319)*

28. **(E)** Acupuncture went through a wave of popularity after China opened its doors to the West. Recently, there has been much less publicity. In evaluating the effectiveness of the technique, one must consider the difference in culture and the methods of study. One of the popular films describing the effects of acupuncture shows a person having a thoracotomy under acupuncture. The patient is breathing comfortably and is sipping orange juice. If someone opens your chest cavity, it is going to be difficult to breathe whether you are Chinese or American. *(138:1319)*

PART III

Practice Test

Practice Test

Carefully read the following instructions before taking the Practice Test.

1. This examination consists of 350 questions divided into two test periods. Each test consists of 175 questions and takes 3½ hours.
2. The tests mimic the actual Board exam. You should not carry any extra time from one test over to the other. Any remaining time from either test should be used to review your answers in that test only. You should take a break of 1 or 2 hours at least between the two tests.
3. The test items are explained in the Introduction to this book. We urge you to read the entire Introduction prior to taking this Practice Test.
4. Be sure you have an adequate number of pencils and erasers, a clock, a comfortable setting, and an adequate amount of undisturbed, distraction-free time.
5. After completion of the entire Practice Test, check your answers and assess your areas of weakness.

Questions Part I

DIRECTIONS (Questions 1 through 90): Each of the numbered items or incomplete statements in this section is followed by answers or by completions of the statement. Select the ONE lettered answer or completion that is BEST in each case.

1. If one measured pleural pressure, one would find that the pressure was

   (A) highest at the apex of the lung
   (B) highest at the base of the lung
   (C) equal at all levels
   (D) unrelated to body position
   (E) completely unpredictable from one level to another

2. Myocardial oxygen demand may be decreased by

   (A) tachycardia ↑
   (B) decreased preload
   (C) increased afterload ↑
   (D) increased contractility ↑
   (E) increased wall tension ↑

3. The functional residual capacity (FRC) is defined as the combination of

   (A) tidal volume and residual volume
   (B) tidal volume and expiratory reserve volume
   (C) inspiratory reserve volume and tidal volume
   (D) residual volume and expiratory reserve volume
   (E) residual volume and inspiratory reserve volume

4. The cilia of the respiratory tract

   (A) are part of the type II pneumocytes
   (B) are not affected by drugs
   (C) are inhibited by the presence of an uncuffed endotracheal tube
   (D) propel a double layer of mucus toward the larynx
   (E) are not affected by temperature

5. Slow diastolic depolarization (phase 4) is

   (A) a property of all cardiac muscle
   (B) due to potassium flux
   (C) the process underlying intrinsic rhythmicity in pacemaker cells
   (D) more pronounced in the bundle of His than in the sinoatrial node
   (E) unrelated to rhythmicity

6. Factors contributing to increased airway pressure under anesthesia include all of the following EXCEPT

   (A) an increase in the caliber of the airways
   (B) a decrease in functional residual capacity
   (C) the supine position
   (D) the presence of an endotracheal tube
   (E) pharyngeal obstruction

7. In the adult, the tracheobronchial tree

   (A) divides at an uneven angle, making foreign bodies more apt to go to the left side
   (B) divides into right and left bronchi—the left bronchus being narrower and longer
   (C) is relatively fixed and immovable with respiration
   (D) is lined with squamous epithelium
   (E) is protected by circular cartilaginous rings throughout

8. The addition of hyaluronidase to local anesthesia

   (A) increases the time to onset of action
   (B) decreases the success rate of blocks
   (C) increases the duration of the block
   (D) increases the incidence of toxic reactions
   (E) has no effect

9. The human larynx

   (A) lies at the level of the second through fifth cervical vertebrae
   (B) in the adult, is narrowest at the level of the cricoid cartilage
   (C) is innervated solely by the recurrent laryngeal nerve

(D) is protected anteriorly by the wide expanse of the cricoid cartilage

(E) lies within the thyroid cartilage

10. Humidification of inhaled air or gases is

(A) more efficient with an endotracheal tube in place

(B) increased with the administration of atropine

(C) more efficient in a open system than in a closed system

(D) at its optimum with the patient breathing through the nose

(E) at its optimum with the patient breathing through a tracheostomy

11. Distribution of ventilation in the lung is such that

(A) the apical portions are better ventilated

(B) the diaphragmatic areas are better ventilated

(C) the central or hilar areas are better ventilated

(D) all areas are ventilated equally

(E) ventilation is not affected by position

12. Inspiratory force is

(A) a measurement of reserve of ventilatory effort

(B) dependent on conscious effort

(C) normal if between 5 and 10 cm H_2O below atmospheric pressure

(D) difficult to measure

(E) normal if between 5 and 10 cm H_2O above atmospheric pressure

13. All of the following components contribute to physiologic shunt EXCEPT

(A) bronchial veins

(B) pleural veins

(C) thebesian veins

(D) abnormal arterial-venous communications

(E) nonperfused alveoli

14. During one-lung anesthesia with a double-lumen tube

(A) no shunting occurs in the unventilated lung

(B) no alveoli are in continuity with the proximal airways

(C) CO_2 removal is difficult

(D) insufflation of oxygen leads to decreased shunting

(E) it is not possible to administer oxygen to the collapsed lung

15. After bilateral carotid endarterectomy, a patient will

(A) have no respiratory changes

(B) show no change in arterial carbon dioxide

(C) respond to hypoxia with hyperventilation

(D) be more susceptible to hypoxemia

(E) always develop hypertension

16. Measurement of arterial oxygen tension

(A) Requires use of the Henderson-Hasselbalch equation

(B) uses the Clark electrode

(C) uses the Severinghaus electrode

(D) is not affected by temperature

(E) is performed on clotted blood

17. Mechanisms that may cause hypoxemia under anesthesia include all of the following EXCEPT

(A) hypoventilation

(B) hyperventilation

(C) increase in functional residual capacity (FRC)

(D) supine position

(E) increased airway pressure

18. In a patient with a fixed shunt, a decrease in cardiac output will

(A) decrease the arterial oxygenation

(B) decrease the arterial carbon dioxide tension

(C) have little effect on oxygenation

(D) increase dead space

(E) increase urinary output

19. After a two-hour anesthetic with hyperventilation, a patient breathing room air will

(A) return to normal parameters within 30 minutes

(B) remain hypocarbic for 2 hours

(C) become hypoxemic if not treated with oxygen

(D) become hypoxemic and hypercarbic

(E) be well oxygenated if the air exchange is unimpaired by drugs

20. Tracheal mucus flow is

(A) impeded by deviation from ambient oxygen tension

(B) decreased in patients with chronic obstructive lung disease

(C) not important as a cleansing mechanism

(D) unrelated to ciliary activity

(E) more active after a patient smokes a cigarette

21. All of the following are true of closing volume EXCEPT that

(A) it is measured by a single-breath nitrogen technique

(B) it is useful in determining disease of small airways

(C) it is decreased at the extremes of age

(D) closing volume plus residual volume equals closing capacity

(E) it is measured at phase IV on the nitrogen washout curve

22. The second heart sound coincides with all of the following EXCEPT

(A) closing of the aortic valve
(B) isometric relaxation of myocardial fibers
(C) closure of the mitral valve
(D) the T wave of the electrocardiogram
(E) closure of the pulmonic valve

23. Breathing 100% oxygen may lead to all of the following EXCEPT

(A) lung damage
(B) decreased volume of air-containing space
(C) retinopathy of prematurity
(D) hyperventilation in the patient with obstructive lung disease
(E) atelectasis

24. The central chemoreceptors responsible for respiratory control are

(A) located in the midbrain
(B) responsive primarily to change in carbon dioxide
(C) responsive primarily to change in hydrogen ion concentration
(D) responsive primarily to hypoxemia
(E) activated by chronic hypercapnia

25. The intrinsic rate of the sinoatrial node is

(A) 20 to 40 beats per minute
(B) 40 to 60 beats per minute
(C) 70 to 80 beats per minute
(D) 80 to 100 beats per minute
(E) 100 to 120 beats per minute

26. Oxygen toxicity (hyperoxia) exhibits all of the following EXCEPT

(A) substernal distress
(B) increased vital capacity
(C) atelectasis
(D) retinopathy of prematurity
(E) tracheobronchitis

27. General anesthesia alters the mechanical properties of the chest wall, leading to

(A) increased functional residual capacity (FRC)
(B) increased lung volume
(C) decreased elastic recoil of the lung
(D) decreased compliance
(E) no change in lung physiology

28. A 35-year-old male enters the hospital with a diagnosis of restrictive pulmonary disease. The pulmonary test result compatible with this diagnosis is

	FORCED VITAL CAPACITY	FEV$_1$	FEV$_1$/FVC%
(A)	normal	decreased	decreased
(B)	decreased	decreased	normal
(C)	decreased	decreased	increased
(D)	increased	increased	normal
(E)	normal	decreased	normal

29. The definitive test of adequacy of ventilation is

(A) listening to the esophageal stethoscope
(B) watching the rise and fall of the chest
(C) analyzing arterial blood gases
(D) measuring tidal volume with a spirometer
(E) using an apnea monitor

30. Pulmonary vascular resistance

(A) is entirely dependent on the cardiac output
(B) is entirely dependent on the pressure in the pulmonary artery
(C) is equal to pressure divided by radius of the artery
(D) depends on the state of vasomotion, flow, and pressure
(E) is not affected by cardiac output

31. Hypoxic pulmonary vasoconstriction

(A) is not important in the intact human being
(B) is active only at high altitude
(C) causes more blood flow to the base of the lung
(D) causes higher dead space/tidal volume (V$_{DS}$/V$_T$) ratio than in the nonhypoxic lung
(E) diverts blood flow from hypoxic to nonhypoxic lung areas

32. Measurements that can be obtained by spirometry include all of the following EXCEPT

(A) tidal volume
(B) closing volume
(C) expiratory reserve volume
(D) inspiratory reserve volume
(E) vital capacity

33. Carbon dioxide transport involves all of the following EXCEPT

(A) water
(B) bicarbonate ion
(C) carbonic anhydrase
(D) hemoglobin
(E) carboxyhemoglobin

34. The Bohr effect refers to the

(A) effect of carbonic anhydrase on the uptake of CO$_2$

(B) ability of the blood to pick up more CO_2 when the oxygen tension is low

(C) amount of hydrogen in solution in the blood

(D) effect of Pco_2 on the saturation of oxygen

(E) presence of catalytic enzymes in the blood

35. In zone 2 of the lung

(A) there is good blood flow regardless of ventilation

(B) venous pressure is high

(C) dead space is high

(D) the pulmonary vessels are collapsed

(E) the blood flow is determined primarily by pulmonary artery pressure and alveolar pressure

36. Boyle's law

(A) describes the molecular motion of a liquid

(B) describes the relation of pressure and volume of a gas

(C) describes the relation of pressure and temperature of a gas

(D) describes the diffusion of a gas across membranes

(E) describes the solution of a solid in a liquid

37. The main buffering system of the body is

(A) hemoglobin

(B) bicarbonate

(C) phosphate

(D) sulfate

(E) plasma proteins

38. Recognition of hypoxemia in the recovery room

(A) depends on the detection of cyanosis

(B) depends on the detection of respiratory responses

(C) depends on the detection of circulatory responses

(D) is most dependable with arterial blood gases

(E) is done better with a transcutaneous oxygen monitor than with a pulse oximeter

39. Signs of hypoxemia include all of the following EXCEPT

(A) decreased ventilatory effort in response to chemoreceptor stimulation

(B) increased heart rate in response to sympathetic stimulation

(C) cyanosis

(D) decreased heart rate due to direct effect of hypoxia on the heart

(E) increased blood pressure due to sympathetic stimulation

40. During apneic ventilation

(A) the time elapsed before desaturation occurs is independent of the patient's oxygen status before the onset of apnea

(B) all arrhythmias are due to hypoxemia

(C) the carbon dioxide tension is not important

(D) the carbon dioxide level rises about 3 torr/minute

(E) pulse oximetry is not helpful

41. All of the following are important in oxygen transport EXCEPT

(A) oxygen content

(B) oxygen tension

(C) cardiac output

(D) hemoglobin level

(E) carboxyhemoglobin level

42. To ensure an accurate indirect blood pressure measurement, the

(A) average width of the inflatable bladder for an adult should be 12 to 14 cm

(B) length of the bladder should be sufficient to encircle the arm

(C) length of the bladder is more important than the width

(D) inflatable bladder need not be over the artery

(E) manometer must read near zero to start

43. In the normal upright lung

(A) the blood flow is greatest at the apex

(B) the ventilation is greatest at the apex

(C) the ventilation/perfusion (V/Q) ratio is higher at the apex

(D) the level of lung area is not critical to ventilation

(E) the Po_2 is lower at the apex

44. The cuff of an endotracheal tube should be inflated to what pressure to prevent aspiration while not causing underlying ischemia?

(A) 20 torr

(B) 30 torr

(C) 40 torr

(D) 50 torr

(E) 60 torr

45. As one moves from the apex of the lung to the dependent portions

(A) the alveoli become larger

(B) the caliber of the air passages becomes larger

(C) pleural pressure decreases

(D) compliance becomes greater

(E) ventilation of the alveoli lessens due to decreased compliance

$CPP = DBP - LVEDP$

46. Coronary perfusion is increased as a result of

    (A) increased diastolic blood pressure
    (B) increased left ventricular end-diastolic pressure
    (C) systolic hypertension
    (D) tachycardia
    (E) hypocapnia

47. Baroreceptor reflex activity is

    (A) unimportant as a circulatory regulator
    (B) responsive to oxygen content
    (C) located primarily in the carotid body
    (D) inversely proportional to age
    (E) responsive to CO_2 concentration

48. Afterload of the left ventricle is

    (A) related only to the aortic valve
    (B) dependent on the distensibility of the large arteries
    (C) best measured by estimating the mean arterial pressure
    (D) increased by vasodilators
    (E) unrelated to ventricular size

49. Observation of the direct blood pressure display can give the following information

    (A) relative strength of left ventricular contraction
    (B) estimate of stroke volume
    (C) estimate of systemic vascular resistance
    (D) heart rate
    (E) all of the above

50. As a flow-directed catheter is inserted, you would expect to see all of the following EXCEPT

    (A) a right atrial pressure of 15 mm Hg
    (B) a right ventricular systolic pressure of 30 mm Hg
    (C) a pulmonary artery pressure of 20 mm Hg
    (D) a pulmonary artery diastolic pressure higher than right ventricular diastolic pressure
    (E) a wedge pressure of 12 mm Hg

51. The standard electrocardiogram records the correct electrical potentials when leads are placed such that

    (A) lead I reads left arm–left leg
    (B) lead I reads right arm–right leg
    (C) lead II reads right arm–left leg
    (D) lead III reads right arm–left leg
    (E) lead II reads right arm–left arm

52. Electrocardiographic monitoring is indicated during anesthesia to detect all of the following EXCEPT

    (A) efficacy of pump function

    (B) arrhythmias
    (C) ischemia
    (D) electrolyte disturbance
    (E) pacemaker function

53. dP/dt is a measure of

    (A) myocardial oxygen demand
    (B) rate of change of ventricular pressure with time
    (C) right atrial pressure
    (D) renal perfusion
    (E) blood pressure

54. The coronary circulation responds to hyperventilation with

    (A) no change
    (B) an increase in flow
    (C) a decrease in flow
    (D) a transient increase followed by an intense vasodilatation
    (E) intense vasoconstriction

55. Myocardial oxygen consumption is most closely tied to

    (A) heart rate
    (B) blood viscosity
    (C) cardiac outputs
    (D) stroke volume
    (E) F_{IO_2}

56. Venous pressure in the median basilic vein of the arm is

    (A) equal to right atrial pressure
    (B) above right atrial pressure
    (C) below right atrial pressure
    (D) not related to blood volume
    (E) independent of arm position

57. The microcirculation

    (A) is under the control of the autonomic nervous system
    (B) contains no musculature
    (C) is always open
    (D) consists only of capillaries
    (E) contains at least 20% of the blood volume

58. Pulmonary edema may result from all of the following EXCEPT

    (A) altered permeability
    (B) decreased pulmonary capillary pressure
    (C) decreased oncotic pressure
    (D) increased negative airway pressure
    (E) head injury

59. The Frank–Starling mechanism refers to the relationship of

(A) the left and right ventricles
(B) the left and right atria
(C) preload and stroke volume
(D) afterload and ventricular volume
(E) stroke volume and afterload

60. Heat production in the body is decreased by

(A) shivering
(B) hunger
(C) activity
(D) secretion of epinephrine
(E) anorexia

61. If the size of the ventricle increases

(A) wall tension needed to pump the same amount of blood is less
(B) less oxygen is needed to pump blood
(C) the heart becomes more efficient
(D) wall tension will increase proportionally with the radius
(E) wall tension will be proportional to wall thickness

62. Pulmonary artery pressure

(A) increases passively with increases of cardiac output
(B) remains constant with change of cardiac output
(C) is not important to pulmonary vascular resistance
(D) is not dependent on the radius of the vessels
(E) depends entirely on cardiac output

63. Defibrillation is

(A) indicated in all instances of cardiac arrest
(B) delivered at an energy level of 400 joules in all patients
(C) always successful if used early
(D) the initial step is resuscitation of the unwitnessed arrest
(E) best attempted with an energy level of 200 joules in an adult

64. The most potent of the inhalation anesthetics is

(A) halothane
(B) cyclopropane
(C) nitrous oxide
(D) enflurane
(E) methoxyflurane

65. A large nerve fiber associated with transmission of deep touch and temperature is the

(A) A-alpha fiber
(B) A-beta fiber
(C) A-gamma fiber
(D) B fiber
(E) C fiber

66. The temperature-regulating mechanism is in the

(A) forebrain
(B) pons
(C) thalamus
(D) hypothalamus
(E) cerebellum

67. Total body water in an adult constitutes

(A) 20% of body weight
(B) 30% of body weight
(C) 40% of body weight
(D) 50% of body weight
(E) 60% of body weight

68. Magnesium

(A) concentration is related to irritability of nervous tissue
(B) concentration is low intracellularly
(C) is not excreted in the urine
(D) is not present in bile
(E) is not present in gastric juice

69. Ringer's lactate solution contains all of the following ions EXCEPT

(A) sodium
(B) potassium
(C) chloride
(D) calcium
(E) bicarbonate

70. Hydrogen ion (H^+)

(A) is secreted by the proximal and distal renal tubules
(B) is not actively transported across the renal tubular cell
(C) is exchanged for bicarbonate
(D) is not related to the movement of other ions
(E) movement is unrelated to HCO_3^- in the kidney

71. The enterohepatic circulation

(A) describes the storage of bile in the gallbladder
(B) is most important for the reabsorption of bile salts
(C) is unimportant in the liver metabolism of drugs
(D) allows all the reabsorbed substances to avoid the systemic circulation
(E) is possible only with conjugated compounds

72. The condition that is referred to as meralgia paresthetica is caused by entrapment of the

(A) peroneal nerve
(B) sciatic nerve
(C) lateral femoral cutaneous nerve
(D) median nerve
(E) posterior tibial nerve

73. A local anesthetic that is an ester derivative is

(A) bupivacaine
(B) etidiocaine
(C) mepivacaine
(D) lidocaine
(E) procaine

74. Broca's area is

(A) in the dominant hemisphere
(B) an area in the cerebellum
(C) in the sensory cortex
(D) in the lateral spinal tract of the cord
(E) an area associated with speech

75. The first-pass effect refers to

(A) the biotransformation of a drug in its vehicle of administration
(B) the change of a drug by enzymes in muscle
(C) biotransformation of a drug as it passes through the intestinal mucosa and liver
(D) the drug lost by urinary excretion
(E) the drug lost by being passed with feces

76. The cardiovascular effects of isoflurane are characterized by

(A) stable cardiac rhythm
(B) sensitization of the heart to epinephrine
(C) a slowing of the heart rate
(D) increased stroke volume
(E) decreased cardiac output

77. The foramen of Monro connects the

(A) lateral ventricles
(B) 3rd ventricle to the lateral ventricle
(C) 3rd ventricle to the 4th ventricle
(D) 4th ventricle to the spinal arachnoid system
(E) cisterna magna to the 4th ventricle

78. The electroencephalographic (EEG) waveform with a frequency range of 8 to 10 Hz is associated with

(A) alpha activity
(B) beta activity
(C) theta activity
(D) delta activity
(E) gamma activity

79. Administration of ketamine causes

(A) decreased heart rate
(B) increased heart rate
(C) decreased cardiac output
(D) no change in cardiac output
(E) no change in heart rate

80. Renal clearance of a drug

(A) is usually of little importance
(B) has no relationship to creatinine clearance
(C) is constant for a given drug
(D) varies with pH, urine flow rate, and renal blood flow
(E) may exceed renal blood flow

81. Halogenation of a hydrocarbon

(A) usually increases its flammability
(B) increases its narcotic activity
(C) has no effect
(D) makes it more of a cardiac irritant
(E) makes it explosive

82. Halothane structurally is

(A) an ether
(B) a methane compound
(C) an ethane compound
(D) an ethane compound substituted with fluorine, chlorine, and iodine
(E) An ethane compound substituted with fluorine, bromine, and iodine

83. Sevoflurane

(A) is an ether compound
(B) has a blood gas coefficient of 1.7
(C) has a vapor pressure of 214
(D) is irritating to the airway
(E) contains no fluoride molecules

84. The action of thiopental after injection is terminated by

(A) its elimination unchanged by the kidneys
(B) its biotransformation by the liver
(C) its being bound to proteins
(D) its redistribution
(E) being taken up in fatty tissues

85. Thiopental is contraindicated in

(A) porphyria congenita
(B) porphyria cutanea tarda
(C) acute intermittent porphyria
(D) myotonia
(E) chorea

86. In an adult patient with severe pain, administration of thiopental 80 mg

(A) will produce sleep
(B) will have an antianalgesic action
(C) will have no effect
(D) will sedate the patient but not induce sleep
(E) is more effective if given alone

87. After the inadvertent injection of 15 ml 2% thiopental into the epidural space, you would expect

(A) immediate complaint of severe pain
(B) onset of drowsiness
(C) complete paralysis
(D) arachnoiditis
(E) cauda equina syndrome

88. A patient has been given an injection of ketamine in a dose calculated to be sufficient for anesthesia. His eyes remain open, and there is slight nystagmus and occasional purposeless movements. This is an indication that

(A) the dose is inadequate
(B) more ketamine should be given to stop the movements
(C) the dose is excessive
(D) the dose is adequate for anesthesia
(E) the patient is having a seizure

89. The rigidity occasionally seen with Innovar injection is

(A) more likely to occur after intramuscular injection
(B) noted chiefly in the leg muscles
(C) due to droperidol
(D) due to fentanyl
(E) seen only after large doses

90. Local anesthetics in the injectable form are

(A) salts
(B) acids
(C) bases
(D) proteins
(E) lipids

DIRECTIONS (Questions 91 through 175): For each of the items in this section, ONE or MORE of the numbered options is correct. Choose the answer

A if only 1, 2, and 3 are correct,
B if only 1 and 3 are correct,
C if only 2 and 4 are correct,
D if only 4 is correct,
E if all are correct.

91. Positive end-expiratory pressure (PEEP)

(1) always improves oxygenation
(2) increases lung volume at end-expiration (FRC)
(3) decreases lung compliance
(4) increases ventilation/perfusion (V/Q) ratio

92. Increased dead space ventilation may occur during anesthesia due to

(1) deliberate hypotension
(2) short rapid ventilations
(3) pulmonary embolus
(4) decreased airway pressure

93. Vital capacity includes

(1) tidal volume
(2) inspiratory reserve volume
(3) expiratory reserve volume
(4) functional residual capacity (FRC)

94. A patient with hypercapnia will have

(1) decreased levels of epinephrine
(2) increased levels of norepinephrine
(3) respiratory alkalosis
(4) increased plasma potassium

95. Factors leading to pulmonary edema include

(1) increased capillary pressure
(2) decreased oncotic pressure
(3) lymphatic insufficiency
(4) increased capillary permeability

96. In the lateral decubitus position, the lung relationships

(1) are the same as in the semirecumbent position; ie, the apex is in zone 1 and the bases are in zone 3
(2) ventilation is highest at the apex
(3) perfusion is greater in the upright lung
(4) perfusion is greater in the dependent lung

97. The adult trachea is

(1) 15 cm in length
(2) about the size of the patient's index finger in diameter
(3) in the midline of the neck
(4) bifurcates at the level of the 3rd thoracic vertebra

98. Airway resistance

(1) is a dynamic measurement
(2) is measured by dividing volume per second by pressure
(3) depends on the caliber of the airway
(4) is independent of the pattern of air flow, ie, whether it is laminar or turbulent

99. The composition of alveolar gases differs from inhaled gas because

(1) oxygen is being absorbed from the alveoli
(2) carbon dioxide is being added to the alveoli
(3) water vapor is being added
(4) nitrogen is taken up by the alveolar capillaries

100. In describing air flow through a tube

(1) Henry's law is important
(2) radius is a crucial factor
(3) tube length is the important factor
(4) viscosity is more important than density

SUMMARY OF DIRECTIONS				
A	B	C	D	E
1, 2, 3 only	1, 3 only	2, 4 only	4 only	All are correct

101. The factors that influence arterial oxygen tension under anesthesia include

   (1) inspired oxygen concentration
   (2) barometric pressure
   (3) alveolar oxygen tension
   (4) age

[handwritten: $Pa O_2 \downarrow$; $P_{AO_2} =$]

102. Assuming a normal oxyhemoglobin dissociation curve position

   (1) a Po_2 of 90 torr will give a saturation of 96.5%
   (2) a Po_2 of 90 torr will give a dissolved oxygen of 0.27 ml/100 ml blood
   (3) a Po_2 of 90 torr will give a combined oxygen of 19.80 ml/100 ml blood
   (4) a Po_2 of 30 torr will give an oxygen saturation of 30%

[handwritten: A]

103. Calcium administration

   (1) decreases myocardial contractility
   (2) decreases excitability
   (3) can be antagonized by calcium chelating agents, but the effects are too long for clinical use
   (4) may potentiate development of digitalis toxicity

104. Factors that increase P_{50} of hemoglobin include

   (1) increased temperature
   (2) decreased DPG
   (3) increased hydrogen ion concentration
   (4) methemoglobin

[handwritten: R]

105. Neurogenic pulmonary edema

   (1) may follow head injury
   (2) is not associated with hypoxemia
   (3) is resistant to treatment unless intracranial pressure is reduced
   (4) develops only in a denervated lung

[handwritten: $C.O. = V \frac{(T_B - T_i) K_1 K_2}{\int(dt)}$]

106. Left ventricular compliance may be decreased in

   (1) aortic stenosis
   (2) ischemia
   (3) inotrope usage
   (4) the patient on vasodilators

107. The reticular activating system (RAS)

   (1) is a specific area with a specific pathway system

   (2) is located in the cerebral cortex
   (3) has input from the spinal cord only
   (4) produces the conscious, alert state that makes perception possible

108. Deliberate hypotensive technique may affect pulmonary gas exchange by increasing

   (1) respiratory dead space
   (2) the $AaDo_2$ gradient
   (3) ventilation perfusion inequality
   (4) shunting

109. The immediate preoperative preparation of a patient with asthma includes

[handwritten: A]

   (1) bronchodilators
   (2) corticosteroids
   (3) high fluid intake
   (4) cromolyn sodium

110. The tetralogy of Fallot includes

   (1) atrial septal defect (ASD)
   (2) ventricular septal defect (VSD)
   (3) patent ductus arteriosus (PDA)
   (4) pulmonary outflow obstruction

[handwritten: VSD, overriding aorta, pulmonary stenosis]

111. The preoperative electrocardiogram can be used to detect

   (1) chamber enlargement
   (2) ischemic heart disease
   (3) electrolyte disturbances
   (4) heart block

112. Determination of cardiac output with the thermodilution technique

   (1) requires a pulmonary artery catheter with a thermistor
   (2) uses the same principle as the dye-dilution technique
   (3) requires the use of an exact amount of fluid with a known temperature
   (4) requires the measurement of the temperature in the pulmonary artery

113. Correct intracardiac pressure value(s) include

   (1) right atrium: mean 5
   (2) right ventricle: 25/5
   (3) pulmonary artery: 23/9
   (4) wedge pressure: 10

114. Elevation of the intracranial pressure seen with succinylcholine is

[handwritten: A]

   (1) due to increase of Pco_2 from fasciculation
   (2) due to CNS activation from proprioceptors
   (3) not seen in patients who are hyperventilated and given thiopental
   (4) due to tightness of the neck muscles

115. Cardioplegia is an important adjunct, since

(1) oxygen consumption increases with ventricular fibrillation
(2) oxygen consumption is reduced to one quarter with arrest
(3) coronary resistance is reduced
(4) myocardial oxygen consumption varies with rhythm

116. Methods of detecting intraoperative air embolism include

(1) mass spectrometry
(2) end-tidal carbon dioxide determination
(3) Doppler monitoring
(4) measurement of end-tidal oxygen

117. The vasomotor center

(1) is located in the right temporal area of the brain
(2) is affected by the hypothalamus
(3) secretes serotonin
(4) is affected by the cerebral cortex

118. The renin-angiotensin mechanism includes

(1) renin, which is in the liver
(2) converting enzyme, which is in the kidney
(3) the conversion of renin substrate to angiotensin I by the converting enzyme
(4) initiation of the entire process by a decrease in blood volume

119. A pacemaker with the letter code AVTPN

(1) paces the atrium
(2) senses the ventricle
(3) triggers a pacemaker spike on sensing an impulse
(4) is not programmable

120. The liver disease that results from alcohol ingestion

(1) can be prevented by a nutritious diet
(2) is usually present without hematologic involvement
(3) does not involve any gastrointestinal disorders
(4) is usually accompanied by vitamin deficiency

121. After insertion of a flow-directed pulmonary artery catheter, you note the presence of large V waves. This may be due to

(1) tricuspid atresia
(2) aortic valve stenosis
(3) aortic regurgitation
(4) mitral regurgitation

122. Factors that increase the risk of anesthesia include

(1) an S3 gallop
(2) rhythm other than sinus
(3) age >70
(4) emergency operations

123. Methods of detecting ventricular dysfunction include

(1) determination of ejection fraction
(2) wall motion studies
(3) determination of cardiac output
(4) determination of end-diastolic pressure

124. During CPR

(1) a central line is preferable for drug administration
(2) a femoral line is preferable to an antecubital line
(3) lidocaine, atropine, and epinephrine may be administered via the endotracheal tube
(4) intracardiac injections should be attempted before an attempt is made to secure a central line

125. The pericardium

(1) serves as a buffer to the heart at times of acceleration
(2) contains nerve fibers that, when stimulated, will slow the heart rate
(3) minimizes cardiac dilatation
(4) is not essential to cardiac function

126. Clotting factor(s) that are vitamin K dependent is (are)

(1) factor I
(2) factor VII
(3) factor V
(4) factor X

127. Stroke volume is dependent on myocardial fiber shortening, which is determined by

(1) preload
(2) contractility of the myocardium
(3) afterload
(4) heart rate

128. Reabsorption of sodium occurs in the

(1) proximal tubule
(2) ascending loop of Henle
(3) distal tubule
(4) collecting tubule

129. Treatment of hyperkalemia includes

(1) elimination of exogenous sources
(2) correction of cause of endogenous sources
(3) administration of glucose with insulin
(4) administration of acidifying solutions

130. Valvular heart disease brings compensatory mechanism(s) into play, which include

   (1) chamber enlargement
   (2) ventricular hypertrophy
   (3) increased sympathetic outflow
   (4) decreased vascular tone

131. Calculation of systemic vascular resistance requires determination of

   (1) mean arterial pressure
   (2) mean central venous pressure
   (3) cardiac output
   (4) pulmonary artery pressure

132. Hematocrit values in patients with cirrhosis may reflect

   (1) coagulation disorders
   (2) increased plasma volume
   (3) bleeding
   (4) megaloblastic anemia

133. The decreased urinary volume seen in patients on PEEP is due to

   (1) decreased renal blood flow
   (2) increased sympathetic outflow
   (3) release of renin
   (4) ADH release

134. Effect(s) of vasopressin include(s)

   (1) production of dilute urine
   (2) antidiuresis
   (3) decreased urine osmolality
   (4) vasoconstriction

135. The syndrome of inappropriate antidiuretic hormone release (SIADH) includes

   (1) hyponatremia
   (2) low serum osmolality
   (3) excessive renal secretion of sodium
   (4) normal renal function

136. A typical nerve cell has

   (1) numerous dendrites that branch out
   (2) three or four axons to conduct impulses
   (3) a dendritic zone that is a receptor membrane
   (4) a myelin sheath that covers the entire cell

137. A typical reflex arc includes

   (1) a sense organ
   (2) an afferent neuron
   (3) an efferent neuron
   (4) one or more synapses in a central integrating station

138. Osmotic diuresis

   (1) is produced only with agents administered intravenously
   (2) is produced by agents that are filtered but not absorbed
   (3) is caused by increased glomerular filtration rate (GFR)
   (4) may follow if a substance is present in an amount exceeding the reabsorption capacity of the tubule

139. If a patient has increased intracranial pressure and a volatile agent is to be used, methods that can be used to mitigate problems include

   (1) use of an agent with the least potential to elevate cerebral blood flow
   (2) use of hyperventilation before the volatile agent
   (3) use of intravenous drugs to reduce intracranial pressure
   (4) use of as low a dose as possible of the volatile agent

140. In the distribution phase of an intravenous drug

   (1) blood is distributed to the vessel-rich group
   (2) there is an equilibrium between blood and tissues
   (3) a high perfusion causes slow equilibration
   (4) diffusion factors may determine the time to equilibration

141. The loading dose of a drug

   (1) helps reach a tissue concentration in a shorter time
   (2) causes a higher level than needed for a short time
   (3) decreases the time to a steady-state plasma concentration
   (4) may lead to undesirable effects

142. Endogenous catecholamines include

   (1) epinephrine
   (2) norepinephrine
   (3) dopamine
   (4) dobutamine

143. Epinephrine

   (1) stimulates alpha and beta receptors

(2) causes decreased systemic vascular resistance
(3) may lead to cardiac arrhythmias
(4) has strong chronotropic effects

144. Amrinone

(1) is useful orally
(2) causes vasoconstriction
(3) has little effect on heart rate
(4) stimulates phosphodiesterase

145. Preanesthetic anticholinergics

(1) have a predictable effect on gastric pH
(2) have a predictable effect on gastric volume
(3) are all good amnestic drugs
(4) produce an antisialogogue effect

146. Systemic signs of local anesthetic toxicity include

(1) numbness of lips and tongue
(2) tinnitus
(3) difficulty in focusing
(4) drowsiness

147. Vecuronium administered to infants

(1) has the same ED_{50} as in adults
(2) has a longer duration
(3) has an altered effect, since infants are more sensitive
(4) has a greater volume of distribution

148. Halothane sensitizes the heart to catecholamines. This sensitization

(1) is accentuated by hypoxemia
(2) is accentuated by hypercarbia
(3) can be abolished by beta blockers
(4) can be abolished by calcium channel blockers

149. Epinephrine regimen(s) that is (are) relatively safe when halothane is employed include(s)

(1) concentration no greater than 1:100,000
(2) adult dose not greater than 10 ml of 1:100,000 within 10 minutes
(3) adult dose not greater than 20 ml of 1:200,000 within 10 minutes
(4) adult total dose not to exceed 30 ml of 1:100,000 within 1 hour

150. Nitrous oxide

(1) decreases pulmonary vascular resistance
(2) increases cardiac output when given with opioids
(3) decreases blood pressure when administered with isoflurane
(4) increases blood pressure when given with halothane

151. Digitalis toxicity may be manifest by

(1) prolonged P-R interval
(2) nausea and vomiting
(3) multifocal PVCs
(4) tachycardia

152. Esmolol

(1) is an ester
(2) has a longer half-life if succinylcholine is used
(3) can blunt response to intubation
(4) has a prolonged effect

153. A child is brought to the emergency room for evaluation of his disoriented state. This was first noticed after he ate some berries. He is also noted to be very warm, to be flushed, and to have dilated pupils. Your suggested treatment should be

(1) CT scan
(2) aspirin
(3) sponge baths for the fever
(4) physostigmine

154. A patient who has been on steroids within a year preceding surgery

(1) may not have any problem
(2) has little risk with low-dose supplementation
(3) is at risk of having a stress reaction without coverage
(4) should be covered with supplemental steroids

155. You have begun to administer intravenous methicillin when there is a sudden increase in airway pressure, wheezing, tachycardia, and a decreased blood pressure. Your treatment should include

(1) stop the methicillin infusion
(2) administer 100% oxygen
(3) give volume expanders
(4) give a bolus of epinephrine of 5 μg

156. Mannitol

(1) is filtered at the glomerulus
(2) is an osmotic diuretic
(3) causes an immediate increase in intravascular volume
(4) is of value in congestive failure

157. Magnesium deficiency may

(1) be seen in the chronic alcoholic
(2) occur as cardiac arrhythmias
(3) be associated with skeletal muscle spasm
(4) be associated with CNS irritability

SUMMARY OF DIRECTIONS				
A	B	C	D	E
1, 2, 3 only	1, 3 only	2, 4 only	4 only	All are correct

158. Cyanide toxicity from administration of sodium nitroprusside

   (1) occurs at blood levels 100 μg/100 ml
   (2) is aggravated by the previous treatment with captopril
   (3) is seen more often in patients who are nutritionally deprived
   (4) will not occur if the dose is kept under 2 mg/kg/ hour

159. Drug therapy appropriate for ventricular arrhythmias includes

   (1) lidocaine
   (2) procainamide
   (3) bretylium
   (4) magnesium sulfate

160. Ionization of a drug

   (1) is a function of pH of the fluid it is in
   (2) may render a drug inactive
   (3) is a function of the pKa
   (4) may affect the drug's ability to cross membranes

161. The principal disadvantage(s) of methohexital is (are)

   (1) poor solubility
   (2) pain on injection
   (3) low pH
   (4) involuntary muscle movements

162. The rapidly perfused (vessel-rich) tissues include

   (1) heart
   (2) kidney
   (3) central nervous system
   (4) muscle

163. Local anesthetic agents block nerve conduction by

   (1) blocking conduction through the myelin sheath
   (2) forming a salt in the nerve membrane
   (3) depolarizing the membrane
   (4) blocking the ionic movement through membrane pores

164. Systemic toxicity to a local anesthetic is related to the

   (1) dose of drug
   (2) rapidity of injection
   (3) vascularity of the site injected
   (4) inherent toxicity of the drug injected

165. Myoglobinemia

   (1) may occur after a single dose of succinylcholine
   (2) is a well-known but harmless side effect of succinylcholine administration in children
   (3) is more common in children
   (4) is known to result from smooth muscle breakdown

166. Succinylcholine may cause prolonged apnea in patients

   (1) exposed to organophosphate insecticides
   (2) with severe liver disease
   (3) receiving echothiophate eyedrops
   (4) with heterozygous atypical pseudocholinesterease

167. A patient has been receiving lithium for a psychiatric disorder. At the time of surgery, you could expect which of the following drugs to be potentiated?

   (1) pancuronium
   (2) succinylcholine
   (3) gallamine
   (4) D-tubocurarine

168. In an anesthetized patient, hemodynamic responses to neuromuscular blockers may be altered by

   (1) depth of anesthesia
   (2) surgical stimulation
   (3) blood volume
   (4) sex of the patient

169. Injection of succinylcholine may be followed by increased intragastric pressure, which

   (1) will not lead to regurgitation unless the pressure exceeds 75 cm H_2O pressure
   (2) may lead to regurgitation more readily if the patient has a hiatal hernia
   (3) may be accentuated by prior injection of atropine, 0.6 mg, intravenously
   (4) may be attenuated by pretreating the patient with 4 to 6 mg of D-tubocurarine

170. The development of dual (phase II, desensitization) block

   (1) only follows prolonged treatment with high doses of succinylcholine
   (2) is both time and dose dependent
   (3) cannot be detected clinically
   (4) follows a stage of tachyphylaxis

171. Histamine release is associated with

(1) erythema of the upper chest
(2) hypertension
(3) bronchospasm in susceptible patients
(4) bradycardia

172. The enzyme acetylcholinesterase is composed of two subsites, the anionic site and the esteratic site. Inhibitors of the enzyme block either one or both of these sites. The inhibitor(s) that block by forming a carbamylester at the esteratic site is (are)

(1) neostigmine
(2) pyridostigmine
(3) physostigmine
(4) edrophonium

173. Succinylcholine is contraindicated in

(1) amyotrophic lateral sclerosis
(2) massive tissue trauma
(3) paraplegia
(4) burns

174. When reversing nondepolarizing neuromuscular blockers

(1) the peak effect of atropine occurs in 10 to 15 minutes
(2) the peak effect of neostigmine occurs in 10 to 15 minutes
(3) the twitch height is the best indicator of reversal
(4) adequate reversal is more important in patients with renal failure

175. Pyridostigmine, when compared with neostigmine, has

(1) a longer duration of action
(2) greater dependence on the kidneys for elimination
(3) fewer side effects
(4) a more rapid onset of action

Questions Part II

176. Antibiotics that possess neuromuscular blocking properties include all of the following EXCEPT

    (A) neomycin
    (B) kanamycin
    (C) penicillin
    (D) gentamicin
    (E) streptomycin

177. The muscle relaxant metocurine

    (A) causes more histamine release than D-tubocurarine
    (B) causes more ganglionic blockade than D-tubocurarine
    (C) causes more blood pressure depression than D-tubocurarine
    (D) is structurally related to D-tubocurarine
    (E) always causes tachycardia

178. If your patient has a need for a high cardiac output and high systemic blood pressure, the relaxant of choice would be

    (A) D-tubocurarine
    (B) atracurium
    (C) pancuronium
    (D) decamethonium
    (E) succinylcholine

179. Botulinus toxin interferes with neuromuscular transmission by

    (A) preventing synthesis of acetylcholine
    (B) increasing breakdown of acetylcholine
    (C) preventing storage of acetylcholine
    (D) preventing release of acetylcholine
    (E) blocking receptors for acetylcholine

180. Vecuronium

    (A) has an activity of about 2 minutes
    (B) is a depolarizing relaxant
    (C) is difficult to reverse
    (D) has very little cumulative effect
    (E) depends on the kidney for elimination

181. The administration of anticholinesterase drugs will

    (A) prolong all neuromuscular blockade
    (B) always reverse nondepolarizing agents
    (C) shorten the block of a depolarizing agent
    (D) reverse nondepolarizing agents if the plasma concentration of the drug is low enough
    (E) reverse the action of a depolarizing agent if only partial paralysis is present

182. The minimum alveolar concentration (MAC) for isoflurane is

    (A) 0.5
    (B) 1.15
    (C) 2.46
    (D) 3.8
    (E) 8.2

183. Myoglobin is a low-molecular weight hemeprotein

    (A) found only in cardiac muscle
    (B) always found in the serum of children
    (C) always found in serum after administration of succinylcholine
    (D) related to fasciculation
    (E) more commonly found in the blood of children than adults after administration of succinylcholine

184. The gasserian ganglion is associated with the

    (A) second cranial nerve
    (B) third cranial nerve
    (C) fifth cranial nerve
    (D) seventh cranial nerve
    (E) ninth cranial nerve

185. Propofol

    (A) is a halogenated liquid delivered by a vaporizer
    (B) is very soluble in aqueous solutions
    (C) is an intravenous anesthetic agent with a slow onset
    (D) has little analgesic property
    (E) has a longer sleep time than thiopental

186. All of the following are capable of antagonizing neuromuscular block EXCEPT

    (A) edrophonium
    (B) neostigmine
    (C) pyridostigmine
    (D) 4-aminopyridine
    (E) atropine

187. Depolarization block is characterized by all of the following EXCEPT

    (A) muscle fasciculation
    (B) initial absence of fade
    (C) post-tetanic facilitation
    (D) antagonism of block by D-tubocurarine
    (E) potentiation of block by anticholinesterase

188. The Bernoulli theorem states that

    (A) pressure and volume in a pipe are related
    (B) pressure and temperature in a pipe are related
    (C) velocity of flow and lateral pressure are related
    (D) the velocity of a gas is related to flow
    (E) the velocity of a gas is related to its temperature

189. The term MAC refers to

    (A) minimal anesthetic concentration
    (B) anesthesia sufficient to prevent movement in response to a painful stimulus in 100% of subjects
    (C) a measurement not affected by age
    (D) measurement that is pertinent only with thiopental
    (E) minimal alveolar concentration

190. The train-of-four ratio for a depolarizing block is

    (A) variable
    (B) 50%
    (C) 60%
    (D) 75%
    (E) 100%

191. The patient with myasthenia gravis

    (A) has normal reactions to muscle relaxants
    (B) reacts abnormally to relaxants only when the condition is not controlled

    (C) has a low sensitivity to nondepolarizing relaxants
    (D) has an increased sensitivity to nondepolarizing relaxants
    (E) has an increased sensitivity to depolarizing relaxants

192. The maximum acceptable leakage current is

    (A) 10 microamperes
    (B) 10 amperes
    (C) 100 microamperes
    (E) 100 amperes

193. You see a patient preoperatively and note that she is on propranolol 40 mg daily for hypertension. This drug

    (A) should be stopped immediately, and the procedure can be done the next day
    (B) should be stopped and surgery postponed for 2 weeks
    (C) should be continued during surgery and then stopped
    (D) will not affect the anesthetic regimen in any way
    (E) should always be discontinued gradually to avoid a sympathetic stimulation response

194. If a liquid at a given temperature is in a closed container, equilibrium is reached when the number of vapor molecules leaving the liquid equals the number reentering it. This vapor pressure will change under all the following conditions EXCEPT if

    (A) the temperature is raised
    (B) the container is opened
    (C) it is allowed to stand for 2 hours
    (D) the container is compressed
    (E) the container is cooled

195. The drug that has only alpha-agonist effects is

    (A) epinephrine
    (B) norepinephrine
    (C) methoxamine
    (D) isoproterenol
    (E) ephedrine

196. Lidocaine

    (A) is eliminated chiefly by the liver
    (B) is effective orally
    (C) is toxic at levels over 1 μg/ml
    (D) toxicity is noted by the appearance of hematuria
    (E) is useful in supraventricular tachycardia

197. Postspinal headaches are

(A) more frequent with large-bone needles
(B) not lessened by the use of a Whittaker 22-gauge needle
(C) aggravated by the supine position
(D) noted immediately
(E) relieved in 12 hours by an epidural blood patch

198. The calcium channel blocking drugs

(A) are all antiarrhythmics
(B) all have a peak effect in about 3 minutes
(C) are poorly bound to proteins
(D) interfere with the flow of calcium ion through cellular membranes
(E) are all about equally effective

199. As a person ascends to an altitude of 10,000 feet

(A) atmospheric pressure remains the same
(B) inspired oxygen pressure remains the same
(C) inspired carbon dioxide decreases
(D) alveolar carbon dioxide and water vapor pressure are constant
(E) alveolar oxygen pressure increases

200. The drug pentazocine is

(A) a nonaddicting narcotic
(B) a pure narcotic agonist
(C) a mixed agonist–antagonist
(D) a pure narcotic antagonist
(E) useful only orally

201. If a patient is taking monamine oxidase (MAO) inhibitors, which of the following should be avoided?

(A) local anesthetics
(B) halothane
(C) vecuronium
(D) meperidine
(E) aspirin

202. All of the following are adverse effects of furosemide EXCEPT

(A) renin release
(B) ototoxicity
(C) hypokalemia
(D) acidosis
(E) hyperglycemia

203. The most common cause of anesthetic disasters is

(A) aspiration pneumonia
(B) halothane hepatitis
(C) circulatory instability
(D) malignant hyperthermia
(E) hypoxemia

204. Nifedipine is a calcium channel blocker that

(A) is quite effective in supraventricular tachycardia
(B) is used for the treatment of ischemic heart disease
(C) has a half-life of 30 minutes
(D) is a peripheral vasoconstrictor
(E) is an effective drug for ventricular tachycardia

205. The interaction of protamine and heparin to terminate anticoagulation is one of

(A) competition for binding sites
(B) a chemical interaction leading to an inactive compound
(C) pH change
(D) a conformational change
(E) platelet stimulation

206. Echothiophate causes prolongation of succinylcholine by

(A) chemical interaction
(B) interaction at site of absorption
(C) altered protein binding
(D) competition for binding sites
(E) altered metabolism

207. Postoperative nerve deficits following regional anesthesia may be due to all of the following EXCEPT

(A) epinephrine 1:200,000 added to lidocaine
(B) positioning
(C) multiple sclerosis
(D) orthopedic casts
(E) surgical trauma

208. The interaction of phenobarbital and phenytoin can be described as one of

(A) chemical interaction
(B) interaction at site of absorption
(C) altered protein binding
(D) competition for binding sites
(E) altered metabolism

209. The combination of nitrous oxide at 0.5 MAC + isoflurane 0.5 MAC is one of

(A) antagonism
(B) potentiation
(C) additive effect
(D) synergism
(E) no effect

210. The chemical formula for isoflurane is

(A) $CFHCl\text{-}CF_2\text{-}O\text{-}CHF_2$
(B) $CH_3\text{-}O\text{-}CF_2\text{-}CCl_2H$
(C) $CF_3\text{-}CHCl\text{-}O\text{-}CHF_2$
(D) $CHClBr\text{-}CF_3$
(E) $C_2H_5\text{-}O\text{-}C_2H_5$

211. If a nitrous oxide tank is contaminated with water vapor, ice will form on the cylinder valve as a result of the

    (A) latent heat of vaporization
    (B) specific heat
    (C) vapor pressure
    (D) low pressure of the nitrous oxide
    (E) ambient temperature

212. The drug diazepam is a(an)

    (A) isopropylphenol
    (B) butyrophenone
    (C) eugenol
    (D) barbiturate
    (E) benzodiazepine

213. A drug that is a pure narcotic antagonist is

    (A) butorphanol
    (B) levallorphan
    (C) naloxone
    (D) neostigmine
    (E) edrophonium

214. A drug that is associated with pulmonary toxicity is

    (A) doxorubicin
    (B) bleomycin
    (C) vincristine
    (D) methotrexate
    (E) L-asparaginase

215. The number of calories required to raise the temperature of 1 g of a substance by 1°C is

    (A) the kilocalorie
    (B) the specific heat
    (C) the standard temperature
    (D) equal for all liquids
    (E) equal for all metals

216. Fade during tetanic contraction is due to

    (A) inability to transmit electrical impulses
    (B) cellular loss of potassium
    (C) depletion of cellular DNA
    (D) inability of apparatus to show all impulses
    (E) inability of endplate to release acetylcholine

217. The tubercle of Chassaignac is the eponym for the

    (A) horn of the hyoid bone
    (B) anterior portion of the cricoid
    (C) transverse process of the sixth cervical vertebra
    (D) tip of the mastoid
    (E) medial portion of the clavicle

218. A partial rebreathing mask contains a small reservoir bag that

    (A) requires an added oxygen flow
    (B) leads to increased carbon dioxide
    (C) leads to decreased carbon dioxide
    (D) provides a high FIO_2 and conserves oxygen
    (E) has no effect on blood gases

219. When performing a caudal block

    (A) the needle enters through the sacral hiatus
    (B) anomalies are seldom encountered
    (C) the patient should be kept flat
    (D) the patient should be asked to keep his or her heels together
    (E) small volumes of agent are needed, since the volume of the canal is only 8 to 12 ml

220. The dermatome level of the xiphoid is

    (A) T-4
    (B) T-6
    (C) T-10
    (D) S-1
    (E) L-1

221. The total dosage of lidocaine for a child should not exceed

    (A) 1 mg/kg
    (B) 3.5 mg/kg
    (C) 5 mg/kg
    (D) 7 mg/kg
    (E) 10 mg/kg

222. As a patient becomes more deeply anesthetized, the last sense to disappear is

    (A) smell
    (B) vision
    (C) pain
    (D) discomfort
    (E) hearing

223. A patient with mild to moderate systemic disturbance, eg, essential hypertension, would be classified as ASA Physical

    (A) class I
    (B) class II
    (C) class III
    (D) class IV
    (E) class V

224. If nitrous oxide is administered at a constant concentration, the uptake into the bloodstream in milliliters per minute will

    (A) be constant
    (B) increase with time
    (C) decrease with time
    (D) depend on temperature
    (E) be independent of concentration

225. The usual blood loss with a normal delivery is

(A) 200 ml
(B) 400 ml
(C) 600 ml
(D) 800 ml
(E) 1000 ml

226. A patient who develops a corneal abrasion during anesthesia should be treated with all of the following EXCEPT

(A) an eye patch
(B) a topical anesthetic to relieve pain
(C) an antibiotic ointment
(D) a cycloplegic
(E) a mydriatic

227. Complications of criocothyroid membrane puncture include all of the following EXCEPT

(A) subcutaneous emphysema
(B) bleeding
(C) pneumothorax
(D) hoarseness
(E) bronchial tear

228. During delivery, a lower dose of local anesthetic is required for regional anesthesia because

(A) pregnant women have greater pain tolerance
(B) the pain fibers are more superficial in the spinal canal
(C) the epidural and subarachnoid spaces are larger
(D) the epidural and subarachnoid spaces are decreased in size
(E) maternal hyperventilation decreases pain

229. A technique most useful in bronchopleural fistula treatment is

(A) spontaneous breathing with a mask
(B) assisted ventilation with positive pressure
(C) controlled ventilation with a mechanical ventilator
(D) positive end-expiratory pressure
(E) high-frequency ventilation

230. Sulfhemoglobin

(A) can be converted to hemoglobin by methylene blue
(B) is an effective oxygen carrier
(C) cannot be converted to hemoglobin
(D) is converted to hemoglobin by phenacetin
(E) is not associated with cyanosis

231. The blood volume of an infant with a normal hemoglobin is estimated to be

(A) 30 ml/kg
(B) 40 ml/kg
(C) 50 ml/kg
(D) 60 ml/kg
(E) 80 ml/kg

232. If this patient aspirates gastric contents, treatment should consist of all of the following EXCEPT

(A) intubation
(B) suctioning
(C) pulmonary lavage
(D) high F_{IO_2}
(E) artificial ventilation as necessary

233. Nasotracheal intubation has a higher incidence of

(A) sinusitis
(B) sore throat
(C) vocal cord injury
(D) subglottic stenosis
(E) arytenoid cartilage injury

234. Signs of causalgia include

(A) hypoesthesia
(B) coldness or hyperthermia
(C) pain that is of short duration
(D) pliable nails
(E) osteopetrosis

235. Preeclampsia is associated with

(A) hypovolemia
(B) hypernatremia
(C) low hematocrit reading
(D) hyperkalemia
(E) hypotension

236. Urinary output during anesthesia in a child should be

(A) 1 ml/kg/hour
(B) 2 ml/kg/hour
(C) 3 ml/kg/hour
(D) 4 ml/kg/hour
(E) 5 ml/kg/hour

237. The internal jugular approach for placement of central venous catheters

(A) is free of complications
(B) is done without benefit of landmarks
(C) has a high incidence of pneumothorax
(D) is especially fraught with difficulty in obese patients
(E) provides a straighter course into superior vena cava when done on right side

238. A 71-year-old male is admitted with a complaint of hoarseness and sore throat. On indirect laryngo-

scopy, a supraglottic mass is noted with edema of the cords. He is scheduled for a direct laryngoscopy under general anesthesia. The approach to this procedure should be

(A) kept simple, since it is a short procedure
(B) induction, paralysis, and laryngoscopy
(C) induction, paralysis, intubation, and laryngoscopy
(D) paralysis, intubation, induction, and laryngoscopy
(E) to establish an airway before any medication is given or instrumentation done

239. An infant born with a heart rate of 70, a weak cry, good muscle flexion, poor reflexes, and a blue-pale complexion would be given at Apgar score of

(A) 2
(B) 4
(C) 5
(D) 6
(E) 7

240. The lifetime of a canister filling of soda lime

(A) depends on the method of filling
(B) is independent of the volume of CO_2 exhaled
(C) is independent of the location of the relief valve
(D) is prolonged by low gas flows
(E) is shortened by channeling

241. In the closed system, the one measure that must be met is

(A) the tidal volume
(B) the minute volume
(C) the respiratory rate
(D) the oxygen consumption
(E) the needed anesthesia

242. Postpuncture headache

(A) is worse in the supine position
(B) is of higher incidence following puncture with a 25-gauge needle
(C) is more prevalent in nonpregnant patients
(D) will be worse with a larger dural hole
(E) is lessened if the patient is dehydrated

243. The muscle power for spontaneous delivery is provided by the

(A) abdominal muscles alone
(B) perineal muscle
(C) abdominal muscles and uterine muscles, the abdominal being dominant
(D) abdominal muscles and uterine muscles, the uterine being dominant
(E) abdominal and back muscle

244. The most significant risk of a free-standing vaporizer is

(A) using the wrong agent
(B) tipping
(C) foaming of the agent
(D) leakage
(E) overfilling

245. An infant under anesthesia loses body heat by all of the following routes EXCEPT

(A) the metabolism of brown fat
(B) breathing dry gases
(C) conduction to cold surroundings
(D) cold preparation solutions
(E) exposure of abdominal contents

246. The only early sign of malignant hyperthermia in an anesthetized infant is

(A) rapid rise in body temperature
(B) tachycardia
(C) hot skin
(D) arrhythmia
(E) hot circle absorber

247. Aerosol therapy is useful in providing for all of the following EXCEPT

(A) improved bronchial hygiene
(B) humidification
(C) a means to deliver medication
(D) decreased coughing
(E) expectoration promotion

248. The usual inspiratory-expiratory (I:E) ratio during spontaneous breathing is

(A) 1:1
(B) 2:1
(C) 1:2
(D) 1:3
(E) 1:4

249. The vapor pressure of a liquid is most dependent on

(A) the atmospheric pressure
(B) the specific heat of the container
(C) the temperature
(D) the conductivity of the container
(E) the partial pressure of the gas

250. The Bain circuit is a modification of the

(A) Mapleson A system
(B) Mapleson B system
(C) Mapleson C system
(D) Mapleson D system
(E) Mapleson E system

251. A 5-year-old patient is admitted with an open eye secondary to severe globe laceration. He had eaten 1 hour before his accident. General anesthesia is required for the repair The intubation should be accomplished

(A) by an awake intubation
(B) after injection of 100 mg of succinylcholine
(C) after D-tubocurarine followed by succinylcholine
(D) after vecuronium administration
(E) after deep halothane by inhalation induction

252. If either the Fluomatic or Fluotec Mark II vaporizer is tipped over

(A) the wick will become saturated
(B) the vaporizer must be returned to the factory
(C) the concentration of the vapor will be higher than calculated
(D) a low concentration will result
(E) the vaporizer should be righted and put into use

253. The Vapor 19.1 vaporizer is temperature compensated as a result of a(n)

(A) bimetallic band
(B) copper element
(C) expansion element to the vaporizing chamber
(D) sintered disc
(E) heating element that keeps the vaporizer at a constant temperature

254. A patient is undergoing transurethral resection under general anesthesia. The urologist is heard to complain to the circulating nurse that the irrigation device is not working properly. The anesthesiologist notices loss of relaxation and irregular respirations. You should immediately think of

(A) massive hemoptysis
(B) electrolyte disturbance
(C) a perforation
(D) increased blood loss
(E) pulmonary embolus

255. The pumping effect in reference to a vaporizer

(A) leads to a decreased concentration of the agent
(B) refers to a method of filling the vaporizer
(C) refers to a method of cleaning the vaporizer
(D) leads to a decreased flow through the vaporizer
(E) is more pronounced at low flow rates

256. The statistical term for the spread of individual values is

(A) mean
(B) median
(C) variance

(D) standard deviation
(E) standard error of the mean

257. The preanesthetic use of atropine in patients with glaucoma

(A) is contraindicated
(B) is of more danger in the patient with open-angle glaucoma
(C) should not precipitate glaucoma
(D) may cause miosis
(E) will decrease the intraocular pressure significantly

258. An example of a central pain state is

(A) postoperative incision pain
(B) gallbladder pain
(C) phantom limb pain
(D) bone fracture pain
(E) headache

259. If a patient has prerenal failure, the urine will

(A) be dilute
(B) be concentrated
(C) have a specific gravity of 1.010
(D) be excreted in large amounts
(E) have a reddish tinge due to presence of red blood cells

260. A patient underwent a thyroidectomy at 0800, and a 2200 he complained to the nurse of difficulty in breathing. She took his blood pressure, which was moderately elevated above previous determinations, but she also noticed that his wrist flexed when the blood pressure cuff remained inflated. The cause of the stridor is probably

(A) vocal cord paralysis
(B) partial cord paralysis
(C) laryngeal edema
(D) cervical hematoma
(E) hypocalcemia

261. The time required for a patient to develop adrenal suppression from cortisone treatment is

(A) 2 weeks
(B) 4 weeks
(C) 8 weeks
(D) 12 weeks
(E) unknown

262. The most important goal in the treatment of the diabetic patient undergoing anesthesia is to

(A) keep blood sugar in the normal range
(B) prevent glycosuria
(C) prevent hypoglycemia

(D) prevent ketoacidosis

(E) prevent acetonuria

263. The clamping of the thoracic aorta in aneurysm repair is followed by

(A) immediate hypotension

(B) immediate hypertension

(C) cardiac standstill

(D) no change

(E) loss of blood pressure in the right arm

264. A complication of aortic surgery is paraplegia that is due to

(A) pressure on the spinal cord during surgery

(B) long periods of hypotension

(C) hypothermia associated with the surgery

(D) spinal cord ischemia

(E) loss of cerebrospinal fluid

265. Treatment of the neurosurgical patient with mannitol may be followed by all of the following EXCEPT

(A) initial hypervolemia

(B) decreased urine volume

(C) hypovolemia

(D) decreased venous pressure

(E) a fall in arterial pressure

266. The cement substance, methylmethacrylate

(A) is a liquid hydrocarbon

(B) generates considerable heat while setting

(C) is associated with hypertension

(D) is always mixed preoperatively

(E) is used only for hip fractures

267. Clinical manifestations of fat emboli include all of the following EXCEPT

(A) petechiae

(B) hypoxemia

(C) confusion

(D) bradycardia

(E) cyanosis

268. Mannitol may lead to subdural hematoma by

(A) causing cerebral edema

(B) affecting clotting mechanisms

(C) leading to cortical vein disruption

(D) causing hypertension

(E) leakage through the vein wall

269. The Glasgow Coma Score is based on

(A) response to eye opening, verbal response and motor response

(B) assessment of knee jerk

(C) assessment of pupil size

(D) assessment of respiration

(E) assessment of EEG

270. The major intracranial buffer against increased intracranial pressure is the

(A) dural sinus

(B) cerebrospinal fluid

(C) white matter

(D) gray matter

(E) glial cells

271. The most profound chemical stimulus for cerebral autoregulation is

(A) metabolic alkalosis

(B) hypothermia

(C) hyperthermia

(D) carbon dioxide

(E) acidosis

DIRECTIONS (Questions 272 through 350): For each of the items in this section, ONE or MORE of the numbered options is correct. Choose the answer

A if only 1, 2, and 3 are correct,

B if only 1 and 3 are correct,

C if only 2 and 4 are correct,

D if only 4 is correct,

E if all are correct.

272. The myasthenic syndrome (Eaton–Lambert syndrome) is a condition in which

(1) patients show sensitivity to depolarizing muscle relaxants

(2) the neuromuscular block is readily reversed by neostigmine

(3) sensitivity to nondepolarizing relaxants is increased

(4) resection of the tumor does not effect a cure

273. The effects of acetylcholine that are accentuated by the use of neostigmine include

(1) bradycardia

(2) sweating

(3) skeletal muscle stimulation

(4) urinary retention

274. Tetanus is a disease characterized by muscle stiffness and paroxysmal spasms. In the treatment

(1) sedation with diazepam may also relieve the spasm

(2) D-tubocurarine is helpful to relieve the spasm

(3) labetalol may relieve the sympathetic overactivity

(4) pancuronium may increase heart rate and cause hypertension

SUMMARY OF DIRECTIONS				
A	**B**	**C**	**D**	**E**
1, 2, 3 only	1, 3 only	2, 4 only	4 only	All are correct

275. The alveolar concentration of a gas

    (1) is independent of the lung volume
    (2) will vary with alveolar ventilation
    (3) will vary with the type of soda lime used
    (4) is dependent on uptake of the blood

276. Uptake of an agent by blood is determined by

    (1) passage across the alveolar membrane
    (2) the Ostwald coefficient
    (3) the cardiac output
    (4) the type of system being used

277. The addition of nitrous oxide to a halothane anesthetic

    (1) will have the greatest effect early in the course of the anesthesia
    (2) will have its greatest effect at deeper levels of anesthesia
    (3) may cause antagonism of halothane
    (4) will cause intense vasodilatation

278. The circulatory effects of halothane are

    (1) insignificant at 0.5%
    (2) due to a single mechanism
    (3) essentially the same at 1% and 2%
    (4) all due to its central action

279. A patient is breathing a nitrous oxide–oxygen mixture and has an endotracheal tube cuff filled with a gas. You would expect an increase in

    (1) volume of the cuff if it is filled with air
    (2) volume of the cuff if it is filled with a nitrous oxide–oxygen mixture
    (3) volume and pressure of a large volume cuff
    (4) pressure but not volume of a small volume cuff

280. A diabetic patient is to undergo anesthesia for a vein stripping. On the morning of surgery, he receives one-half dose of his insulin requirement and his usual morning dose of 40 mg of propranolol. Anesthesia is maintained with isoflurane. In the recovery room 4 hours later, his blood sugar is 52 mg/dl. The cause of this could be

    (1) stress of surgery
    (2) propranolol
    (3) isoflurane
    (4) insulin

281. The drug propanidid is

    (1) a barbiturate
    (2) a premedicant administered intramuscularly
    (3) hepatoxic
    (4) short-acting

282. Microshock hazard is increased in patients

    (1) with a pacemaker in place
    (2) who are in rooms with isolation transformers
    (3) with a central venous line in place
    (4) in mechanically operated beds

283. The flow rate of fluid flowing smoothly through a tube is

    (1) proportional to the pressure gradient
    (2) proportional to the fourth power of the radius of the tube
    (3) inversely proportional to the viscosity of the fluid
    (4) proportional to the temperature of the tube

284. A transducer is a device used to

    (1) convert a nonelectric parameter to an electric signal
    (2) measure heart voltages in the electrocardiogram
    (3) measure temperature using the thermistor
    (4) measure electrical activity in the electroencephalograph

285. Turbulent flow is

    (1) characterized by irregular lines of flow
    (2) characterized by parallel lines of flow
    (3) noted at branches, obstructions, or roughness of the conduit
    (4) proportional to volume flow

286. Pulse oximeters

    (1) are based on Beer's law
    (2) will not read carboxyhemoglobin
    (3) will read methemoglobin
    (4) provide a heart rate but do not need pulsatile flow

287. The viscosity of a fluid

    (1) depends on its density
    (2) affects its specific gravity
    (3) does not affect resistance to flow
    (4) is the intrinsic property that affects its laminar flow

288. The relationship of the femoral nerve in the inguinal area is that it lies

    (1) superficial to the inguinal ligament
    (2) lateral to the femoral artery

(3) medial to the femoral vein
(4) lateral to the lacunar ligament

289. When performing a lumbar puncture, the spinal needle passes through the

(1) supraspinal ligament
(2) interspinal ligament
(3) ligamentum flavum
(4) pia mater

290. Anesthesia for surgery on the medial malleolus requires block of the

(1) femoral nerve
(2) obturator nerve
(3) sciatic nerve
(4) inguinal nerve

291. Structures lying medially on the anterior aspect of the wrist include the

(1) median nerve
(2) ulnar nerve
(3) radial nerve
(4) ulnar artery

292. When administering a spinal anesthetic, the solution and technique to be used are influenced by the

(1) duration of anesthesia desired
(2) intraabdominal pressure of obesity
(3) height of the patient
(4) sex of the patient

293. Which of the following statements is (are) correct when comparing spinal to epidural anesthesia of equal degree?

(1) hypotension is less profound with spinal anesthesia
(2) there is a greater loss of peripheral resistance with epidural anesthesia
(3) there are few systemic effects of the local anesthesia with epidural anesthesia
(4) systemic effects of epinephrine are more evident with epidural anesthesia

294. In the patient with an acute injury at the C4-5 level, you would expect

(1) a major loss of diaphragmatic power
(2) no breathing
(3) grossly impaired alveolar ventilation
(4) disturbance of heart rate

295. To ascertain proper placement of the endotracheal tube, the

(1) cords should be visualized
(2) tube should be seen to pass between the cords

(3) thorax should be auscultated
(4) end-tidal carbon dioxide should be detected on the monitor

296. Tracheal stenosis is a serious complication of long-term ventilation. It can be avoided best by the use of

(1) hourly cuff deflation
(2) minimal leak
(3) frequent suctioning
(4) low-pressure cuff

297. A patient has a right-sided internal jugular catheterization done while under anesthesia. Complications that may occur include

(1) hematoma
(2) arrhythmias
(3) air embolism
(4) chylothorax

298. Administering humidified gases and mist therapy to a patient may result in

(1) lung infection
(2) loss of heat
(3) water load
(4) increased airway resistance

299. Patients with acromegaly are more prone to airway obstruction because of

(1) thickening of the vocal cords
(2) laryngeal stenosis
(3) large tongue
(4) receding chin

300. Hypocalcemia occurring during blood transfusion

(1) follows rapid transfusion
(2) is of no clinical significance
(3) is aggravated by hypothermia
(4) need not be treated

301. Complications of nasotracheal intubation include

(1) sinusitis
(2) nosebleed
(3) nasal necrosis
(4) broken teeth

302. After a spinal anesthetic, the parturient woman becomes hypotensive. The drug(s) of choice for treatment is (are)

(1) norepinephrine
(2) methoxamine
(3) phenylephrine drip
(4) ephedrine

SUMMARY OF DIRECTIONS				
A	**B**	**C**	**D**	**E**
1, 2, 3 only	1, 3 only	2, 4 only	4 only	All are correct

303. Gastric changes associated with pregnancy include

(1) decreased acid secretion
(2) decreased gastric emptying time
(3) the downward displacement of the pylorus
(4) incompetence of the gastroesophageal sphincter

304. Maternal changes associated with preeclampsia include

(1) increased cardiac output
(2) decreased renal blood flow
(3) decreased cerebral blood flow
(4) increased hepatic blood flow

305. Anesthesia for emergency cesarean section can be provided by

(1) general anesthesia
(2) local infiltration
(3) subarachnoid block
(4) spinal epidural block

306. Halothane is not often used in obstetrics because

(1) it is not of sufficient solubility to give fast relief
(2) it is not a good analgesic
(3) of its liver toxicity
(4) it produces myometrial depression even in low concentrations

307. Treatment of postspinal headache includes

(1) orders to keep NPO
(2) reassurance
(3) subarachnoid injection of the patient's blood
(4) codeine or aspirin

308. Pulmonary vascular resistance in newborns decreases because of

(1) closure of the ductus
(2) lung expansion
(3) decreased pH
(4) improved oxygenation

309. Drugs are handled differently by neonates because of differences in

(1) absorption
(2) total body water
(3) albumin levels
(4) metabolism

310. The work of breathing in a newborn infant

(1) involves overcoming elastic forces
(2) involves overcoming resistive forces
(3) is least when the infant breathes at 35 times per minute
(4) is less if the child is breathing very rapidly

311. Racemic epinephrine administered by aerosol

(1) is a mixture of epinephrine and norepinephrine
(2) is a potent alpha and beta stimulant
(3) causes mucosal edema
(4) is a mild bronchodilator

312. Aerosol therapy may cause

(1) lower airway obstruction
(2) fluid overload
(3) contamination of the airway
(4) decreased bronchospasm

313. The pulmonary changes characteristic of the post-operative period include

(1) decreased total lung capacity
(2) decreased functional residual capacity (FRC)
(3) decreased residual volume
(4) increased compliance

314. The Cole tube

(1) has a lower resistance when compared to a tube of similar size
(2) is the tube of choice for nasotracheal intubation
(3) carries less likelihood of endobronchial intubation
(4) should be inserted to the maximum distance possible to get a good fit

315. The Macintosh laryngoscope blade

(1) has a straight spatula
(2) has no flange
(3) has a pointed tip
(4) is manufactured in various sizes

316. Nasopharyngeal airways are contraindicated in the patient with

(1) nasal polyps
(2) sepsis of the nasopharynx
(3) a very low platelet count
(4) the jaw wired shut

317. The oxygen analyzer

(1) is a good disconnect alarm
(2) should be placed on the exhalation side of the circuit
(3) is unaffected by humidity
(4) should be placed on the fresh gas side of the circuit

318. The reaction of carbon dioxide and soda lime produces

(1) $CaCO_3$
(2) Na_2CO_3
(3) H_2O
(4) HCl

319. Soda lime granules

(1) are manufactured to be smooth and round
(2) are of a size 4 to 8 mesh
(3) of a small size give a lower resistance
(4) of a small size give better absorption function

320. The function of the reservoir bag is to

(1) accumulate gas during expiration
(2) provide a means for assisting or controlling respiration
(3) serve as a monitor of ventilation
(4) serve as a pressure buffer because of its compliance

321. General anesthesia is indicated for computed tomography (CT) scanning when the patient

(1) is very young
(2) is restless
(3) has involuntary movements
(4) is febrile

322. The doctrine of *res ipsa loquitur* is applicable where the

(1) accident is of a kind that usually does not happen without negligence
(2) apparent cause of the accident is within the control of the defendant
(3) plaintiff could not have contributed to the accident
(4) defendant wants to settle out of court

323. If it is discovered at the end of a procedure that a tooth is missing, the anesthesiologist should

(1) awaken the patient as usual
(2) check the oropharynx and nasopharynx
(3) ask the family about the tooth when the patient is in the recovery room
(4) get x-rays of the head, chest, and abdomen

324. Drugs affecting intraocular pressure include

(1) acetazolamide
(2) succinylcholine
(3) mannitol
(4) atropine

325. A patient with obstructive lung disease develops a causalgia syndrome involving the right arm after a nerve injury. Treatment of the syndrome may involve

(1) stellate ganglion block
(2) physical therapy
(3) application of moist heat
(4) axillary block

326. The placebo effect occurs

(1) only in patients who are emotionally unstable
(2) with normal individuals
(3) only in those who are faking pain
(4) with pharmacologically active substances

327. Anesthetic agents and adjuncts acceptable for renal transplantation include

(1) halothane
(2) gallamine
(3) thiopental
(4) enflurane

328. The patient who absorbs fluid during transurethral surgery is in danger of pulmonary edema as a result of

(1) increased intravascular pressure
(2) position on the operating table
(3) decreased osmotic pressure
(4) increased sodium concentration

329. The irrigating fluids for prostatic resection should be

(1) nonhemolytic
(2) close to water in composition
(3) isoosmolar
(4) electrolyte solutions

330. Insulin should be administered to a diabetic patient during surgery

(1) by adding it to the container of intravenous fluids
(2) only when monitoring urine and blood for sugar
(3) in the usual daily dosage
(4) only if glucose is being infused

331. Hormones secreted by the adrenal cortex include

(1) mineralocorticoids
(2) glucocorticoids
(3) sex hormones
(4) norepinephrine

332. A patient with a thyroid tumor develops hypertension during the procedure. This may be due to

(1) light anesthesia
(2) pheochromocytoma
(3) hypercarbia
(4) myxedema

SUMMARY OF DIRECTIONS				
A	B	C	D	E
1, 2, 3 only	1, 3 only	2, 4 only	4 only	All are correct

333. Anesthetic agents must be used with caution in patients with cardiac tamponade to avoid cardiac depression, and

 (1) compensatory mechanisms must be preserved
 (2) the heart should be kept full
 (3) the heart rate should be kept high
 (4) peripheral vasculature should be kept constricted

334. In a patient who has had a heart transplant, you would expect heart rate changes with

 (1) atropine
 (2) pancuronium
 (3) neostigmine
 (4) propranolol

335. The primary determinant(s) of myocardial oxygen supply is (are)

 (1) the oxygen-carrying capacity of the blood
 (2) F_{IO_2}
 (3) coronary blood flow
 (4) age

336. Mannitol given to a head-injured patient

 (1) may lead to hyperosmolar coma
 (2) removes water from the normal brain tissue
 (3) may lead to cerebral edema if the blood–brain barrier is impaired
 (4) is effective in doses of 0.25 g/kg

337. Air embolism may be a fatal complication, depending on

 (1) the amount of air present
 (2) the site of entry
 (3) the rate of entry
 (4) whether a Swan-Ganz catheter is in place

338. Anesthetic agents that increase intracranial pressure in the neurosurgical patient include

 (1) fentanyl
 (2) halothane
 (3) thiopental
 (4) nitrous oxide

339. The blood–brain barrier is

 (1) relatively impermeable to morphine
 (2) readily permeable to glucose
 (3) readily permeable to carbon dioxide
 (4) readily permeable to bicarbonate

340. Causes of arrhythmias associated with neurosurgical procedures include

 (1) orbital decompression
 (2) carotid ligation
 (3) tonsillar herniation
 (4) trigeminal nerve surgery

341. During a cerebral aneurysm procedure, sodium nitroprusside was infused. You can expect

 (1) short duration of action
 (2) bradycardia
 (3) acidemia
 (4) nitric acid toxicity

342. The incidence of hepatitis after blood transfusion

 (1) is usually due to non-A, non-B hepatitis
 (2) is 1/100 units transfused
 (3) is lower if blood donation is limited to volunteers
 (4) is higher after transfusion of red cells

343. Vitamin K-dependent coagulation factors are

 (1) II
 (2) VII
 (3) IX
 (4) X

344. Surgical procedures and conditions known to predispose to a bleeding diasthesis include

 (1) abruptio placentae
 (2) prostate surgery
 (3) portacaval shunt
 (4) small bowel resection

345. Wilson's disease is an inborn error of copper metabolism. Anesthetic implications include

 (1) possible hepatic involvement
 (2) drug metabolism
 (3) possible prolongation of neuromuscular blockade
 (4) renal tubular disease

346. Marfan's syndrome (arachnodactyly) is not always diagnosed before a disastrous event. Many of these patients have another illness. Anesthetic considerations include

 (1) avoidance of hypertension to avoid dissection
 (2) aortic stenosis
 (3) difficult intubations
 (4) short stature, making airway management difficult

347. If anesthesia is required for a patient who chronically smokes marijuana, you would expect

 (1) withdrawal symptoms
 (2) bronchitis
 (3) hepatic dysfunction
 (4) tachycardia

348 If patients with multiple myeloma require general anesthesia, it is important to have preoperative documentation of

 (1) serum calcium
 (2) renal studies
 (3) bone involvement
 (4) serum chloride

349. Autonomic hyperreflexia

 (1) occurs with a lesion above T-5
 (2) is initiated only by bladder distention
 (3) is accompanied by severe hypertension
 (4) is accompanied by tachycardia

350. The Pierre Robin syndrome presents anesthetic difficulty because of the prevalence of

 (1) heart problems
 (2) lung problems
 (3) renal problems
 (4) intubation problems

Answers and Explanations

1. **(B)** Pleural pressure increases 0.25 cm H_2O every centimeter down the lung. Thus it is lowest at the apex and highest at the base. The pleural pressure is related to body position in that in different positions, different areas will be dependent.

2. **(B)** Myocardial oxygen consumption is increased by tachycardia. It causes increased demand for oxygen at the same time that it leads to decreased oxygen supply by decreasing coronary blood flow. Increased afterload leads to increased wall tension, both of which require more oxygen. Increases of contractility require more oxygen.

3. **(D)** The FRC is composed of expiratory reserve volume and residual volume. Tidal volume plus inspiratory reserve volume comprise the inspiratory capacity. The other options are not designated capacities.

4. **(D)** The cilia of the respiratory tract move a double layer of mucus toward the larynx. There is an inner layer of thin mucus and an outer layer of thick mucus that is able to trap particulate matter or microorganisms. The cilia are part of the columnar cells lining the trachea. Body temperature does have an effect on ciliary motility.

5. **(C)** The process of slow diastolic depolarization is a property of pacemaker cells and is the process causing intrinsic rhythmicity. The process is due to calcium changes. The higher the pacemaker, the more pronounced is the process. Therefore, it is seen less in the His bundle.

6. **(A)** All of the factors cited except for an increase in the caliber of the airways will lead to increased airway resistance. The supine position will cause increased resistance due to decreased lung volume. The presence of an endotracheal tube increases resistance, and this may be aggravated by secretions and kinking.

7. **(B)** The bronchial tree divides into right and left bronchi, the left bronchus being narrower and longer. Foreign bodies are more apt to go to the right side. The trachea moves during respiration and with movement of the head. It is lined with pseudostratified columnar epithelium. The rings of cartilage do not completely encircle the trachea.

8. **(D)** Hyaluronidase increases the incidence of toxic reactions by allowing more widespread distribution of the drug, thereby increasing the uptake of the drug. This spread also increases the success rate of the block and decreases the duration of the block. The time of onset of the block is decreased.

9. **(E)** The larynx lies at the level of the third through sixth cervical vertebrae, and in the adult, the narrowest portion is at the level of the vocal cords. The larynx is supplied by the recurrent laryngeal nerve and the superior laryngeal nerve. It lies within the thyroid cartilage. The wide margin of the cricoid cartilage is posterior.

10. **(D)** Humidification of inhaled gases is at its optimum with the patient breathing through the nose. Atropine will dry out secretions. Endotracheal tubes and tracheostomies bypass the humidification process of the nose. A closed system will keep humidity in the system.

11. **(B)** The dependent areas are better ventilated, since the alveoli in the dependent areas expand more per unit pressure change than do nondependent alveoli.

12. **(A)** Inspiratory force is a measurement of reserve of ventilatory effort. It is a simple method that does not depend on patient cooperation. Therefore, it is particularly useful in the unconscious or anesthetized patient. A pressure in excess of 20 cm H_2O below atmospheric pressure is considered minimum to show adequate reserve.

13. **(E)** All of the options contribute to physiologic shunt except nonperfused alveoli, which produce increased dead space.

14. **(D)** Insufflation of oxygen to the unventilated lung will decrease the shunt and attenuate the desaturation. This implies that some alveoli are in continuity with the proximal airways. Shunting does occur in the unventilated lung. CO_2 removal is not usually a problem.

15. **(D)** After bilateral carotid endarterectomy, a patient will be more susceptible to hypoxemia because of denervation of the carotid body. The patient will not respond to hypoxemia with hyperventilation. In addition, the resting P_{CO_2} is elevated, and the response to small doses of narcotics may be accentuated. Hypertension is not a constant finding in these patients.

16. **(B)** The measure of oxygen tension requires the Clark electrode. This measurement is affected by temperature. The Severinghaus electrode is used for the measurement of carbon dioxide and uses the Henderson-Hasselbalch equation to relate pH to carbon dioxide.

17. **(C)** Anesthesia usually causes a decrease in FRC, which leads to hypoxemia. All of the other options can lead to hypoxemia: hypoventilation by decreased FRC and increased shunt, hyperventilation by shift of the oxyhemoglobin dissociation curve and decreased cardiac output, supine position by decreased ventilation and decreased FRC, and increased airway pressure by change in the ventilation/perfusion relationship.

18. **(A)** When venous admixture and oxygen remain constant, a decrease in cardiac output will decrease arterial oxygen. This is because the blood passing through the shunt circuit will be more desaturated due to the decreased cardiac output. This leads to more desaturation in the tissues. Urinary output usually decreases with decreased cardiac output.

19. **(C)** Patients who are hyperventilated for long periods of time have their carbon dioxide stores depleted. Postoperatively, these patients hypoventilate in an effort to restore their carbon dioxide and, in so doing, may become hypoxic if not given supplemental oxygen.

20. **(A)** Tracheal mucus flow and, necessarily, ciliary activity are impeded by deviation from ambient oxygen tension. Tracheal mucus flow is increased in patients with obstructive lung disease. Tracheal mucus flow is an important cleansing mechanism. Mucus flow and ciliary activity are depressed by cigarette smoke.

21. **(C)** Closing volume is increased in the small baby and in the elderly. Measurement of closing volume will detect changes in the small airways before they would become apparent by spirometry.

22. **(C)** At the time of the second heart sound, the mitral valve is opening. The closing of the aortic and pulmonic valves, isometric relaxation, and the T wave are all coincident.

23. **(D)** A high concentration of oxygen may be harmful to many organ systems. It is especially harmful to the patient with obstructive lung disease who is functioning on a hypoxic drive to ventilation.

24. **(C)** The medullary center located in the pons and medulla respond primarily to hydrogen ion concentration. Although this is related to the level of carbon dioxide, the primary stimulant is hydrogen ion Chronic hypercapnia depresses the centers.

25. **(C)** The intrinsic rate of the sinoatrial node is 70 to 80 beats per minute. Since it has a faster rate, it is the dominant pacemaker. As you progress down the conduction system, the rates are slower. The AV node, eg, has an intrinsic rate of 40 to 60 beats per minute.

26. **(B)** Vital capacity is decreased when the exposure is more than 12 hours. All of the other options are true.

27. **(D)** General anesthesia leads to an alteration of chest wall mechanics, resulting in decreased FRC. Breathing at the lower lung volume may also affect the lung mechanics, leading to increased elastic recoil and decreased compliance.

28. **(B)** The patient with restrictive disease will have a decrease in FVC. The FVC_1 may be decreased also, but the FVC_1/FVC is usually normal.

29. **(C)** All of the factors cited are presumptive evidence of ventilation. The only good measure of those listed is the analysis of blood gases, especially carbon dioxide.

30. **(D)** Pulmonary vascular resistance is the result of cardiac output, the state of vasomotion and pressure. A change in cardiac output will be followed by changes in the radius of the vessels to allow maintenance of normal pressure. The resistance is equal to pressure divided by flow.

31. **(E)** Hypoxic pulmonary vasoconstriction causes diversion of blood flow from hypoxic to nonhypoxic lung tissue. In the usual circumstance, blood is diverted to areas where flow is decreased, eg, to the apices. This causes a decrease in the V_{DS}/V_T.

32. (B) Closing volume requires nitrogen washout or the use of a tracer gas. It is not possible by spirometry. The other values are available by spirometry.

33. (E) Carboxyhemoglobin is involved in the transport of carbon monoxide. The other options are intimately involved in the transport of carbon dioxide.

34. (D) The Bohr effect describes the effect of carbon dioxide on the uptake of oxygen. Option B describes the Haldane effect. Carbonic anhydrase, hydrogen ion, and catalytic enzymes are not involved.

35. (E) In zone 2, the blood flow is dependent on arterial pressure and the alveolar pressure. These change with the status of ventilation. Venous pressure is still not a determinant of blood flow in this zone.

36. (B) Boyle's law states that the volume of a gas at a constant temperature is inversely proportional to the pressure. The other options are not appropriate.

37. (B) The main buffer in the body is the bicarbonate system. It is not the only system, and the other options are involved in the other buffering systems.

38. (D) Analysis of arterial blood gases is the most reliable method of documenting hypoxemia. Detection of cyanosis, respiratory responses, and circulatory responses is subjective and may not be accurate. The pulse oximeter has improved the detection of hypoxemia, and it responds faster than transcutaneous oxygen readings.

39. (A) Chemoreceptor stimulation leads to an increased ventilatory effect. Many rely on bradycardia as the only sign of hypoxia, but the response is a complex one.

40. (D) Carbon dioxide tension rises under apneic ventilation and may contribute to the problems seen. It will rise more quickly in one in whom there is lung disease. All arrhythmias are not due to hypoxemia but may be due to increased catecholamines. These, in turn, may be increased due to increased carbon dioxide. Pulse oximetry has been of definite value in these procedures.

41. (E) Carboxyhemoglobin is not usually involved in the transport of oxygen. The other factors are important.

42. (A) The width of the inflatable bladder need encircle only one-half the arm. In the average adult, the width of 12 to 14 cm is appropriate. In the person who is not average, spurious readings may result if a standard adult cuff is used. This is particularly true in the child, and the need for an assortment of cuffs is apparent. The manometer should be calibrated on a routine basis to ascertain that it is giving true readings. The reading should always start at zero.

43. (C) The V/Q ratio is higher at the apex. The blood flow and ventilation are greatest at the base. The Po_2 is higher at the base.

44. (A) The cuff of an endotracheal tube should be inflated enough to prevent aspiration and still allow capillary flow in the underlying trachea. A pressure of 20 torr will allow this in a high-volume, thin-walled cuff.

45. (D) Compliance becomes better as one moves down the lung. The alveoli become smaller, and pleural pressure increases. Ventilation of the alveoli increases due to increased compliance.

46. (A) Coronary perfusion occurs for the most part during diastole. The perfusion pressure (CPP) relationship is

$$CPP = DBP - LVEDP$$

where DPB is the diastolic blood pressure and LVEDP is left ventricular end-diastolic pressure. As DBP rises or LVEDP falls, the flow will increase. Tachycardia decreases time of perfusion, since diastole is shortened. Systolic hypertension decreases perfusion, since the ventricle contracts harder, allowing less perfusion during systole.

47. (C) The baroreceptors are located principally in the carotid body. These are important to the regulation of circulation. The baroreceptors respond to pressure, not to carbon dioxide or oxygen.

48. (B) Afterload is dependent on the distensibility of the arteries into which the ventricle ejects the blood. The best measure of afterload is the systemic vascular resistance (SVR). The calculation of SVR takes mean blood pressure into account. Afterload involves the aortic valve but not solely. Vasodilators decrease afterload. Ventricular size is related to afterload but is not an important consideration.

49. (E) Observation of the direct display of arterial pressure will give all of the information cited. However, in reference 57, Barash disputes whether one can accurately assess changes in systemic vascular resistance.

50. (A) The drawing in reference 57 (p. 574) shows the typical tracing familiar to anyone who has inserted a flow-directed catheter. The right atrial pressure is about 5 mm Hg. The step-up in diastolic pressure shows the entry into the pulmonary artery.

51. **(C)** The correct lead placement is right arm–left leg in lead II. The other leads are right arm–left arm in lead I and left arm–left leg in lead III.

52. **(A)** The ECG cannot detect efficacy of pump function. The ECG may show a normal sinus rhythm during electromechanical dissociation when the pump is not working effectively at all. The tracing can be observed for changes in electrolyte disturbance, especially calcium and potassium. Ischemia is detected by changes in the tracing. Pacemaker function is checked by observing the tracing. Arrhythmias are detected by the electrocardiogram.

53. **(B)** dP/dt is a measure of ventricular contractile force over time. The other options are incorrect.

54. **(C)** Coronary circulation reacts to carbon dioxide in a manner similar to cerebral circulation. Although this may be salutary in the instance of head trauma, in the patient with chest pain and ischemia, hyperventilation may lead to further decrease of coronary flow. The decrease is not an intense vasoconstriction.

55. **(A)** Myocardial oxygen consumption is closely and directly related to cardiac rate over wide ranges. The rate–pressure product is also closely related to myocardial oxygen consumption. An increase in stroke volume does not cause as much of an increase in oxygen as an increase in pressure.

56. **(B)** Since blood flow to the heart runs along pressure gradients in the upper extremities, the blood in the basilic vein runs from a site of higher pressure to a site of lower pressure, the right atrium. In the lower extremities, blood flow is assisted by valves and muscular activity.

57. **(A)** The microcirculatory beds are not always open but in a constantly changing state of flow. This flow is regulated by the autonomic nervous system and local factors, including the state of oxygenation. The amount of muscular investment varies with the specific structure, being higher in arteriole than in metarteriole and even less in the venules. The capillary beds, although small, hold a great amount of the blood volume at any one time.

58. **(B)** Pulmonary edema results from an increase in pulmonary capillary pressure. Pulmonary edema may also result from neurologic injury. Reports of negative airway pressure pulmonary edema have been reported in the patient with airway obstruc-

tion who is breathing against a closed glottis or an occluded endotracheal tube.

59. **(C)** The Frank–Starling law of the heart is the underlying principle in the use of ventricular function curves. It relates preload and stroke volume. As more volume is presented, more output will occur, assuming that the heart is normal.

60. **(E)** Heat production in the body is decreased by anorexia. Shivering, hunger, and activity lead to an increase in temperature. Epinephrine increases temperature by leading to vasoconstriction, which conserves heat.

61. **(D)** As the size of the ventricle increases, the radius increases, and the wall tension increases. The law of LaPlace states that more tension is needed to generate the same pressure as the radius increases. This makes the heart more inefficient and requires more oxygen to pump blood.

62. **(A)** As the cardiac output increases, pulmonary artery pressure increases. Other factors also are involved in pulmonary artery pressure, eg, the radius of the vessels. Vasoconstriction and vasodilatation of the pulmonary vessels occur with changes of cardiac output to regulate pulmonary vascular resistance.

63. **(E)** The current recommendation (no pun intended) is to attempt defibrillation with an energy level of 200 joules in an adult. If that is unsuccessful, a second attempt is made with 200 to 300 joules; if that is unsuccessful, a third attempt with 360 joules is made. It is not always indicated, and it is not always successful.

64. **(E)** The MAC for methoxyflurane is 0.16 at 1 atm, making it the most potent of the inhalation anesthetics. In comparison, enflurane has a MAC value of 1.7.

65. **(B)** The A-beta fibers are large fibers that are involved with deep touch and temperature.

66. **(D)** The temperature setting mechanism is in the hypothalamus. This structure controls the set point for temperature.

67. **(E)** The total body water in the adult constitutes 60% of the body weight.

68. **(A)** Magnesium concentration is related to the irritability of nervous tissue. It has a high intracellular concentration. It is excreted in the urine even in the face of a low concentration in the blood. It is present in the bile and the gastric juice.

69. (E) Ringer's lactate solution contains sodium, potassium, chloride, and calcium. It does not contain bicarbonate ions.

70. (A) Hydrogen ion is secreted by the proximal and distal tubules. It is actively transported and exchanged for sodium. The ion movement is interrelated, the hydrogen ion coming from the carbonic acid breakdown into hydrogen and bicarbonate.

71. (B) The enterohepatic circulation is the mechanism whereby some substances are reabsorbed from the gut into the portal blood and then from the liver back into the gut. The mechanism is most important for bile salts. It is of importance in the use of drugs that undergo this mechanism. The mechanism can function whether or not the substance is conjugated.

72. (C) Meralgia paresthetica is a condition marked by paresthesia on the anterior and lateral surfaces of the thigh. This condition is of importance to an anesthesiologist because it may develop following herniorrhaphy. It may also follow positioning in the lithotomy position if the legs are pushed back over the body trapping the lateral femoral cutaneous nerve.

73. (E) Procaine is the only choice that is an ester. All of the other options are amide derivatives.

74. (E) Broca's area is an area in the nondominant hemisphere associated with speech. It is in the frontal area.

75. (C) The first-pass effect is the biotransformation of a drug as it passes through the intestinal mucosa and liver. In some cases, much of the effective concentration is lost at this point, leaving little of the drug to have its desired effect. Some drugs are poorly soluble and never diffuse through the mucosa to be picked up in the bloodstream. There are other sites where drugs are altered, but this effect is important for the drugs that are administered orally.

76. (A) Isoflurane is characterized by a stable cardiac rhythm that is maintained in the face of epinephrine injection in conservative doses. A tachycardia is noted that leads to a decrease in stroke volume. Cardiac output is maintained.

77. (B) The foramen of Monro connects the lateral ventricle to the 3rd ventricle. The 3rd and 4th ventricles are connected by the sylvian aqueduct. From the 4th ventricle, the fluid passes into the cisterna and from the cisterna into the subarachnoid space of the spinal cord through foramina of Magendie and Luschka.

78. (A) Alpha activity has a frequency range of 8 to 10 cycles per second. Beta activity has a frequency of 18 to 30 cycles per second. Theta rhythm has an activity of 4 to 7 cycles per second. Delta rhythm has an activity of 4 cycles per second.

79. (B) Ketamine administration is associated with changes in cardiovascular parameters similar to those seen with sympathetic stimulation. Therefore, the heart rate is increased, and there is an increase in cardiac output.

80. (D) Renal clearance of a drug in an individual with normal renal function may vary from patient to patient and from time to time, depending on the variables stated. The excretion is correlated with renal blood flow. Drug elimination is correlated with creatinine clearance, and one may use changes in creatinine clearance to gauge how doses must be altered.

81. (B) Halogenation decreases flammability and increases anesthetic potency. Cardiac irritation is not increased.

82. (C) Halothane is a halogenated hydrocarbon of the ethane series. The halogen substitutions are fluorine, chlorine, and bromine.

83. (A) Sevoflurane is a fluorinated ether. The blood gas coefficient is 0.6, and the vapor pressure is 160. The vapor is not irritating.

84. (D) The action of thiopental is terminated by its redistribution. The drug is bound to protein, and the binding may be interfered with by various concomitant drugs. It is taken up in fatty tissues, but that is not the mechanism of terminating the effect.

85. (C) Thiopental is contraindicated in patients with acute intermittent porphyria. The other porphyrias listed as options are not associated with drug induction. Two others are: variegate porphyria and hereditary copraporphyria. Thiopental also should be avoided in those.

86. (B) Thiopental is known to have an antianalgesic effect. If given in small doses for sedation to one who is experiencing severe pain, the pain will be aggravated. The drug is a poor choice for sedation in this type of patient.

87. (B) After the inadvertent injection of thiopental into the epidural space, the patient would become drowsy but would have no complaints of severe pain, nor would paralysis, arachnoiditis, or cauda equina syndrome follow. The fact that the patient becomes drowsy suggests that significant absorption occurs through the epidural vessels. This refer-

ence also points up the fact that we must always identify what we are injecting.

88. **(D)** Traditional signs of the anesthetic state are not seen with ketamine administration. Purposeless movements are seen, and these do not indicate the need for more anesthesia.

89. **(D)** The chest wall rigidity seen with Innovar injection is due to the fentanyl component. The rigidity can be seen with fentanyl alone, and although usually seen with large doses, it may be seen with small doses. The rigidity usually is seen in the muscles of the chest wall and may make ventilation difficult.

90. **(A)** Local anesthetics in the free base form are poorly soluble and are prepared as hydrochloride salts in water or saline. The acid solutions help the solutions that contain epinephrine, since basic solutions promote the breakdown of catecholamines.

91. **(C)** PEEP does increase FRC and V/Q ratio. It may not improve oxygenation, and it increases lung compliance.

92. **(A)** Increased dead space may result from hypotension, short, rapid ventilation, and pulmonary embolus. Increased airway pressure leads to increased dead space.

93. **(A)** Vital capacity includes tidal volume, inspiratory and expiratory reserve volumes, but not all of FRC. FRC includes residual volume.

94. **(C)** The patient with hypercapnia has increased catecholamines, respiratory acidosis, and increased plasma potassium. The potassium comes from the liver and other tissues.

95. **(E)** All of these factors my lead to pulmonary edema in the awake patient or the patient under anesthesia. It is important to know the reason for the pulmonary edema so that treatment is directed accordingly.

96. **(D)** In the lateral position, lung relationships change. The perfusion is now greater in the dependent lung.

97. **(A)** The trachea is a midline structure about 15 cm in length and about the diameter of a person's index finger. It bifurcates at the level of the 5th thoracic vertebra!

98. **(B)** Airway resistance is a dynamic measurement obtained by dividing pressure by flow. It is dependent on the caliber of the airway and on the pattern of flow.

99. **(A)** The composition of alveolar gas differs by the first three options. Nitrogen remains constant, since an equilibrium is established.

100. **(C)** Air flow through a tube is dependent on the radius and length of the tube, the radius being more important. Viscosity is more important than density.

101. **(E)** All of these factors are important in providing the proper amount of oxygen to the anesthetized patient. Since oxygen is so important and changes so subtle, monitoring the oxygenation of the anesthetized patient are becoming a standard of care

102. **(A)** The first three statements are true, but the fourth is false: a P_{O_2} of 30 gives a saturation of 60%

103. **(D)** Calcium administration increases myocardial contractility and increases excitability. The effect of calcium can be antagonized by calcium chelating agents, but the effect is too short for clinical use Calcium may predispose to digitalis toxicity.

104. **(B)** Increased body temperature and increased hydrogen ion concentration both shift the oxyhemoglobin dissociation curve to the right, thereby increasing the P_{50}. Methemoglobin is a hemoglobin molecule in which the iron is in the ferric state and is unable to combine with oxygen.

105. **(B)** Neurogenic pulmonary edema may follow head injury or other cause of increased intracranial pressure. It is resistant to treatment unless the pressure is reduced. It will lead to hypoxemia. It is known that it will not develop in a denervated lung.

106. **(A)** Left ventricular compliance is decreased in the patient with aortic stenosis or ischemia and the patient receiving inotropes. It is increased in the patient on vasodilators. The typical aortic stenosis patient has a normal sized cavity with a large myocardial mass. Small increases in fluid lead to a large increase in pressure.

107. **(D)** The RAS is a nonspecific area in the brainstem that is responsible for maintaining the conscious, alert state. It receives input from above and below

108. **(A)** Deliberate hypotension was carried out with sodium nitroprusside and halothane. No shunt was noted in these studies. Miller cites one article in which shunt was increased.

109. **(A)** Cromolyn has no place in the immediate preparation, since it does not relieve bronchospasm. It would be helpful in the long-term preparation.

110. **(C)** The tetralogy of Fallot includes a VSD, pulmonary outflow obstruction, overriding of the aorta, and right ventricular hypertrophy. An ASD or PDA is not part of the complex.

111. **(E)** The preoperative ECG can be used for detection of all the options. Chamber enlargement is seen readily in the tracing, as are some electrolyte disturbances, especially changes in calcium and potassium. Heart block and ischemic changes are seen.

112. **(E)** Cardiac output determination with the thermodilution technique uses a dilution calculation just as does the dye-dilution technique. A thermistor measures the change in temperature in the pulmonary artery. In the dye-dilution technique, changes in dye concentration are determined. Attention to detail is important, including the injection of an exact amount at a known temperature.

113. **(E)** The values are all correct.

114. **(A)** The elevation of intracranial pressure seen with succinylcholine is due to the transient increase in P_{CO_2} seen with fasciculation and to CNS propriceptors. If the patient is hyperventilated and give thiopental, the effect is not seen. This concept is important in intubating the patient who has increased intracranial pressure. If the patient has a full stomach, one may not want to wait the time necessary for a nondepolarizer to act. If thiopental is given, the patient is hyperventilated and then intubated, further damage should be mitigated. The fasciculation and tightness of neck muscles are not involved.

115. **(E)** Cardioplegia has improved the success rate of cardiac procedures, since it provides a relaxed heart. This factor leads to a decrease in oxygen consumption and coronary resistance. Oxygen consumption is about doubled with ventricular fibrillation.

116. **(E)** All the options are methods of detecting air embolism. Measurement of end-tidal oxygen is not a good method. In the presence of air embolism, end-tidal oxygen will rise. Doppler monitoring will detect small amounts of air. Mass spectrometry measures levels of nitrogen. End-tidal carbon dioxide, which decreases with air embolism, is sensitive but requires some decrease in pulmonary blood flow before a change is noted. The esophageal stethoscope is not sensitive.

117. **(C)** The vasomotor center, located in the reticular formation of the medulla and lower pons, receives input from the cortex and the hypothalamus. It secretes norepinephrine.

118. **(D)** The renin-angiotensin system includes renin, which is secreted by the kidney. Renin acts on plasma angiotensinogen to form angiotensin I, which is converted to angiotensin II by converting enzyme in the lung. The entire process is set into motion by decreased blood volume.

119. **(A)** There is a standard code for pacemakers:

1st letter:	The chamber paced
2nd letter:	The chamber sensed
3rd letter:	Mode of response
4th letter:	Programmable features
5th letter:	Dysrhythmia treatment

When treating a patient who has a pacemaker, it is important to know what kind of pacer is involved.

120. **(D)** Alcohol ingestion in large amounts will lead to liver disease in spite of good nutrition. Hematologic disorders are due to clotting deficiencies and to the alcohol itself. Gastrointestinal problems, including pancreatitis, are common.

121. **(D)** The presence of large V waves is due to some influence affecting left atrial filling. Large V waves may show evidence of mitral regurgitation. Aortic valve and tricuspid valve abnormalities should not be reflected in the measurements. It would be very difficult to insert a pulmonary artery catheter into a patient with tricuspid atresia.

122. **(E)** The Goldman study showed a correlation between all the factors listed and increased risks of anesthesia. There is not complete agreement among anesthesiologists concerning the implications of the Goldman study, but it has stimulated many studies on outcome.

123. **(E)** Ventricular dysfunction may be detected by the several methods outlined. Ejection fraction is a relatively better predictor of survival. If the ejection fraction is 40%, there is a worse prognosis. One of the problems is that there is no good, early method of evaluating ventricular dysfunction.

124. **(B)** Injection of medications at the time of cardiac arrest is usually problematic. If a deep line is in place, it should be used. If no line is in place, an antecubital line should be attempted first. This will allow drug administration and not interrupt resuscitation procedures. If no line is available, lidocaine, atropine, and epinephrine can be administered through the endotracheal tube.

125. **(E)** The pericardium is not necessary for life, as is evidenced in the many patients who function after open heart surgery without one. The function of the pericardium is to buffer the heart from sudden

movement, provide lubrication between the myocardium and adjacent structures, and minimize cardiac dilatation.

126. **(C)** The vitamin K-dependent factors are II, VII, IX, and X.

127. **(A)** Preload, contractility, and afterload are important for determination of stroke volume. Stroke volume and heart rate are the determinants of cardiac output.

128. **(E)** Sodium conservation is important to homeostasis. Sodium is reabsorbed throughout the tubule system so that only about 1% of the filtered sodium is excreted by the kidney.

129. **(A)** Hyperkalemia may be treated by the administration of glucose-insulin solutions, eliminating exogenous sources (one of the major causes), and correcting causes of endogenous sources. Treatment entails alkalinizing the blood, not acidifying it.

130. **(A)** Mechanisms of compensation for valvular disease include chamber enlargement and ventricular hypertrophy. These are efforts to increase the contractile force. In addition, there is increased sympathetic outflow. This increases vascular tone.

131. **(A)** The calculation requires mean arterial pressure, mean central venous pressure, and cardiac output. Pulmonary pressure is not needed.

132. **(E)** A decreased hematocrit in the patient with cirrhosis may reflect many factors: coagulation defect leading to bleeding, increased plasma volume leading to dilution of the red cells, megaloblastic anemia, and increased hemolysis. Many of these factors are interrelated.

133. **(A)** Decreased urinary output in the patient being ventilated with PEEP is due to decreased cardiac output, increased sympathetic output, and release of renin. Most believe that ADH is not involved, but there those who think that ADH secretion is important.

134. **(C)** Vasopressin causes a concentrated urine and antidiuresis. In addition, the urine has a high osmolality. Vasoconstriction also occurs.

135. **(E)** Inappropriate secretion of ADH is seen often after surgery. It includes hyponatremia and low serum osmolality. The kidneys excrete an excessive amount of sodium under the influence of ADH. The renal function is normal.

136. **(B)** The typical nerve cell has numerous dendrites that branch out and a dentritic zone that is a recep-

tor membrane. The nerve cell has only one axon The myelin sheath covers the axon only.

137. **(E)** All of the options are present in the reflex arc Many problems in patients under anesthesia are attributed to a reflex. It is very difficult to describe the pathways in these reflexes. One should try to determine the cause before assuming all problems are related to some ill-defined refex.

138. **(C)** Osmotic diuresis may follow ingestion of substances that are filtered by the kidney but not absorbed or if the substance is in an amount exceeding the capacity of the kidney to reabsorb it. Increased GFR is not involved.

139. **(E)** If it is necessary to use a volatile agent for a procedure, steps should be taken to decrease the effect as much as possible. Intravenous drugs, such as thiopental, should be administered when practical, and hyperventilation and as low a dose as possible should be used. The choice of an agent with the least effect on cerebral blood flow is also helpful

140. **(D)** After injection of a drug, there is a rapid mixing of the drug in the blood and vessel-rich group. In the distribution phase, the drug equilibrates with the lesser perfused tissues. High perfusion increases the rate of equilibration. Diffusion factors may affect the speed of equilibration.

141. **(E)** The loading dose of a drug is the dose given to achieve a faster blood concentration. This decreases the time needed to achieve a steady state. In some drugs, the larger dose can have detrimental effects, eg, a larger dose of relaxants may lead to a longer time of paralysis or cardiovascular effects.

142. **(A)** Endogenous catecholamines are epinephrine, norepinephrine, and dopamine. Dobutamine is a synthetic drug.

143. **(E)** Epinephrine is the most widely used catecholamine. It has many uses due to its effects on alpha and beta receptors. Arrhythmias have been noted. There are strong chronotropic effects that may limit its use as an inotrope.

144. **(B)** Amrinone is an orally effective inotrope that has little effect on heart rate. It causes some vasodilatation. Amrinone is a phosphodiesterase inhibitor that causes an increase in cyclic AMP.

145. **(D)** Antisialogogue effects are consistent, although of varying degree, among the anticholinergics. Amnestic effects and effects on gastric volume and pH are not consistent among this group of drugs.

146. **(E)** Systemic signs of local anesthetic toxicity involve all of the options. When a block is being administered, it is important to look for these signs.

147. **(E)** Vecuronium effects in the infant are complex. Although the ED_{50} is the same as in adults, infants have a greater sensitivity to the drug. The volume of distribution of vecuronium in the infant is larger, and the drug lasts longer.

148. **(E)** Halothane sensitization of the heart is increased with hypoxemia and hypercarbia. This effect is abolished by both alpa and beta blockers and by calcium channel blockers.

149. **(E)** The question is asked: How much epinephrine can I use? The options, taken together, give a good regimen to have in mind. Although this is not guaranteed to avoid problems, it gives a good guideline to follow. The dose that is allowable for use with isoflurane is even greater.

150. **(D)** Nitrous oxide increases blood pressure when it is given with halothane. Nitrous oxide increases pulmonary vascular resistance. When given with opioids, nitrous oxide causes decreases in cardiac output. When given with isoflurane, the blood pressure increases because of the increase in systemic vascular resistance.

151. **(A)** Digitalis toxicity is manifest as nausea and vomiting, visual disturbances, prolonged P-R interval, and arrhythmias, especially multifocal PVCs. A bradycardia is common.

152. **(B)** Esmolol is an ester that is broken down by an esterase that is distinct from the one that breaks down succinylcholine. Therefore, there should be no prolongation of the effect with the use of succinylcholine. Esmolol is of short duration. The drug can be used to blunt the effect of intubation.

153. **(D)** The patient has all the symptoms of the central anticholinergic syndrome that may follow the ingestion of jimson weed. The typical symptoms of "blind as a bat, red as a beet, hot as a hare, and mad as a hatter" are due to antimuscarinic effects of drugs that can pass the blood-brain barrier. Physostigmine also can pass the blood-brain barrier and will counteract its effects. Administration of this drug will treat all of the symptoms, and the CT scan, aspirin, and sponge baths will not be necessary.

154. **(E)** The patient who has been on steroids is at risk of having a reaction and should be covered. The patient may get by without any trouble at all, but the risk of giving the steroids is less than the risk of the stress reaction. Smaller doses suited to the procedure should be used.

155. **(E)** A patient with the symptoms indicated may be having an anaphylactic reaction. Your first reaction should be to stop the suspected offender. The treatment is to ensure oxygenation, to improve the relative volume status, and to improve the blood pressure. Antihistamines also may be administered.

156. **(A)** Mannitol is filtered at the glomerulus. It is an osmotic diuretic and will acutely increase the blood volume. It may be a hazard in congestive failure, since the blood volume may be increased, making the failure worse until the diuresis takes effect.

157. **(E)** Magnesium deficiency may occur as muscle spasm, arrhythmia, or CNS irritability. It should be suspected in the chronic alcoholic and in anyone who is nutritionally deprived.

158. **(B)** Cyanide toxicity must be avoided in the use of sodium nitroprusside. Captopril given before the nitroprusside is started has been shown to be effective in decreasing the amount needed to give the desired hypotension. Patients more at risk are those who are nutritionally deprived due to a deficiency of vitamin B_{12}. Miller cites the safe dose as under 0.5 mg/kg/hour.

159. **(E)** All of the drugs listed are antidysrhythmics or can be used for ventricular arrthythmias. Magnesium sulfate is not a drug that is used often, but in arrhythmias that are resistant to therapy, it may be life saving.

160. **(E)** Ionization of a drug is important in the drug's function, since charged particles do not cross membranes well. The ionization is a function of the pH and the pKa.

161. **(C)** The principal disadvantages of methohexital are pain on injection and involuntary muscle movements. Hiccoughs are frequent. The pH is high, and the solubility is not low.

162. **(A)** The vessel-rich group includes those organs that receive the bulk of circulation. It includes the heart, kidneys, and the central nervous system. Muscles are not included.

163. **(C)** Local anesthetics block conduction by blocking pores in the cell membrane. The local anesthetics do not deplorarize the membrane. The drugs exist as salts.

164. **(E)** The toxicity of the local anesthetic drugs can be altered by adjusting the options cited. Limiting

the dose, injecting over a longer period of time, and avoiding sites of high vascularity when possible will lessen the risk of toxicity.

165. **(B)** Myoglobinemia may occur after a single dose of succinylcholine and is more common in children. It is not necessarily harmless, since there may be renal failure to the deposition of the myoglobin in the kidneys. Myoglobin is released from skeletal muscle, not smooth muscle.

166. **(A)** Succinylcholine effect may be prolonged in the patient on echothiophate eyedrops and in those exposed to organophosphate insecticides. The patient with liver disease may have low cholinesterase levels. A patient who has a heterozygous atypical pseudocholinesterase should have no problem with succinylcholine.

167. **(A)** In a study reported by Hill, the lithium potentiated the block by pancuronium and succinylcholine but not the block of gallamine or D-tubocurarine. The reason for the difference is difficult to explain.

168. **(A)** The hemodynamic response to a relaxant will be altered by depth of anesthesia. A patient deeply anesthetized may have a more pronounced vasodilatation and more sympathetic blockade. Surgical stimulation may lead to more sympathetic stimulation. Blood volume changes may make the effect of the relaxants a more pronounced (in hypovolemia) or less pronounced (hypervolemia). The sex of the patient should have no effect.

169. **(C)** The increase in intragastric pressure is well documented. Regurgitation may occur if the pressure exceeds 25 cm H_2O. Any condition that relaxes the esophageal sphincter, eg, hiatal hernia, will predispose to regurgitation. Atropine will not block the pressure rise, but pretreatment with curare will.

170. **(C)** The development of dual block follows a stage of tachyphylaxis. It is both time and dose dependent. It may occur with doses as low as 2 to 4 mg/kg. It is difficult to detect clinically.

171. **(B)** Histamine release is followed by bronchospasm in some cases and by upper chest erythema. Hypotension is usually seen along with a tachycardia.

172. **(A)** The drugs, neostigmine, pyridostigmine, and physostigmine, form a chemical complex at the esteratic site of the acetylcholinesterase molecule. In contrast, edrophonium forms an electrostatic bond at the anionic site and has hydrogen bonding at the esteratic site.

173. **(E)** Succinylcholine is relatively contraindicated in all of these cases, but factors that must be taken into consideration are the extent of burn, time of the burn, and the amount of muscle wasting. In most cases, another method is available to provide relaxation, and my policy is that if I have to consider the problems, I use another drug.

174. **(C)** The peak effect of neostigmine is at 10 to 15 minutes. Adequate reversal is more important in the patient with renal disease, since complete excretion of the drug may not have taken place. The peak effect of atropine is about 5 minutes, whereas its onset is faster. This matches the onset time of edrophonium. The best indicator of full recovery is not the assessment of a single twitch height but the lack of fade with the train-of-four.

175. **(A)** Pyridostigmine has a longer duration of action and a greater dependence on the kidneys for excretion. The onset of action is slower. In general, there is little advantage in the use of pyridostigmine.

PART II

176. **(C)** Penicillin does not have neuromuscular blocking properties. The aminoglycoside-type antibiotics are associated with decreased muscle function or potentiation of muscle relaxants in a dose-related fashion. This is probably due to a prejunctional inhibition of acetylcholine release.

177. **(D)** Metocurine is related structurally to D-tubocurarine but causes less histamine release. It also has a less pronounced effect on the autonomic nervous system, with less ganglionic blockade and blood pressure depression.

178. **(C)** Churchill-Davidson makes the point that we should choose a relaxant that is consistent with our needs in regard to hemodynamics and relaxation. D-tubocurarine is associated with decreased pressure due to histamine release, and succinylcholine may cause heart rate drops that may affect pressure. Atracurium also may be associated with histamine release.

179. **(D)** Botulinus toxin leads to muscular weakness by preventing the release of acetylcholine at the nerve endings. The release of acetylcholine is necessary for muscle function. Calcium and cyclic AMP also are involved in the release of acetylcholine at the nerve ending.

180. **(D)** Vecuronium has little cumulative effect. It is a nondepolarizing relaxant with an activity of about

30 minutes. It is not difficult to reverse. Vecuronium is eliminated chiefly in the bile.

181. **(D)** Administration of anticholinesterase drugs will reverse the block of a nondepolarizing agent only if the drug is in low enough concentration. It may prolong the block produced by depolarizers. If there is free succinylcholine in circulation, administration of an anticholinesterase will prolong the block.

182. **(B)** The minimum alveolar concentration for isoflurane is 1.15.

183. **(E)** Myoglobin is more commonly found in the serum of children than adults after the administration of succinylcholine. The reason is not definitely known. It is found in skeletal muscle, and its appearance in the serum is due to loss of integrity of the muscle cell.

184. **(C)** The gasserian ganglion is associated with the fifth (trigeminal) cranial nerve.

185. **(D)** Propofol is an intravenous agent with a fast onset and short time to awakening. It is essentially insoluble in water. There is very little analgesic effect. When compared to thiopental, the sleep time is shorter.

186. **(E)** Atropine is part of the regimen to reverse a neuromuscular blockade but in itself has no ability to reverse a block. Edrophonium, neostigmine, and pyridostigmine are all cholinesterase inhibitors. 4-Aminopyridine does not inhibit cholinesterase but has its effect by facilitating calcium entry into the nerve ending.

187. **(C)** A depolarization block does not have any post-tetanic facilitation. The block is characterized by fasciculation and is antagonized by nondepolarizers and potentiated by anticholinesterase compounds. There is no fade initially, but fade may appear with the onset of a phase II block.

188. **(C)** The Bernoulli theorem states that the velocity of flow and lateral pressure are related. If a liquid is flowing through a pipe, the lateral wall pressure decreases if the flow velocity increases.

189. **(E)** The term MAC refers to minimal alveolar concentration. It is measured as an anesthetic concentration sufficient to prevent movement in response to a painful stimulus in 50% of the subjects. It is affected by age. The dose of thiopental is not measured in this way, since it is not an inhalation agent.

190. **(E)** The train-of-four ratio for a depolarizing block is 100%, since there is no fade. The fourth twitch will be as high as the first.

191. **(D)** The patient with myasthenia gravis has an altered sensitivity to relaxants. These patients are more sensitive to nondepolarizing agents. This sensitivity is present with or without control of the disease.

192. **(A)** The maximum acceptable leakage current is 10 microamperes. This is a small current, but it does not take a great amount of current to cause ventricular fibrillation in a patient with lines directly into the heart. There was little discussion of leakage current until it became technically possible to place lines into the heart and pacemakers became commonplace.

193. **(E)** Propranolol should not be terminated suddenly, since a withdrawal syndrome has been reported with sudden termination. In general, most antihypertensive agents should be continued, and the induction planned around them. This makes heart rate and blood pressure easier to control.

194. **(C)** The vapor pressure is subject to change with increases in temperature, since more molecules will leave the liquid. If the container is opened, the space above the liquid will be expanded, and it will take longer for equilibrium to be reached. If the container is compressed, more molecules will be in the liquid phase (as in a soda bottle).

195. **(C)** Methoxamine is the drug with pure alpha effects. Epinephrine, norepinephrine, and ephedrine have mixed effects. Isoproterenol has all beta effects.

196. **(A)** Lidocaine is eliminated chiefly by the liver. It is not effective orally. The toxic level is at 5 μg/ml The symptoms of toxicity are usually CNS stimulation. Lidocaine is useful in ventricular arrhythmias.

197. **(A)** Postspinal headaches are less frequent with small-bore needles and with the 22-gauge Whittaker needle. The typical headache must be posturally dependent, being relieved by the supine position and aggravated by standing. It is relieved immediately by an epidural blood patch.

198. **(D)** The calcium channel blockers have an effect by interfering with the flow of calcium through membranes. All are highly bound to protein. The peak effect is about 20 minutes. Some are good for treatment of arrhythmias; others are poor.

199. **(D)** Carbon dioxide is a function of body metabolism and, therefore, will remain essentially constant. Water vapor is essentially dependent on body temperature, and, therefore, it also will remain constant. Levels of both of these gases may be altered by the hyperventilation that usually accompanies the ascent to altitude.

200. **(C)** Pentazocine is a mixed narcotic agonist–antagonist that is useful both orally and parenterally. Although originally thought to have no addiction potential, it has been found to cause dependence in some people.

201. **(D)** Drugs that release histamine, eg., meperidine and morphine, should be avoided. Local anesthetics, halothane, vecuronium, and aspirin should not cause problems.

202. **(D)** Use of furosemide leads to alkalosis. Renin release follows decreased volume. Hypokalemia is one of the most common problems in the patient on diuretics. Hyperglycemia is not as common as with thiazides. Ototoxicity usually is seen with chronic treatment in high doses. It is probably related to changes in the endolymph.

203. **(E)** The most common cause of anesthetic disasters is hypoxemia. Hypoxemia is the end point of other problems, eg., esophageal intubation, low blood pressure, and machine problems. For this reason, it is important to monitor carefully and do machine checks carefully.

204. **(B)** Nifedipine is a drug effective for coronary vasospasm. It has no antiarrhythmia effect. It is a vasodilator. The half-life is about 4 hours.

205. **(B)** The combination of protamine and heparin results in a compound with no anticoagulation effect. There is no other mechanism involved.

206. **(E)** Echothiophate treatment leads to a prolongation of succinylcholine effect by altering the metabolism. This occurs because echothiophate is a cholinesterase inhibitor with a prolonged effect. Since pseudocholinesterase is needed for the breakdown of succinylcholine, problems may arise in patients who are taking these eyedrops.

207. **(A)** Postoperative nerve deficits following anesthesia are rare. Epinephrine is not a known cause. There are many causes, including positioning as well as preoperative neurologic disease.

208. **(E)** The interaction of phenytoin and phenobarbital is one of altered metabolism due to enzyme induc-

tion. If a patient has a stable drug level, this can be changed by starting another drug that may induce the enzyme system that metabolizes the drug.

209. **(C)** The combination of nitrous oxide in 0.5 MAC concentration and isoflurane in 0.5 MAC concentration will lead to an anesthetic combination of 1 MAC potency. For all practical purposes, nitrous oxide and a halogenated agent are the only agents that are administered together, but if two halogenated agents could be used together, their effect would be additive.

210. **(C)** Isoflurane is an ether compound with 3 fluorine substitutions on the 1st carbon atom.

211. **(A)** The nitrous oxide tank contains a liquid, and in order for it to become vaporized, heat must be supplied. As the cylinder is opened, heat is removed from the cylinder and from the air in the immediate vicinity. The temperature falls, causing condensation.

212. **(E)** Diazepam is a benzodiazepine derivative.

213. **(C)** Naloxone is a pure narcotic antagonist, meaning that the drug has no narcotic effect of its own. Butorphanol and levallorphan are both mixed agonist–antagonists. Neostigmine and edrophonium are cholinesterase inhibitors.

214. **(B)** Bleomycin is associated with pulmonary toxicity. This is manifest as pulmonary fibrosis, sometimes long after the drug has been stopped. Doxorubicin has cardiac toxicity. Vincristine is associated with myelosuppression. Methotrexate toxicity is manifest as immunosuppression. L-Asparaginase is associated with hepatic toxicity.

215. **(B)** The number of calories required to raise the temperature of 1 g of a substance by 1° C is its specific heat. The specific heat varies for different substances.

216. **(E)** The endplate become depleted with tetanic stimulation. The apparatus is not at fault, nor is the ability to transmit electrical impulses. Potassium and DNA are not involved.

217. **(C)** The transverse process of the sixth cervical vertebra is referred as Chassaignac's tubercle.

218. **(D)** The partial rebreathing mask provides an increased F_{IO_2} and conserves oxygen. The oxygen flow can be decreased. Oxygen tension in the blood should be increased. There is no effect on carbon dioxide.

219. **(A)** The needle for the caudal block enters through the sacral hiatus. Anomalies in the sacral region are frequent. The patient should be prone, with the hips on a pillow and the toes pointed in. Even though the caudal canal is of low volume, there is leakage through the foramina requiring injection of a larger volume.

220. **(B)**

221. **(D)** The dose of lidocaine in a child should not exceed a total dose of 7 mg/kg. This dose, as all doses, depends on the route and the speed of administration. If a dose of lidocaine is given intravenously, 7 mg/kg will be excessive. For infiltration of a laceration, the dose would be appropriate.

222. **(E)** This is an important point, since we have all heard operating room personnel say things that they would not want the patient to hear. Since hearing is the last sense to be lost, the patient may be aware of the operating room sounds longer than we think.

223. **(B)** A patient with a moderate disease that is not incapacitating would be ASA physical status II.

224. **(C)** Since nitrous oxide is a relatively insoluble agent, the uptake will decrease over time as equilibrium is reached. The uptake is dependent on concentration, being greater with a higher concentration.

225. **(C)** The usual blood loss for a normal vaginal delivery is 400 to 600 ml.

226. **(B)** Corneal abrasions are very painful and should be adequately treated. The use of topical anesthesia is not recommended by all authors because of its tendency to retard regeneration of the corneal epithelium. In addition, if a topical anesthetic is placed in the eye and the patient rubs the eye emerging from anesthesia, further damage may be incurred. In some publications, the use of local anesthetic is still recommended.

227. **(E)** Bronchial tear should not occur, since the bronchi are more distal. The other options are possible, and the patient should be warned that they may occur, especially hoarseness.

228. **(D)** Less local anesthetic is needed in the later stages of pregnancy, since the epidural space is decreased in size. This is due to the venous congestion caused by the weight of the uterus. In addition, there are studies showing that the nerves are more sensitive to the local anesthetics. This is thought to be a hormonal effect.

229. **(E)** The patient with a bronchopleural fistula requires a method of ventilation that does not increase the flow across the fistula. Spontaneous ventilation with a mask is seldom sufficient, and methods employing positive pressure may not be able to accomplish ventilation because of loss of inspired air through the fistula. In these patients, the use of high-frequency ventilation may be life saving.

230. **(C)** Sulfhemoglobin cannot be converted to hemoglobin by methylene blue or any known medication. Sulfhemoglobin is not an effective oxygen carrier. Cyanosis may be present if sulfhemoglobin is at levels as low as 0.5 g/dl.

231. **(E)** The normal blood volume in an infant is 80 ml/ kg. A premature infant has a higher volume per unit of weight.

232. **(C)** Treatment of aspiration includes intubation, suctioning, high F_{IO_2} (if needed), and artificial ventilation if needed. Pulmonary lavage is not useful unless there is particulate matter. Most studies have found that lavage is not useful and is potentially harmful.

233. **(A)** Sinusitis is more common with nasotracheal intubation due to blockage of the sinus drainage. This must be considered in the febrile patient who has a nasotracheal tube in place. Sore throat, vocal cord injury, subglottic stenosis, and arytenoid damage are of equal incidence with orotracheal intubation.

234. **(B)** The signs of causalgia are hyperesthesia, extremities that may be cold or warm, pain that is long-lasting, and trophic changes. These may include brittle nails and osteoporosis.

235. **(A)** In spite of the fact that patients may exhibit edema and weight gain, they are hypovolemic due to the vasoconstriction that is part of the disease. They have hypertension, hyponatremia, increased hematocrit (due to the vasoconstriction and hypovolemia), and hypokalemia.

236. **(B)** Urinary output for a child should be 1 ml/kg/ hour. This should be monitored if appropriate for the procedure.

237. **(E)** Internal jugular cannulation is done with landmarks that are definite. There are risks with the procedure, including pneumothorax and bleeding. These should be in low incidence with experienced operators. The vessels are more superficial in the obese, and the vessels should be easy to cannulate if the landmarks are followed. The right side gives a straight course to the superior vena cava.

238. (E) In any patient with hoarseness and a documented supraglottic mass, it is mandatory to establish the airway before proceeding with the anesthesia. Any other approach is likely to make the airway maintenance difficult if not impossible.

239. (C) The baby would get 1 point for heart rate, 1 for a weak cry, 2 for muscle tone, 1 for reflexes, and no points for color.

240. (E) Channeling of the airflow shortens the life of soda lime by allowing passage of the exhaled gas along channels of low resistance. This expends the soda lime along the channels, and carbon dioxide will flow through the system without being absorbed. The method of filling does not affect the length of soda lime usefulness. The relief valve position does have an effect. The valve should be placed to vent the air that has the highest concentration of carbon dioxide. The higher the gas flow, the longer the soda lime will last.

241. (D) In any anesthesia system, the one factor that must be provided for is oxygen. All other considerations are secondary.

242. (D) The typical postspinal puncture headache is worse in the upright position and relieved by the recumbent position. It is more prevalent in the obstetric female. A smaller needle makes a smaller dural hole, and there is a lower incidence of headache. Dehydration aggravates the headache.

243. (D) The muscle power is provided by both the uterus and the abdominal muscles. The uterine muscle is the more important. The perineal muscle does not have any effect in pushing the child through the birth canal. Relaxation of the perineum will help in the birth.

244. (B) The most troublesome problem with free-standing vaporizers is the danger of tipping, which can lead to very high concentrations of the agent. Use of the wrong agent, foaming, leaking, and overfilling are problems seen with all vaporizers and are not specific for the free-standing vaporizers.

245. (A) The metabolism of brown fat is a heat-producing mechanism. All of the other options are common methods of losing heat in an operating room. The temperature must be monitored, and methods must be initiated to prevent heat loss.

246. (B) Tachycardia is an early sign of malignant hyperthermia. If one waits for the development of fever, hot skin, and hot absorber, the syndrome has already developed quite far.

247. (D) An increase in cough after mobilizing the secretions is one of the aims of aerosol therapy. This leads to improved bronchial hygiene. The aerosol also may be used to deliver medication.

248. (C) The normal I:E time is 1:2. The longer expiratory time allows the airways to clear the inhaled gases. The patient with obstructive lung disease has prolonged expiratory times. We must be concerned with the ratio, since efficient ventilation requires that the times be adjusted to the individual patient.

249. (C) The vapor pressure of a liquid is most dependent on the temperature. It is independent of the atmospheric pressure. The heat conductivity of the container may affect the temperature, but it does not directly affect the vapor pressure. The specific heat of the container and the partial pressure of the gas are not determinants.

250. (D) The Bain circuit is a modification of the Mapleson D system. This system has a fresh gas inlet at the patient end, a piece of corrugated tubing that connects the inflow to the relief valve. The relief valve is adjacent to the reservoir bag.

251. (C) There is no consensus in answering this question. Succinylcholine alone is not good. An awake intubation is not good. If starting an intravenous line will cause such anxiety in a child that the intraocular pressure increases due to his thrashing around, that is unacceptable. In a given situation, I have used a gas induction with cricoid pressure successfully. The intravenous line was started after the child was asleep, and then vecuronium was given. Cricoid pressure was maintained until the airway was secure. I have also started an intravenous line with no difficulty with the child and then used vecuronium. If one chooses to use succinylcholine, the fasciculations must be blocked. It is important to explain the problem to the parents before the procedure. Let them know that there is a serious problem.

252. (C) If a vaporizer tips over, liquid agent may find its way into the tubing. This will cause an increased concentration of anesthetic agent in the system. If tipping occurs, it is not necessary to return the vaporizer to the factory, but it must be righted and allowed to air out. It should not be put into immediate use.

253. (C) The Vapor 19.1 vaporizer accomplishes temperature compensation by virtue of an expansion element that extends into the vaporizing chamber. Older vaporizers used the bimetallic band. No heating elements are involved.

254. **(C)** Perforation is a possibility with transurethral resection. An electrolyte disturbance is possible, and the patient may have had a pulmonary embolus, but the most likely problem with the situation cited is a perforation.

255. **(E)** The pumping effect refers to the increase in anesthetic concentration from a vaporizer during assisted or controlled ventilation. This effect is more pronounced at low flow rates.

256. **(D)** The statistical term for the spread of individual values is the standard deviation. The mean is the average of the data, and the standard error of the mean is a precision factor. Variance is the difference of each value from the mean.

257. **(C)** In the dosage needed for premedication, atropine should not cause problems in the patient with glaucoma. The theoretical problem is in the patient with closed-angle glaucoma. Atropine can cause mydriasis. Atropine does lower intraocular pressure due to its smooth muscle relaxation, but it is not significant. If given in large doses and there is a problem precipitated, the pressure will increase.

258. **(C)** Phantom limb pain is an example of central pain. Another example is postherpetic neuralgia. The other options are examples of somatic pain. Central pain is usually amenable to the same treatment as somatic pain.

259. **(B)** When trying to diagnose the cause of renal failure, one should obtain a urine specimen before treatment is begun. The urine will be concentrated in the patient with prerenal failure and will have a higher specific gravity. The urine need not be blood tinged. Oliguria is present.

260. **(E)** Stridor occurring 14 hours after thyroidectomy and accompanied with signs of tetany is most likely due to hypocalcemia. This patient has an airway problem, and that should be given priority in management. All of the options may be correct. The patient should be observed and intubated if necessary to protect the airway.

261. **(E)** There are many estimates of time to development of adrenal suppression, but the definite time is not known. For this reason, many will cover anyone who has been on steroids within the previous 6 months.

262. **(C)** The most important goal is to prevent hypoglycemia. One can monitor glucose levels and try to keep them in a normal range, but this should not be done at the risk of hypoglycemia. Many regimens are proposed to handle the sugar and insulin, but

the one thing that is necessary is to avoid hypoglycemia.

263. **(B)** Clamping of the thoracic aorta leads to an immediate increase in blood pressure. Assuming the heart can withstand the markedly increased afterload, there should not be standstill or hypotension. Blood pressure readings are lost in the left arm, but the pulse in the right arm should be present, depending on the placement of the clamp relative to the take-off of the vessels to the arms.

264. **(D)** A complication of aortic surgery is spinal cord ischemia due to the compromise of the radicular arteries. These arteries are not constant, and the large artery to the spine, the artery of Adamkiewitz, may be compromised, leading to ischemia. Pressure on the cord can lead to ischemia. Hypothermia may be protective. Loss of cerebrospinal fluid is not a factor. Long periods of hypotension may lead to ischemia.

265. **(B)** Urinary volume will increase with mannitol administration. The patient may become hypervolemic at first but may become hypovolemic after diuresis. The venous pressure and arterial pressure may fall.

266. **(B)** Methylmethacrylate is an acrylic cement. It does generate heat when setting. It is mixed at the time of usage. Placement may lead to hypotension. It is a glue used for many types of fractures.

267. **(D)** Fat emobli may be seen with fractures. The emboli are associated with petechiae, hypoxemia, and confusion. Cyanosis may be apparent. There is usually a tachycardia.

268. **(C)** Mannitol may lead to vein disruption, leading to hematoma. This may be more of a problem in the elderly. Mannitol may also lead to cerebral edema but that does not lead to hematoma. This drug may leak through vein walls and may cause hypervolemia, but these factors do not contribute to the development of hematomas.

269. **(A)** The Glasgow Coma Score is based on the ability to open the eyes, the verbal response, and the motor response. Responses to knee jerk, pupil size, respiration, and EEG are assessed in a general neurologic workup but are not part of the Glasgow Coma Score.

270. **(B)** The major buffer against increases in intracranial pressure is the cerebrospinal fluid. The dural sinuses that contain blood also are a buffer. The other options are tissue, which do not act as buffers.

271. **(D)** The most profound stimulus to cerebral auto-regulation is carbon dioxide. Changes in electrolytes and acid-base balance may have an effect, but the predominant effect is from CO_2.

272. **(B)** Patients with the Eaton–Lambert syndrome have a sensitivity to both depolarizing and nondepolarizing relaxants. The block is not readily reversed. Resection of the tumor does effect a cure.

273. **(A)** The effects of neostigmine include bradycardia, sweating, and skeletal muscle stimulation. The bladder is stimulated to contract.

274. **(E)** Tetanus is a rare disease, but we may be consulted for the treatment. The muscle spasm may be treated by diazepam, and relaxation may be needed for artificial ventilation. Labetalol may be employed to control the sympathetic overactivity. If pancuronium is used, it may lead to hypertension and increased heart rate; therefore, some recommend that it not be used.

275. **(C)** The alveolar concentration of a gas is independent of lung volume. The type of soda lime is not important. Both alveolar ventilation and uptake by the blood will affect the concentration.

276. **(A)** Uptake of an agent is dependent on the passage across the alveolar membrane. The Ostwald coefficient is an expression of the solubility of an agent that has an effect of the uptake. Cardiac output also is important. The type of system does not affect the uptake.

277. **(B)** When nitrous oxide is added to halothane, there is a sympathetic stimulating effect seen. This may antagonize halothane to some degree. The effect is seen early in the anesthesia and at light levels. The sympathetic stimulation causes vasoconstriction.

278. **(B)** The circulatory effect of halothane is due to multiple factors. The classic article by Price showed, in dogs, little effect at 0.5% and about the same at 1% and 2%. The effects are due to action on the heart, the ganglia, and peripheral resistance.

279. **(B)** The cuff on the endotracheal tube acts as an air-containing pocket acts anywhere else in the body. It will be distended with nitrous oxide just as air in the bowel. If the cuff is filled with nitrous oxide, there will be no gradient and no inflow of nitrous oxide.

280. **(C)** Propranolol causes hypoglycemia, as does insulin. Isoflurane has little effect on blood sugar, and the stress of surgery should cause an increase.

281. **(D)** Propanidid is a nonbarbiturate induction agent. It is an intravenous agent that is short-acting and has no hepatotoxic effect.

282. **(B)** Any direct entry into the heart is a pathway for microshock. Mechanical beds should have no electrical hazard. Isolation transformers serve to protect the patient from underground equipment.

283. **(A)** The flow rate through a tube of a smoothly flowing liquid is proportional to the pressure gradient and the fourth power of the radius. There is an inverse relationship to viscosity. The temperature of the tube is not involved.

284. **(B)** A transducer converts a nonelectric parameter into an electrical signal that can be recorded. Temperature is such a parameter. Electrocardiograms and electroencephalograms measure electrical signals and, therefore, do not need transducers.

285. **(B)** Turbulent flow is characterized by irregular lines of flow. It is mainly noted at branches, obstructions, and roughness of the tubes. Parallel lines of flow are seen with laminar flow.

286. **(B)** Pulse oximeters are based on technology that follows Beer's law, which relates the concentration of a solute to the intensity of light transmitted through the solution. The oximeter will read both carboxyhemoglobin and methemoglobin. In the currently used pulse oximeters, a pulsatile wave form is needed, since they analyze the pulsatile component of absorbance.

287. **(D)** The viscosity of a fluid is an intrinsic property that affects it laminar flow characteristics. It is not dependent on density and does not affect its specific gravity. It does affect resistance to flow.

288. **(C)** The femoral nerve lies lateral to the femoral artery and lateral to the lacunar ligament. The femoral vein lies medial to the artery.

289. **(A)** The needle does not pass through the pia meter, the covering immediately investing the spinal cord. It does pass through the supraspinal ligament, the interspinal ligament (unless the lateral approach is used), and the ligamentum flavum.

290. **(B)** A sciatic–femoral block may be used for procedures below the knee that do not require the use of a tourniquet. The obturator nerve and the inguinal nerve need not be blocked.

291. **(C)** The ulnar nerve and ulnar artery lie medially on the anterior aspect of the wrist. The median

nerve lies in the central part of the wrist, and the radial nerve lies laterally.

292. (A) A spinal anesthetic will vary with the duration of the agent, the presence of increased abdominal pressure, and the height of the patient. The sex of the patient has no effect.

293. (C) Hypotension is more profound with spinal anesthesia. Peripheral resistance decreases to a greater degree with epidural anesthesia. Since more drug is used for epidural anesthesia, more systemic effects are to be expected. The systemic effects of epinephrine are more likely.

294. (B) There would be no disturbance of heart rate unless hypoxemia occurred. The diaphragmatic innervation is by the phrenic nerve, which arises from cervical segments 3-5. This patient would have severe ventilatory problems.

295. (E) Proper placement of the endotracheal tube is necessary to avoid ventilatory problems. The advent of the end-tidal carbon dioxide monitor has been a great advance. With this monitor, one can show that the tube placement is correct. Before, we had several presumptive methods. Carbon dioxide demonstration is definitive.

296. (C) The use of a low-pressure cuff will decrease trauma to the trachea. Other techniques, eg., using a high-pressure cuff with a leak, frequent suctioning, and hourly deflation, are not helpful. Frequent suctioning may cause more damage to the trachea.

297. (D) Chylothorax should not occur with right internal jugular cannulation. Air embolism may occur if air is allowed to enter the catheter. Hematoma is a possibility. Arrhythmias may occur if the catheter enters the heart and stimulates the sensitive areas of the right ventricle.

298. (E) Administration of humidified gases is of benefit to some patients. The risks are that the humidifier may become contaminated, that the body will have to expend heat to warm the humidified gases, that the patient will receive a water load, and that the airway resistance will increase. These are not insurmountable problems: the mist can be heated to avoid patient heat loss, the fluid load can be compensated for by decreasing other fluids, and contamination can be avoided with good technique.

299. (A) Patients with acromegaly present problems for the anesthesiologist in addition to their large structures. The upper airway is different in that they have thickening of the vocal cords, often laryngeal stenosis, and macroglossia. The chin is prognathic. Intubation may be difficult.

300. (B) Hypothermia will aggravate the problem of hypocalcemia by decreasing the rate of metabolic clearance of exogenous citrate. This is another good reason to warm blood when it is given rapidly.

301. (E) Nasotracheal intubation has the usual possibility of broken teeth and, in addition, the problems of sinusitis, nosebleed, and nasal necrosis.

302. (D) Ephedrine increases the blood pressure without decreasing uterine blood flow. Drugs with pure alpha action will increase uterine resistance and decrease uterine blood flow.

303. (D) Gastric changes seen with pregnancy include incompetence of the gastroesophageal sphincter, increased acid secretion, increased gastric emptying time, and the upward displacement of the pylorus. These make the pregnant patient more susceptible to aspiration.

304. (A) Maternal changes seen with preeclampsia include increased cardiac output, decreased renal blood flow, and decreased cerebral blood flow. The last two are reasons for some of the complications. Hepatic flow is decreased in the preeclamptic patient.

305. (A) Anesthesia for an emergency cesarean section requires fast onset. Therefore, a spinal epidural block is not appropriate. Since time is of the essence in these situations, a room with all equipment is left ready at all times.

306. (C) Halothane, although a good anesthetic agent in general, provides little analgesia and leads to depression of the uterus. This may be a positive characteristic in some procedures, but in most obstetric procedures, it is unwanted. The drug has been associated with liver problems, but that is not the reason for avoiding it in the obstetric patient. Halothane solubility is not a reason to avoid it.

307. (C) Treatment of a postspinal headache includes reassurance and analgesics. In addition, the patient should have fluids and, if necessary, an epidural not subarachnoid blood patch.

308. (C) Pulmonary vascular resistance decreases with lung expansion and improved oxygenation. A decrease in pH will increase pulmonary vascular resistance. The closure of the ductus does not affect vascular resistance.

309. (E) Infants differ from adults in drug handling in absorption. The infant stomach has a higher pH, leading to increased absorption of some drugs. The total body water is greater in the infant, making

distribution different. The albumin levels are lower, leading to more unbound drug. The immaturity of the liver leads to decreased metabolism of some drugs.

310. (A) The work of breathing involves overcoming both elastic and resistive forces. As the child breathes very fast the work is increased, since turbulent flow is more prevalent. The optimal rate is 35 breaths per minure.

311. (D) Racemic epinephrine is a mild bronchodilator. This drug is a 50/50 mixture of the levo- and dextro- isomers of epinephrine. Compared with epinephrine, the drug has little alpha and beta effects. It is a good mucosal decongestant.

312. (A) Aerosol therapy can cause obstruction of the lower airway due to swelling of the retained secretions that are present. The secretions swell, since they take up the water that is used in the aerosol. Any aerosol can lead to fluid overload if the fluid delivered is not considered in the overall fluid plan. Contamination of respiratory therapy equipment is a constant threat. Aerosols may lead to bronchospasm due to irritation of the airways.

313. (A) The postoperative period is marked by a decreased lung capacity, a decrease in the FRC, and decreased residual volume. Respiratory therapy maneuvers in the postoperative period are aimed at increasing these volumes. The compliance is decreased.

314. (B) The Cole tube is a tube with a small diameter at the distal end but a larger proximal end. The supposed advantage is that the tube cannot be place in an endobronchial position. The resistance is lower, since the diameter is larger for part of the tube. There is no guarantee that endobronchial intubation will not occur. The tube should be advanced to a distance judged to be correct for the patient, not to the maximum distance.

315. (D) The Macintosh blade is manufactured in various sizes. It has a flat tip, a curved spatula, and a flange.

316. (A) Any instrumentation of the nose should be done after a history to ascertain the absence of a condition likely to precipitate problems. Nasal polyps that may bleed or be sheared off, a low platelet count, and sepsis of the nasal areas and contraindications to the use of a nasopharyngeal airways. A wired jaw, in itself, is not a contraindication to a nasopharyngeal airway.

317. (D) The oxygen analyzer should be placed on the fresh gas side of the system. It is not a good discon-nect alarm, since the time lag is too great. Analyzers may be affected by humidity and become nonfunctional.

318. ((B) The reaction of carbon dioxide and soda lime yields calcium carbonate, sodium carbonate, and water. No hydrochloric acid is formed.

319. (C) Soda lime granules are in the size of 4 to 8 mesh. Smaller granules give a larger absorptive surface for the number of granules but cause more resistance. The irregular shape is better to give more absorptive area.

320. (E) The reservoir bag on the machine has the function, besides being a reservoir, of a monitor, a ventilation assist device, and a pressure buffer. The reservoir of gases must be present to accommodate the needs of the inspiratory flow rate.

321. (A) Most CT scans can be done without anesthesia. There are situations in which the patient cannot or will not hold still to get a good study. In those situations, anesthesia is helpful. In our hospital, even the very young are done with sedation. Little general anesthesia is employed. Fever is not an indication for general anesthesia.

322. (A) The doctrine of *res ipsa loquitur* (the thing speaks for itself) is invoked if the accident usually does not happen without negligence, the plaintiff was not a factor, and the defendant usually has control of whatever caused the accident. Settling out of court is not a factor.

323. (C) If it is discovered that a tooth is missing, immediate steps should be taken to ascertain the location. First, make sure that it was there when the case started. Examine the oropharynx and nasopharynx. This can be done visually and by x-ray. If the tooth is in the trachea, a bronchoscopy should be done immediately.

324. (E) All the options may cause changes in intraocular pressure. Azetazolamide lowers pressure in glaucoma. Mannitol will lead to decreased intraocular pressure. One must be sure that the patient has good renal function. Atropine may increase the pressure in patients with glaucoma, or it may decrease the pressure by relaxing smooth muscle.

325. (E) All of the options listed are important for the patient with causalgia. In the patient with obstructive lung disease, one may want to avoid the stellate ganglion approach, since there is a possibility of pneumothorax, which could be life threatening.

326. (C) The placebo effect is present in all therapeutic situations. It is seen not only in those who are

unstable or who are faking symptoms but also in normal patients.

327. (B) Halothane and thiopental should cause no problem to the kidney. Gallamine may not be excreted in a timely fashion. Enflurane may lead to fluoride ion increases on metabolism and should be avoided on theoretical grounds.

328. (B) The syndrome of fluid absorption may lead to pulmonary edema due to increased intravascular pressure and to decreased osmotic pressure. The serum sodium will fall. The position on the table is not a factor.

329. (B) The irrigating fluids should be nonhemolytic and isoosmolar. (Glycine is hypoosmolar. Cytal is isoosmolar.) The composition should not be close to water, since water is hypoosmotic. Electrolyte solutions interfere with the cautery.

330. (C) Administration of insulin should be carefully monitored during surgery. Blood sugar should be followed closely. The intravenous line containing the insulin should not be the primary line but should be piggy-backed into another line. There is concern that some of the insulin will be absorbed to the intravenous tubing. The dosage should be titrated to needs.

331. (A) Mineralocorticoids, glucocorticoids, and sex hormones are secreted by the cortex. Norepinephrine is secreted by the medulla.

332. (A) Hypertension may be caused by many factors. In this case, the first three options are correct. Myxedema is not associated with hypertension. Pheochromocytoma is possible if the tumor is part of the multiple endocrine adenoma syndrome.

333. (E) In caring for the patient with tamponade, the heart is kept full, the heart rate fast, the periphery constricted, and the compensatory mechanisms intact. This patient is living on compensatory mechanisms.

334. (D) Surgery for the patient with a transplanted heart will be rare and in most cases will be done in centers where the transplant was done. The transplanted heart is essentially denervated. Drugs that usually work directly have more effect.

335. (A) The primary determinants of myocardial oxygen supply are blood flow and the oxygen-carrying capacity of the blood. Age is not a primary determinant. F_{IO_2} affects oxygen supply by increasing the amount of dissolved oxygen in the blood.

336. (E) Mannitol may lead to hyperosmolar coma if given in large doses. The drug has its effect by removing water from the normal tissues. If the blood–brain barrier is impaired, mannitol may pass into the cells and cause cerebral edema. The drug is effective in doses as low as 0.25 gm/kg.

337. (B) Factors of importance in air embolism are amount and rate of entry. The site of entry is not important. A pulmonary artery catheter may be useful for the monitoring aspects, but the port is too small to be very helpful in the withdrawal of air.

338. (C) Fentanyl and thiopental do not increase intracranial pressure. Halothane and nitrous oxide do increase the pressure.

339. (A) The blood–brain barrier is readily permeable to drugs that have an affinity for the membrane lipid. Morphine, glucose, and carbon dioxide pass through. Bicarbonate does not.

340. (E) Any one of these procedures may be associated with arrhythmias.

341. (B) Sodium nitroprusside is of short duration. It may cause an acidemia. It is usually associated with a tachycardia. The toxicity is cyanide toxicity.

342. (A) Hepatitis may follow transfusion of blood products. The most common type is non-A, non-B. The incidence is lower if the donor pool is volunteers. Transfusion of red cells does not carry a higher risk. Current data list the risk as 1/100 units transfused.

343. (E) Vitamin K-dependent factors are II, VII, IX, and X.

344. (A) Small bowel resections does not have any increased incidence of bleeding. The other options are all associated with bleeding.

345. (A) Wilson's disease is a metabolic derangement of copper metabolism. Hepatic involvement may affect drug metabolism. The action of neuromuscular blocking agents may be prolonged if the liver disease is severe. The kidneys are not involved.

346. (B) Marfan's syndrome is associated with aortic changes making dissection more common. Hypertension should be avoided. The high-arched palate may make intubation more difficult. Aortic stenosis is not seen, but aortic insufficiency is common. The patients do not have short stature but are tall with long extremities.

347. (C) The chronic use of marijuana leads to bronchitis and tachycardia. There is not a withdrawal

syndrome to marijuana alone. The liver is not involved unless other drugs are involved.

348. (A) The patient with multiple myeloma has hypercalcemia. Bone pain is common and the patient is subject to easy bone fractures. Renal failure may occur due to the deposition of the abnormal protein in the tubules. Serum chloride levels are not usually deranged.

349. (B) Autonomic hyperreflexia occurs with spinal lesions above T-5. Any stimulation, eg., urinary catheter stimulation, will lead to hypertension accompanied by sweating and bradycardia. The anesthesiologist must be prepared to treat the hypertension immediately.

350. (D) The Pierre Robin syndrome presents problems because of the recessed chin. Intubation may be very difficult. Tracheostomy may be necessary to avoid airway obstruction. There are usually no associated renal, cardiac, or lung problems.